Approaches and Applications of Deep Learning in Virtual Medical Care

Noor Zaman
Taylor's University, Malaysia

Loveleen Gaur
Amity University, Noida, India

Mamoona Humayun
Jouf University, Saudi Arabia

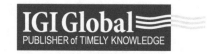

A volume in the Advances in Healthcare
Information Systems and Administration (AHISA)
Book Series

Published in the United States of America by
    IGI Global
    Medical Information Science Reference (an imprint of IGI Global)
    701 E. Chocolate Avenue
    Hershey PA, USA 17033
    Tel: 717-533-8845
    Fax: 717-533-8661
    E-mail: cust@igi-global.com
    Web site: http://www.igi-global.com

Library of Congress Cataloging-in-Publication Data

Names: Zaman, Noor, 1972- editor. I Gaur, Loveleen, editor. I Humayun,
    Mamoona, editor.
Title: Approaches and applications of deep learning in virtual medical care
    / Noor Zaman, Loveleen Gaur, and Mamoona Humayun, editor.
Description: Hershey, PA : Medical Information Science Reference, [2022] I
    Includes bibliographical references and index. I Summary: "The book will
    focus on Innovative approaches for medical sensor/image data analysis,
    event detection, segmentation, and abnormality detection, object/lesion
    classification, organ/region/landmark localization, object/lesion
    detection, organ/substructure segmentation, lesion segmentation, and
    medical image registration using deep learning"-- Provided by publisher.

Identifiers: LCCN 2021035208 (print) I LCCN 2021035209 (ebook) I ISBN
    9781799889298 (hardcover) I ISBN 9781799889304 (ebook)
Subjects: MESH: Diagnostic Techniques and Procedures I Deep Learning I
    Telemedicine I Models, Statistical
Classification: LCC RC71.3 (print) I LCC RC71.3 (ebook) I NLM W 26.5 I
    DDC 616.07/5--dc23
LC record available at https://lccn.loc.gov/2021035208
LC ebook record available at https://lccn.loc.gov/2021035209

This book is published in the IGI Global book series Advances in Healthcare Information Systems and Administration (AHISA) (ISSN: 2328-1243; eISSN: 2328-126X)

British Cataloguing in Publication Data
A Cataloguing in Publication record for this book is available from the British Library.

All work contributed to this book is new, previously-unpublished material. The views expressed in this book are those of the authors, but not necessarily of the publisher.

For electronic access to this publication, please contact: eresources@igi-global.com.

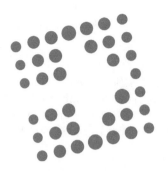

Advances in Healthcare Information Systems and Administration (AHISA) Book Series

Anastasius Moumtzoglou

Hellenic Society for Quality & Safety in Healthcare and P. & A. Kyriakou Children's Hospital, Greece

ISSN:2328-1243
EISSN:2328-126X

MISSION

The **Advances in Healthcare Information Systems and Administration (AHISA) Book Series** aims to provide a channel for international researchers to progress the field of study on technology and its implications on healthcare and health information systems. With the growing focus on healthcare and the importance of enhancing this industry to tend to the expanding population, the book series seeks to accelerate the awareness of technological advancements of health information systems and expand awareness and implementation.

Driven by advancing technologies and their clinical applications, the emerging field of health information systems and informatics is still searching for coherent directing frameworks to advance health care and clinical practices and research. Conducting research in these areas is both promising and challenging due to a host of factors, including rapidly evolving technologies and their application complexity. At the same time, organizational issues, including technology adoption, diffusion and acceptance as well as cost benefits and cost effectiveness of advancing health information systems and informatics applications as innovative forms of investment in healthcare are gaining attention as well. **AHISA** addresses these concepts and critical issues.

COVERAGE

- Role of informatics specialists
- IS in Healthcare
- Management of Emerging Health Care Technologies
- Rehabilitative Technologies
- Virtual health technologies
- E-Health and M-Health
- IT Applications in Health Organizations and Practices
- Nursing Expert Systems
- IT security and privacy issues
- IT Applications in Physical Therapeutic Treatments

IGI Global is currently accepting manuscripts for publication within this series. To submit a proposal for a volume in this series, please contact our Acquisition Editors at Acquisitions@igi-global.com or visit: http://www.igi-global.com/publish/.

The Advances in Healthcare Information Systems and Administration (AHISA) Book Series (ISSN 2328-1243) is published by IGI Global, 701 E. Chocolate Avenue, Hershey, PA 17033-1240, USA, www.igi-global.com. This series is composed of titles available for purchase individually; each title is edited to be contextually exclusive from any other title within the series. For pricing and ordering information please visit http://www.igi-global.com/book-series/advances-healthcare-information-systems-administration/37156. Postmaster: Send all address changes to above address. © © 2022 IGI Global. All rights, including translation in other languages reserved by the publisher. No part of this series may be reproduced or used in any form or by any means – graphics, electronic, or mechanical, including photocopying, recording, taping, or information and retrieval systems – without written permission from the publisher, except for non commercial, educational use, including classroom teaching purposes. The views expressed in this series are those of the authors, but not necessarily of IGI Global.

Titles in this Series

For a list of additional titles in this series, please visit: http://www.igi-global.com/book-series/advances-healthcare-information-systems-administration/37156

Prospects of Blockchain Technology for Accelerating Scientific Advancement in Healthcare
Malaya Dutta Borah (National Institute of Technology (NIT), India) Peng Zhang (Belmont University, USA) and Ganesh Chandra Deka (Ministry of Skill Development and Entrepreneurship, Government of India, India)
Medical Information Science Reference • © 2022 • 315pp • H/C (ISBN: 9781799896067) • US $285.00

Quality of Healthcare in the Aftermath of the COVID-19 Pandemic
Anastasius Moumtzoglou (P&A Kyriakou Children's Hospital, Greece)
Medical Information Science Reference • © 2022 • 403pp • H/C (ISBN: 9781799891987) • US $325.00

Handbook of Research on Applied Intelligence for Health and Clinical Informatics
Anuradha Dheeraj Thakare (Pimpri Chinchwad College of Engineering, Savitribai Phule Pune University, India) Sanjeev J. Wagh (Shivaji University, India) Manisha Sunil Bhende (Dr. D.Y. Patil Institute of Engineering, Management, and Research Akurdi, India & Savitribai Phule Pune University, India) Ahmed M. Anter (Beni-Suef University, Egypt) and Xiao-Zhi Gao (University of Eastern Finland, Finland)
Medical Information Science Reference • © 2022 • 470pp • H/C (ISBN: 9781799877097) • US $425.00

Developing Maternal Health Decision Support Systems in Developing Countries
Vincent Mzazi (University of South Africa, South Africa)
Medical Information Science Reference • © 2021 • 286pp • H/C (ISBN: 9781799839583) • US $265.00

Cloud-Based M-Health Systems for Vein Image Enhancement and Feature Extraction Emerging Research and Opportunities
Kamta Nath Mishra (Birla Institute of Technology, India) and Subhash Chandra Pandey (Birla Institute of Technology, India)
Medical Information Science Reference • © 2021 • 246pp • H/C (ISBN: 9781799845379) • US $195.00

The NHS and Contemporary Health Challenges From a Multilevel Perspective
Louise Dalingwater (Sorbonne Université, France)
Medical Information Science Reference • © 2020 • 261pp • H/C (ISBN: 9781799839286) • US $265.00

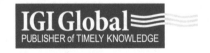

701 East Chocolate Avenue, Hershey, PA 17033, USA
Tel: 717-533-8845 x100 • Fax: 717-533-8661
E-Mail: cust@igi-global.com • www.igi-global.com

Editorial Advisory Board

Table of Contents

Chapter 10
Soobia Saeed, Universiti Teknologi Malaysia, Malaysia
Habibullah Bin Haroon, Universiti Teknologi Malaysia, Malaysia
Mehmood Naqvi, Mohawk College, Canada
Noor Zaman Jhanjhi, Taylor's University, Malaysia
Muneer Ahmad, National University of Science and Technology, Pakistan
Loveleen Gaur, Amity University, Noida, India

Detailed Table of Contents

    Preeti Sharma, Manipal University Jaipur, Jaipur, India
    Devershi Pallavi Bhatt, Manipal University, Jaipur, Jaipur, India

Medical imaging applications like MRI, CT scan, x-ray, PET, ultrasound, etc. provide health experts fast and comprehensive information of the internal organs and tissues of the human body. MRI of the brain is used to get inside information of any sort of brain injury, tumor, stroke, or wound in a blood vessel. The complex structure of the brain makes it a challenging responsibility for the researcher to design a model to precisely segment the brain region from the skull and to find any abnormality in the tissue. This chapter helps to understand the importance of deep learning to perform segmentation on MRI (magnetic resonance imaging) scans of the brain by reviewing previous studies and also presents brief knowledge of different brain imaging techniques, digital image segmentation techniques, and deep learning.

    Soobia Saeed, Taylor's University, Malaysia
    Noor Zaman Jhanjhi, Taylor's University, Malaysia
    Mehmood Naqvi, Mohawk College, Canada
    Mamoona Humyun, Jouf University, Saudi Arabia
    Muneer Ahmad, School of Electrical Engineering and Computer Science (SEECS), National
        University of Science and Technology, Pakistan
    Loveleen Gaur, Amity University, Noida, India

Breast cancer is the most common cancer in women aged 59 to 69 years old. Studies have shown that early detection and treatment of breast cancer increases the chances of survival significantly. They also demonstrated that detecting small lesions early improves forecasting and results in a significant reduction in death cases. The most effective screening diagnostic technique in this case is mammography. However, interpretation of mammograms is difficult due to small differences in tissue densities within mammographic images. This is especially true for dense breasts, and this study suggests that screening mammography is more effective in fatty breast tissue than in dense breast tissue. This study focuses on breast cancer diagnosis as well as identifying risk factors and their assessments of breast cancer as well as premature detection of breast cancer by analyzing 3D MRI mammography methods and segmentation of mammographic images using machine learning.

Chapter 3

Smita Das, MBB College, India
Swanirbhar Majumder, Tripura University, India

Diabetic retinopathy (DR) detection techniques is a biometric modality that deserves systematic review and analysis of the connected algorithms for further improvement. The ophthalmologist uses retinal fundus images for the early detection of DR by segmenting the images. There are several segmentation algorithms reported as earlier. This chapter presents a comprehensive review of the methodology associated with retinal blood vessel extraction presented to date. The vessel segmentation techniques are divided into four main categories depending on their underlying methodology as pattern recognition, vessel tracking, model based, and hybrid approaches. A few of these methods are further classified into subsections. Finally, a comparative analysis of a few of the DR detection techniques will be presented here based on their merits, demerits, and other parameters like sensitivity, specificity, and accuracy and provide detailed information about its significance, present status, limitations, and future scope.

Chapter 4

Gauri Sharma, Manipal University, Jaipur, India

Over the past few decades, chronic illnesses have been on a continuous rise of which epilepsy has been the most common neurological disorder. However, due to the recent progress that has been made by medical science, epilepsy can be controlled for about 70% of the cases. To diagnose epilepsy, EEG, CT scan, MRI, etc. are some of the most common ways, but in this chapter, diagnosis using EEG shall be most focused upon. Although EEG can be considered a good way to decide upon the results of epilepsy proving whether a person is epileptic or not, it is not a completely reliable method. Hence, for its accurate detection we must use sophisticated techniques like CNN and LSTM that will provide a timely and correct diagnosis, reducing the chances of frequent epileptic seizures and SUDEP. Using anti-epileptic drugs cannot guarantee epilepsy prevention, and even if they do, these drugs come with some serious side effects, so people must look back to yoga for a probable permanent treatment.

Chapter 5

Rohit Rastogi, Dayalbagh Educational Institute, India & ABES Engineering College, India
Sheelu Sagar, Amity University, Noida, India
Neeti Tandon, Vikram University, Ujjain, India
Bhavna Singh, G.S. Ayurved Medical College and Hospital, Pilkhuwa, India
T. Rajeshwari, Gayatri Chetna Kendra, Kolkata, India

The happiness programs and seeking their various means are popular across the globe. Many cultures and races are using them in different ways through carnivals, festivals, and occasions. In India, the Yajna,

Mantra, Pranayama, and Yoga-like alternate therapies are now drawing attention of researchers, socio behavioral scientists, and philosophers by their scientific divinity. The chapter is an honest effort to identify the logical progress on happiness indices and reduction in radiation of electronic gadgets. The visualizations propound evidence that the ancient Vedic rituals and activities were effective in maintaining the mental balance. The data set was collected after a specified protocol followed and analyzed through various scientific data analysis tools.

Chapter 6

Khalid A. Al Afandy, National School for Applied Science (ENSA), Abdelmalek Essaadi University, Tetouan, Morocco

Hicham Omara, Faculty of Science (FS), Abdelmalek Essaadi University, Tetouan, Morocco

Mohamed Lazaar, ENSIAS, Mohammed V University, Rabat, Morocco

Mohammed Al Achhab, National School for Applied Science (ENSA), Abdelmalek Essaadi University, Tetouan, Morocco

This chapter provides a comprehensive explanation of deep learning including an introduction to ANNs, improving the deep NNs, CNNs, classic networks, and some technical tricks for image classification using deep learning. ANNs, mathematical models for one node ANN, and multi-layers/multi-nodes ANNs are explained followed by the ANNs training algorithm followed by the loss function, the cost function, the activation function with its derivatives, and the back-propagation algorithm. This chapter also outlines the most common training problems with the most common solutions and ANNs improvements. CNNs are explained in this chapter with the convolution filters, pooling filters, stride, padding, and the CNNs mathematical models. This chapter explains the four most commonly used classic networks and ends with some technical tricks that can be used in CNNs model training.

Chapter 7

Soobia Saeed, Universiti Teknologi Malaysia, Malaysia

Habibullah Bin Haroon, University Technology Malaysia, Malaysia

Noor Zaman Jhanjhi, Taylor's University, Malaysia

Mehmood Naqvi, Mohawk College, Canada

Muneer Ahmad, National University of Science and Technology, Pakistan

Low-grade tumor or CSF fluid, the symptoms of brain tumour and CSF liquid, usually requires image segmentation to evaluate tumour detection in brain images. This research uses systematic literature review (SLR) process for analysis of the different segmentation approach for detecting the low-grade tumor and CSF fluid presence in the brain. This research work investigated how to evaluate and detect the tumor and CSF fluid, supervised machine learning algorithm and segmentation method (3D and 4D segmentation process, supervised segmentation process, Fourier transformation, and Laplace transformation), and mentioned the details of publication selection with the publishing digital libraries bodies. Furthermore, this research discusses selected segmentation techniques to detect the low-grade tumor and CSF fluid in systematic mapping through systematic literature review (SLR) process.

Chapter 8

Soobia Saeed, Department of Software Engineering, UniversitiTeknologi Malaysia, Malaysia
Afnizanfaizal Abdullah, UniversitiTeknologi Malaysia, Malaysia
Noor Zaman Jhanjhi, Taylor's University, Malaysia
Mehmood Naqvi, Mohwak College, Canada
Muneer Ahmad, National University of Science and Technology, Pakistan

Brain metastases are the most prevalent intracranial neoplasm that causes excessive morbidity and mortality in most cancer patients. The current medical model for brain metastases is focused on the physical condition of the affected individual, the anatomy of the main tumor, and the number and proximity of brain lesions. In this paper, a new hybrid Metastases Fast Fourier Transformation with SVM (MFFT-SVM) method is proposed that can classify high dimensional magnetic resonance imaging as tumor and predicts lung cancer from given protein primary sequences. The goal is to address the associated issues stated with the treatment targeted at unique molecular pathways to the tumor, together with those involved in crossing the blood-brain barrier and migrating cells to the lungs. The proposed method identifies the place of the lung damage by the Fast Fourier Technique (FFT). FFT is the principal statistical approach for frequency analysis which has many engineering and scientific uses. Moreover, Differential Fourier Transformation (DFT) is considered for focusing the brain metastases that migrate into the lungs and create non-small lungs cancer. However, Support Vector Machine (SVM) is used to measure the accuracy of control patient's datasets of sensitivity and specificity. The simulation results verified the performance of the proposed method is improved by 92.8% sensitivity, of 93.2% specificity and 95.5% accuracy respectively.

Chapter 9

Navirah Kamal, Amity University, Noida, India
Pragati Sharma, Amity University, Noida, India
Rangana Das, Amity University, Noida, India
Vipul Goyal, Amity University, Noida, India
Richa Gupta, Amity University, Noida, India

In this chapter, a deep study of dysgraphia and its various available technical aids is discussed. A person suffering from dysgraphia struggles to carry out day-to-day activities like schoolwork, paperwork, and other writing activities. A suitable aid is required to overcome the hurdles due to the suffering. This literature establishes the various effects of dysgraphia in adults and children. An analysis of various effective tools is carried out in the study. Some tools are directly designed to tackle the inconveniences that come along with this disability; others provide a more general aid for writing. The literature also identifies the patterns and quirks commonly found in the handwriting. Algorithms for handwriting recognition is discussed to lay the foundation of aids present for dysgraphia. The objective of the chapter is to provide foundation work to create aids for dysgraphia by categorizing the various related key points.

Chapter 10
    Soobia Saeed, Universiti Teknologi Malaysia, Malaysia
    Habibullah Bin Haroon, Universiti Teknologi Malaysia, Malaysia
    Mehmood Naqvi, Mohawk College, Canada
    Noor Zaman Jhanjhi, Taylor's University, Malaysia
    Muneer Ahmad, National University of Science and Technology, Pakistan
    Loveleen Gaur, Amity University, Noida, India

Low-grade tumor or CSF fluid, the symptoms of brain tumor and CSF liquid, usually require image segmentation to evaluate tumor detection in brain images. This research uses systematic literature review (SLR) process for analysis of the different segmentation approach for detecting the low-grade tumor and CSF fluid presence in the brain. This research work investigated how to evaluate and detect the tumor and CSF fluid, improve segmentation method to detect tumor through graph cut hidden markov model of k-mean clustering algorithm (GCHMkC) techniques and parameters, extract the missing values in k-NN algorithm through correlation matrix of hybrid k-NN algorithm with time lag and discrete fourier transformation (DFT) techniques and parameters, and convert the non-linear data into linear transformation using LE-LPP and time complexity techniques and parameters.

Preface

It gives us immense pleasure to put forth the book *Approaches and Applications of Deep Learning in Virtual Medical Care*. The virtual healthcare market has been growing exponentially in recent years. The coronavirus pandemic has pushed the necessity for virtual healthcare services even further, with most nations executing constraints that persuade the public to stay at home. Advanced technologies like artificial intelligence (AI) and deep learning (DL) are essential to enhancing these experiences for both practitioners and patients. Healthcare corporations of all dimensions, sorts, and disciplines are becoming more fascinated by how artificial intelligence or deep learning technologies can assist superior patient care while reducing costs and enhancing efficacies. Telehealth and virtual consults are transforming how medical care is provided. Virtual care is a technique that incorporates the medication of patients enduring routine healthcare concerns using video, audio, or transcribed message.

AI's ability in reforming healthcare is very encouraging, the sub-domains of AI, like computer vision, beat experts in precise diagnosis in many areas such as brain signals translation helps in recuperating failed physical functions such as speech due to stroke or other neurological illnesses. DL has revolutionary applications in pharma and medicine, varying from disease diagnosis to epidemic forecast. DL an extension of machine learning is extensively trendy and pertinent in analyzing complex patterns from huge complex data (e.g., medical illustrations). Advanced DL variations such as convolution neural networks (CNN), recurrent neural networks (RNN) can investigate high-dimensional data broadly embraced in medical applications.

This book is very appropriate in these exceptional times. It comes at a moment of great global turbulence in the healthcare sector. Healthcare presently is about contemporary thoughts, innovative approaches, and the latest technology. Approaches and Applications of Deep Learning in Virtual Medical Care considers the applications of deep learning in virtual medical care and delves into complex deep learning algorithms, calibrates models, and improves the predictions of the trained model on medical imaging. In this book, we attempted to discuss all the latest approaches, experiments, and evaluate actual and potential contributions with deep learning algorithms in dealing with challenges primarily related to virtual medical care. We strongly believe that this critical reference source is ideal for researchers, academicians, medical practitioners, hospital workers, and students.

CHAPTER 1: IMPORTANCE OF DEEP LEARNING MODELS IN THE MEDICAL IMAGING FIELD

This chapter focuses on the importance of deep learning to perform segmentation on MRI (Magnetic Resonance Imaging) scans of the brain by reviewing various previous studies and presents brief knowledge of different brain imaging techniques, digital image segmentation techniques, and deep learning. Medical Imaging applications like MRI, CT scan, X-ray, PET, Ultrasound, etc., provide health experts fast and comprehensive information on the internal organs and tissues of the human body. MRI of the brain is used to get inside information of any sort of brain injury, tumor, stroke, and wound in a blood vessel. The complex structure of the brain makes it's a challenging responsibility for the researcher to design a model to precisely segment the brain region from the skull part and to find any abnormality in the tissue part.

CHAPTER 2: OPTIMIZED BREAST CANCER PREMATURE DETECTION METHOD WITH COMPUTATIONAL SEGMENTATION – A SYSTEMATIC REVIEW MAPPING

This chapter focuses uses a systematic literature review (SLR) process for analysis of the different segmentation approach for detecting the low-grade tumor and CSF fluid present in the brain. Low-Grade tumor or CSF fluid, the symptoms of brain tumor and CSF liquid usually require image segmentation to evaluate tumor detection in brain images. This research work investigated how to evaluate and detect the tumor and CSF fluid: (a) supervised machine learning algorithm and segmentation method (3D and 4D segmentation process, supervised segmentation process, Fourier transformation, and Laplace transformation), (b) mentioned the details of publication selection with multiple the publishing digital libraries bodies. Furthermore, this research discusses all selected segmentation techniques to detect the low-grade tumor and CSF fluid in systematic mapping through a systematic literature review (SLR) process. This systematic analysis of the latest literature on low-grade tumor and CSF fluid includes detail on the MRI images with multiple segmentation techniques and their characteristics.

CHAPTER 3: OVERVIEW AND ANALYSIS OF PRESENT-DAY DIABETIC RETINOPATHY (DR) DETECTION TECHNIQUE

Diabetic Retinopathy (DR) detection Techniques is a biometric modality that deserves systematic review and analysis of the connected algorithms for further improvement. The Ophthalmologist uses retinal fundus images for the early detection of DR by segmenting the images. There are several segmentation algorithms reported as earlier. This chapter presents a comprehensive review of the methodology associated with retinal blood vessel extraction presented to date. The vessel segmentation techniques are divided into four main categories depending on their underlying methodology as pattern recognition, vessel tracking, model-based and hybrid approaches. Few of these methods are further classified into subsections. Finally, a comparative analysis of a few of the DR detection techniques will be presented here based on their merits, demerits, and other parameters like Sensitivity, Specificity, and Accuracy, etc, and provide detailed information about its significance, present status, limitations, and future scope.

CHAPTER 4: APPLICATION OF DEEP LEARNING IN EPILEPSY – A CATALYST IN BETTER DIAGNOSIS OF EPILEPTIC SEIZURES AND PREVENTION

Over the past few decades, chronic illnesses have been on a continuous rise of which Epilepsy has been the most common neurological disorder. However, due to the recent progress that has been made by medical science Epilepsy can be controlled for about 70% of the cases. To diagnose Epilepsy, EEG, CT scan, MRI, etc are some of the most common ways but in this chapter, diagnosis using EEG shall be most focused upon. Although EEG can be considered as a good way to decide upon the results of Epilepsy proving whether a person is Epileptic or not, it is not a completely reliable method. Hence for its accurate detection, we must use sophisticated techniques like CNN and LSTM that will provide a timely and correct diagnosis, reducing the chances of frequent Epileptic seizures and SUDEP. Using Anti-Epileptic drugs cannot guarantee Epilepsy prevention and even if they do these drugs come with some serious side effects, so people must look back to Yoga for a probable permanent treatment.

CHAPTER 5: COMPUTATIONAL STATISTICS ON STRESS PATIENTS WITH HAPPINESS AND RADIATION INDICES BY VEDIC HOMA THERAPY – A KNOWLEDGE-BASED APPROACH TO GET INSIGHTS IN THE GLOBAL PANDEMIC

The happiness Programs and seeking its various means are popular across the globe. Many cultures and races are using it in different ways through Carnivals, festivals, and occasions. In India, the Yajna, Mantra, Pranayama, and Yoga-like alternate therapies are now drawing the attention of researchers, socio-behavioral scientists, and philosophers by their scientific divinity. The present manuscript is an honest effort to identify the logical progress on happiness indices and reduction in the radiation of electronic gadgets. The visualizations propound pieces of evidence that the Ancient Vedic Rituals and Activities were much effective in maintaining the mental balance. The data set was collected after a specified protocol followed and analyzed through various scientific data analysis tools available.

CHAPTER 6: DEEP LEARNING

This chapter provides a comprehensive explanation of deep learning, including an introduction to deep learning, the ANNs, Improving the deep NNs, the CNNs, the Classic Networks, and some technical tricks for image classification using deep learning. The ANNs, mathematical models for one node ANN, and multi-layers/multi-nodes ANNs have explained then the ANNs training algorithm followed by the loss function, the cost function, the activation functions with its derivatives, and the back-propagation algorithm. This chapter also outlines the most common training problems with the most common solutions and ANNs improvements. The CNNs are explained in this chapter with the convolution filters, pooling filters, stride, and padding, with numerical examples, and the CNNs mathematical models. This chapter explains the four most used classic networks and ends with some technical tricks that can be used in CNN's model's training.

CHAPTER 7: A SYSTEMATIC MAPPING STUDY OF LOW-GRADE TUMOR OF BRAIN CANCER AND CSF FLUID DETECTING IN MRI IMAGES THROUGH MULTI-ALGORITHM TECHNIQUE

Low-Grade tumor or CSF fluid, the symptoms of brain tumour and CSF liquid usually requires image segmentation to evaluate tumour detection in brain images. This research uses systematic literature review(SLR) process for analysis the different segmentation approach for detecting the low-grade tumor and CSF fluid presence in the brain. This research work investigated how to evaluate and detect the tumor and CSF fluid: (a) supervised machine learning algorithm and segmentation method (3D and 4D segmentation process, supervised segmentation process, Fourier transformation, and Laplace transformation), (b) mentioned the details of publication selection with multiple the publishing digital libraries bodies. Furthermore, this research discusses all selected segmentation techniques to detect the low-grade tumor and CSF fluid in systematic mapping through a systematic literature review (SLR) process.

CHAPTER 8: OPTIMIZED HYBRID PREDICTION METHOD FOR LUNG METASTASES

Low-Grade tumor or CSF fluid, the symptoms of brain tumor and CSF liquid usually requires image segmentation to evaluate tumour detection in brain images. This research uses systematic literature review (SLR) process for analysis the different segmentation approach for detecting the low-grade tumor and CSF fluid presence in the brain. The aim is to determine and characterize various types of detecting approaches and techniques use for segmentation process. This research work investigated how to evaluate and detecting the tumor and CSF fluid: (a) supervised machine learning algorithm and segmentation method (3D and 4D segmentation process, supervised segmentation process, Fourier transformation and Laplace transformation), (b) mentioned the details of publication selection with multiple the publishing digital libraries bodies. This systematic analysis of the latest literature on low-grade tumor and CSF fluid includes detail on the MRI images with multiple segmentation techniques and their characteristics.

CHAPTER 9: VIRTUAL TECHNICAL AIDS TO HELP PEOPLE WITH DYSGRAPHIA

In this chapter, a deep study of dysgraphia and its various available technical aids is discussed. A person suffering from dysgraphia struggles to carry out day-to-day activities like schoolwork, paperwork, and other writing activities. A suitable aid is required to overcome the hurdles due to the suffering. This literature establishes the various effects of dysgraphia in adults and children. An analysis of various effective tools for carried in the study. Some tools are directly designed to tackle the inconveniences that come along with this disability, others provide a more general aid for writing. The literature also identifies the patterns and quirks commonly found in handwriting. Algorithms for handwriting recognition are discussed to lay the foundation of aids present for dysgraphia. The objective of the paper is to provide foundation work to create aids for dysgraphia by categorizing the various related key points

CHAPTER 10: A SYSTEMATIC MAPPING STUDY OF LOW-GRADE TUMOR OF BRAIN CANCER AND CSF FLUID DETECTING APPROACHES AND PARAMETERS

Low-Grade tumor or CSF fluid, the symptoms of brain tumor and CSF liquid usually require image segmentation to evaluate tumor detection in brain images. This research uses systematic literature review(SLR) process for analyzing the different segmentation approach for detecting the low-grade tumor and CSF fluid presence in the brain. This research work investigated how to evaluate and detect the tumor and CSF fluid: (a) improve segmentation method to detect tumor through Graph Cut Hidden Markov Model of k-mean Clustering Algorithm(GCHMkC) techniques and parameters, (b) Extracting the missing values in k-NN algorithm through Correlation matrix of hybrid k-NN algorithm with time lag and Discrete Fourier transformation (DFT) techniques and parameters. (c) To convert the non-linear data into linear transformation using LE-LPP and Time Complexity techniques and parameters.

The global sphere is progressing, and with it is the landscape of healthcare and patient expectations. Digital technologies such as artificial intelligence, machine learning, deep learning will persist to be a vital part of how healthcare providers provide care to their patients. We are also grateful to the IGI team for giving us the opportunity to publish it. We thank our esteemed authors for having shown confidence in the book and considering as a platform to showcase and share their original work.

Noor Zaman
Taylor's University, Malaysia

Loveleen Gaur
Amity University, Noida, India

Mamoona Humayun
Jouf University, Saudi Arabia

Acknowledgment

We would like to express our thanks to Almighty Allah SWT for his all blessings and then great appreciation to all of those we have had the pleasure to work with during this project. The completion of this project could not have been accomplished without their support. First, the editors would like to express deep and sincere gratitude to all the authors who shared their ideas, expertise, and experience by submitting chapters to this book and adhering to its timeline. Second, the editors wish to acknowledge the extraordinary contributions of the reviewers for their valuable and constructive suggestions and recommendations to improve the quality, coherence, and content presentation of chapters. Most of the authors also served as referees. Their willingness to give time so generously is highly appreciated. Finally, our heartfelt gratitude goes to our family members and friends for their love, prayers, caring, and sacrifices in completing this project well in time.

We dedicate this book to our best friend, Late Dr. G. Suseendran. We lost him recently during the current COVID-19 Pandemic.

Noor Zaman
Taylor's University, Malaysia

Loveleen Gaur
Amity University, Noida, India

Mamoona Humayun
Jouf University, Saudi Arabia

Chapter 1
Importance of Deep Learning Models in the Medical Imaging Field

Preeti Sharma
Manipal University Jaipur, Jaipur, India

Devershi Pallavi Bhatt
Manipal University, Jaipur, Jaipur, India

ABSTRACT

Medical imaging applications like MRI, CT scan, x-ray, PET, ultrasound, etc. provide health experts fast and comprehensive information of the internal organs and tissues of the human body. MRI of the brain is used to get inside information of any sort of brain injury, tumor, stroke, or wound in a blood vessel. The complex structure of the brain makes it a challenging responsibility for the researcher to design a model to precisely segment the brain region from the skull and to find any abnormality in the tissue. This chapter helps to understand the importance of deep learning to perform segmentation on MRI (magnetic resonance imaging) scans of the brain by reviewing previous studies and also presents brief knowledge of different brain imaging techniques, digital image segmentation techniques, and deep learning.

INTRODUCTION

The brain is the main controller organ of the body that regulates the functioning of other organs. The central organ of the nervous system is the brain that is protected by skull bones. The main parts of brain structure are the brainstem, cerebrum, and cerebellum shown in Figure 1. The brain collects, organizes, and distributes information throughout the body. The main functions of the brain are to process the information collected by sense organs, regularization of breathing and blood pressure, and release hormones in the body. A healthy brain works fast and spontaneously. Any kind of problem inside the brain can make the working of the body difficult. The complex structure of the brain makes it difficult to find any kind of abnormality in it. It requires a lot of experience and precise knowledge to diagnose issues in the brain.

DOI: 10.4018/978-1-7998-8929-8.ch001

Medical Imaging applications provide health professionals detail and fast information about the internal organs and tissues of patients. There are so many types of medical imaging technologies that give information about different body parts. Medical imaging techniques help diagnose diseases like pneumonia, brain injuries, cancer, internal bleeding, and many other issues. Large amount of data is generated by medical imaging applications. High quality of imaging can advances medical decision making and can lessen the unnecessary procedures. Anatomical and physiological database are created with help of these techniques. Timely diagnosis of disease plays a very important part for recovery of patient from disease. For early diagnosis and other information that needed of patient's body parts, medical imaging plays significant role here. Medical imaging procedures like X-ray images, Computed Tomography (CT) scans, and MR images are supporting medical teams in diagnosing disease or any kind of abnormality in distinct body parts of patients to determine what procedure should be followed for an early recovery. The Magnetic Resonance Imaging (MRI) technique is practiced in radiology for investigating the human body through MR scans. MR images give specific information of internal tissues that can help in the diagnosis of disease, injury or tumor, etc. The powerful magnetic field is applied to produce pictures through an MRI scanner. MRI-generated pictures are more detailed compare to other techniques, like Ultrasound or CT.

Digital Image processing methods like image classification and segmentation are extremely important techniques to follow in the image processing field. Segmentation is the method of generating distinct sets of pixels in an image with pixels sharing common characteristics included in the same set. In many cases, the entire image is not required for additional processing that is why with the help of the segmentation method the region of interest (ROI) can be acquired within the targeted image, and the useless part is discarded. The complex structure of the brain makes it's quite challenging for detailed segmentation of the brain region for the investigation of pathological tissues. Researchers are attempting to develop automatic image segmentation and classification models to assist the medical team in finding the appearance of any sort of abnormality in scanned images. The feature of self-leaning and fast processing of deep learning technology is raising its use in several fields including the medical field too. There has been a lot of work accomplished on segmentation of brain region and brain tumor detection on brain MRI scans and it's still attracting many researchers to extend their study in this field and develop models with high efficiency. The employment of deep learning models is increasing the performance levels on segmentation of brain MRI in multiple measurement aspects and defeating the performance of many machine learning models.

Figure 1. Three main parts of brain

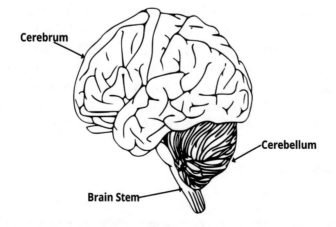

This chapter explicates the significance of deep learning methods in neuroimaging area. This chapter covers previous studies that have been conducting to segment the brain region or detect brain tumor, using deep learning models while MRI scan data sets are common in all elected studies. This chapter also presents a skimpy knowledge of digital image processing, brain imaging techniques and, deep learning technique. This study encourages the readers to know how deep learning models can perform well in image segmentation tasks by examining the previously done works and to provide contribution in the medical imaging field.

The book chapter organization starts with the introduction part. After the introduction of the chapter, different brain imaging techniques have been explained. The next part after introduction explains digital image processing (DIP), its key steps, and its applications. Then, the next part is all about the concept of deep learning technique, its architecture followed by its use in medical science then a brief knowledge of segmentation and its various types is described. After knowing about MRI, deep learning, and segmentation; the importance of deep learning in brain MRI segmentation is explained by reviewing previous studies. Previous studies have been included from year 2015 to 2021. The last section of this chapter is the discussion part.

BRAIN IMAGING TECHNIQUES

The medical imaging technique is a diagnostic imaging process where a series of tests is done to generate images of inner body parts. These techniques are utilized to give the doctors views of the inside picture of the body or the inside areas that remain invisible to naked eyes. These techniques can give view of bones, nerves, muscles, the function of organs, tissues, and internal body parts hidden by skin and bones. The medical professionals that are specialists in imaging are called Radiologists. With the help of imaging, the presence of abnormality in the internal body like disease, damages in tissue, tumor, cracked bone, condition of various important organs like heart, lungs, liver, etc. identified. These techniques also help doctors to monitor the condition of health of patients post disease diagnosis. The X-ray imaging technique is known as the first imaging technique. After the invention of X-ray imaging in 1895, various other imaging techniques have been developed like CT scan, Ultrasound, MRI, Positron Emission Tomography (PET), etc. Each kind of technique works on different methods and is used for different purposes.

Capturing the deep inside view of the brain through imaging techniques is called brain scanning or famously known as Neuroimaging. The physician who performs neuroimaging is called neuro-radiologists. Neuroimaging can be categorized into two types, functional imaging and structural imaging.

1. **Functional Imaging:** This technique is used for the diagnosis of metabolic diseases and brain lesions. This imaging visualizes information processing of the brain. Any activity in the brain area increases metabolism that reflects on scan.
2. **Structural Imaging:** This technique is used to get information about the structure of the brain and is normally used to diagnose tumor or brain injuries.

Imaging techniques that are specifically used for scanning the brain comes under the category of brain imaging techniques. There are various techniques that can display inside information of the brain.

Some of the most important and used brain imaging techniques are PET, MRI, fMRI, and EEG, that give information about the internal side of the brain. These techniques are described as follows:

Electroencephalography (EEG)

In the year 1929, A German psychiatrist Hans Berger discovered Electroencephalography (EEG). Electroencephalography (EEG) is used to observe the activity of the brain under some psychological stages like drowsiness and alertness. Any kind of excessive or lack of activity inside the brain can be diagnosed with EEG. Electrodes present on the EEG headset are put on the scalp of the patient. These electrodes detect the electrical changes of neurons and send the signal to amplifier for the amplification of signals. Amplified signals then transferred to a computer system to produce different maps of the activity that happens inside the brain. The frequency of EEG is varying for walking and sleeping states. This technique is one of the earliest brain imaging techniques. Figure 2 shows an image of EEG.

Figure 2. Electroencephalography
(Nagel, 2019)

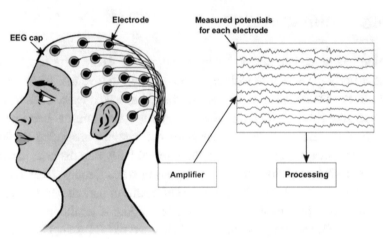

Positron Emission Tomography (PET)

PET is a type of functional imaging developed by Edward J. Hoffman with Michael E. Phelps, in 1974. PET imaging is mostly used in cancer treatment and to diagnose brain and heart diseases. PET technique works with other imaging techniques like CT scan and MRI to observe the brain's functionality. By scanning the place of neural firing, PET measures sugar glucose. For active neurons, glucose works as fuel. This technique helps in locating only generalized areas of brain activity, not any kind of specific location. For diagnosing Alzheimer's disease PET can be helpful. This technique is quite costly and aggressive. Figure 3 shows output images of PET.

Figure 3. Positron emission tomography
(Phelps, 2000)

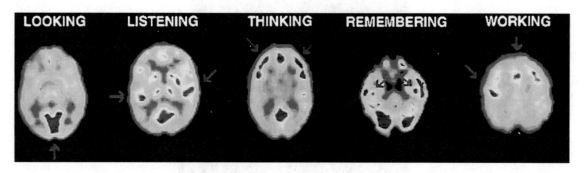

Magnetic Resonance Imaging (MRI)

MRI and functional MRI (fMRI) are mostly used imaging techniques in the area of psychology. An MRI image gives thorough information of internal tissues (Rao et al., 2017). Monitoring of patient's status during treatment is observed through MRI. A strong magnetic field is used to align rotating atomic nuclei to generate pictures through an MRI scanner. MRI-generated pictures are more thorough compare to other techniques. The non-aggressive quality of MRI scan makes them more reliable, and this scan can be used for infants also. The drawback of this scan is that patients need to stay still during the process of scanning. Functional MRI (fMRI) is used to calculate both functional activity and structure of the brain using multiple images. Due to neural activity, signals get changed inside the brain and fMRI calculated these signals.

MRI of the brain gives information of brain injury, tumor, and damage in the blood vessel, stroke, etc. An external strong magnetic field is applied to line up protons disturbed by external Radio Frequency (RF) energy. Different kinds of pictures are produced by a sequence of RF pulses that are applied and collected. Two major terms related to MRI are Repetition time (TR) and Time to Echo (TE). RT is measured among consecutive pulse sequences used on the same slice and TE is the interval of time within delivery of RF pulse and arrival of the echo signal.

The different kinds of relaxation times that can characterize tissues are T1 and T2. T1 is longitudinal relaxation time that is taken during the realigning of spinning protons amidst an outside magnetic field. T2 is transverse relaxation time that is the time occupied by spinning protons to drop the phase coherence.

MRI Sides

Right side and left side are two sides that present the side of the brain shown in Figure 4. When radiology images are analyzed then the initial step is to find out the side of the brain (Preston, 2006).

Figure 4. MR Image showing both right and left side of brain

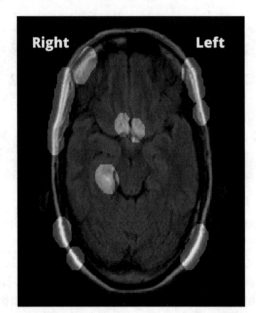

Imaging Planes

In neuroimaging, three main planes of the brain are considered ("The Basics", 2011). These different planes are shown in Figure 5 and described below:

1. **Axial Plane:** Also known as the Transverse plane where an MRI scanner scans the brain from chin to head.
2. **Sagittal Plane:** Also known as lateral view in which images are captured by starting to one ear and moving towards another ear. That is vertical to the axial plane.
3. **Coronal Plane:** Also called frontal view where images are taken from the backside of the head and then move towards the face that is vertical to the lateral view.

Figure 5. Different Imaging planes of MRI
("The Basics", 2011)

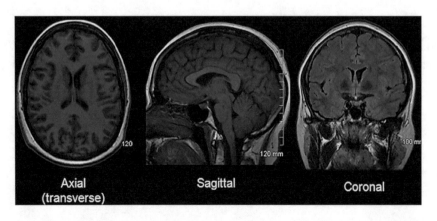

MRI Sequences

An MRI sequence in the form of an MR pulse sequence is applied to get series of images. These sequences are shown in Figure 6 and their comparison is shown in Table 1.

1. **T1:** Weighted pictures are generated by short TR and TE times.
2. **T2:** Weighted pictures are produced by long TR and TE times. T1- weighted sequence and T2-weighted sequences are common kinds of sequences.
3. **Flair (Fluid Attenuated Inversion Recovery):** It is alike T2-weighted images but TR and TE times are longer than T2-weighted.

Figure 6. Different MRI sequences
("The Basics", 2011)

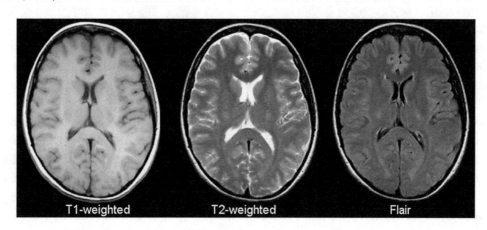

Table 1. Comparison of various MRI sequences with the intensity level

Tissue	T1-weighted	T2-weighted	Flair
White Matter	Light	Dark Gray	Dark Gray
CSF	Dark	Bright	Dark
Cortex	Gray	Light Gray	Light Gray
Fat with bone marrow	Bright	Light	Light
Inflammation	Dark	Bright	Bright

Source: (Saxena et al., 2021)

DIGITAL IMAGE PROCESSING (DIP): DEFINITION, STEPS AND APPLICATIONS

Digital image processing is a method in which digital images are edited to improve pictorial presentation of digital pictures using the support of the computer systems by processing pictures. Processing of pictures is done with the help of software; those are specially developed for image processing. Pictures are captures with the help of a camera. The sensor present in the camera captures the images of the objects of this 3d world. Sunlight works as an energy source here. Sensor, sense the light that is reflected by the object when sunlight falls upon that object and produce sensed data. With the help of sampling and quantization methods, sensed data is converted into digital form. This conversion results in a digital image that is presented in a 2-D matrix form. In the whole process of digital image processing, the input is in form of image while output could be an image or some information associated to input image.

Digital image processing is applied on images to get enhanced images with some processing applied on these images such as making them clearer, removing blur, making the size smaller or larger, etc. These enhanced images help users to get some kind of meaningful information for further processing. Digital image processing methods can be applied on both color and black & white images.

Digital Image Processing Steps

The steps involved in processing of digital images are start with capturing the image through a sensor. After that, some pre-processing steps are applied on digital image to make the image more clearly, remove noise, contrast adjustment, and remove blurriness. Filters are used in pre-processing steps. Further steps involve the segmentation of objects, assign labels to these objects and interpret the objects based on learned features from objects. Steps of digital images processing are described step by step as follows:

1. Image Acquisition: The first stage in DIP is to take a picture with the help of a sensor. Image is caught by a sensor and converted into digital format through an analog-to-digital converter.
2. Pre-processing: Some processing is done on the picture so that the quality of the picture can be enhanced. This step is called the pre-processing step. Noise is removed from the photo in this step, its color is improved, and the contrast is improved, so that the picture can be much bigger and clearer. Filters are applied to the photo in this step. Image pre-processing is the step in which image data is improved to remove noise and improve features. Geometric transformations are performed on the image.
3. Segmentation: A picture contains one or more different objects, these objects can be in different shape and size. Mostly, a specific object of a picture has to be worked on; the process in which the object in the picture is separated from the other objects is called image segmentation. This separation occurs in various ways. Separation of objects can be done either from the boundary or from the object's edges. Also, segmentation can be done by the intensity of the pixel of the picture. This is the procedure of dividing an image into various segments. An image is segmented so that for further processing important segments can be differentiated that required for further processing.
4. Representation and Description: After segmentation, the output of segmented image is represented in form of a boundary or the form of a complete region. Raw data is transformed in a way that could be appropriate for further processing. Two kinds of representations are as follows: External characteristics (boundary) like the shape of the object. Internal characteristics (region) like color and texture of an object. After the representation of segmented objects, a description is done to describe the region that differentiates one class of objects from another class of objects.
5. Recognition and Interpretation: For further processing; the description of the object is taken, and based on this description, the object is identified, after which labels are assigned to these objects. Identified objects are interrupted, narrated, and described. Descriptors provide information about

objects that are further assigned labels in the recognition phase. In the Interpretation phase, recognized objects are assigned meaning.

6. Knowledge Base: The main task of knowledge is to help in efficient processing and inter-module connections. Knowledge base step takes care of efficient processing, and here all the main point has an interconnection so that information can be shared among them. Figure 7 shows the steps of DIP.

Figure 7. Various steps in DIP

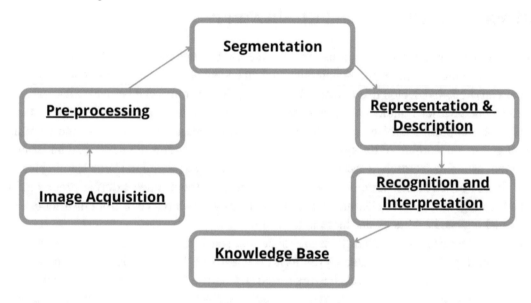

Applications of Digital Image Processing

DIP has impacted almost all technical fields. Some of its applications are:

1. Image Restoration: The process of improving the image is called image restoration. The image is improved or recovered by removing the blur and noise of the original image (Rani, 2016). The main objective of the image restoration is to restoration of a degraded image into the original form of the image captured.

2. Medical Field: The processing of medical images is known as medical image processing. Various image processing procedures are applied on the images captured through different imaging techniques like CT scans, X-rays, MRI, ultrasound, etc. Processing of medical images can help doctors to give a clear picture of internal body parts and to diagnose the diseases. Various image processing methods are used to classify the diseases or to segment the ROI from the original image.

3. Remote Sensing: Data that is collected remotely from objects on the Earth's surface through satellites and aircraft is known as remote sensing. The images are captures to gather pieces of information for weather forecasting, land mapping, monitoring of crops, etc. The image processing method helps to extract information from these images (Fonseca & Costa, 1997).

4.   Transmission: Another application of image processing is related to handling of the size of image data. The large-size images are compressed for the adequate storage and speedy transmission of images. Advancement in image processing techniques has helped in restoring the compressed images without loss of primary data.

5.   Robot Vision: Various robotic machines run on digital image processing methods. Digital image processing is part of robot vision in robotics. With the help of image processing methods, robots can search their ways and hurdles between their ways.

WHAT MAKES DEEP LEARNING STIMULATING?

Artificial intelligence (AI) has brought the world to the forefront of technology. With the assistance of AI, humans can automate the work around them and an endeavor to make machines so intelligent that machines can think and decide like humans. In this way, the machines can be made efficient in doing automatic work. Artificial Intelligence is a dispersed area that has a lot of applications in it. One of the very important applications of these applications is machine learning. Under machine learning, the ability of automatic learning of the system is developed. Such programs are developed under machine learning that uses data themselves and learns on their own. The purpose of machine learning is to make the machine so efficient that it does its automatic learning without much external programming. In machine learning, machines use learning power from their own experience or from instructions so that decision-making can be done by machines in the future.

In machine learning, where algorithms are made that learn from the data, they work on it and do automatic working. Another sub-category of this is deep learning. Before we learn about deep learning, we must know about Artificial Neural Networks (ANN). Geoffrey Hinton in the 1980s created the concept of a "neural network" that is based on the concept to the way the human brain has a lot of neurons that are connected, exchanging narratives and information. Whenever we see an object around us, we can identify that object from our past learned experience. If an object is new to us, then we remember its different features and with the help of these features, we identify that object further. This concept has been introduced in the Artificial Neural Network where multiple neurons are arranged in different layers. These neurons are connected and share information to other layers. If we understand the ANN in a normal way, then it has an input layer that take the input, then the information from the input layer is transferred to hidden layers, processing of the data take place in these hidden layers and the output of hidden layers is transferred to output layer. Neurons in neural networks are basic mathematical functions that are applied on data to get results.

The concept of the artificial neural network is applied in deep learning where multiple neurons are arranged in a layered structure and this structure works like a human brain. Deep learning models have a largely hidden layer so that data processing can be done closely. A deep neural network is trained from a very large database. The more the data used for training, the more the model will work effectively. During training, deep learning models extract features from data and identify objects with these features. Extracting features and learning features on their own makes deep learning models powerful. In machine learning, where the main focus is on the structured data, in deep learning, structured data is not necessary for the artificial neural network.

Architecture of Deep Neural Network

The structure of deep neural network shown in Figure 8 is similar to artificial neural network. The architecture is a layered design. Input layer and output layer is starting and final layer consecutively. Between these layers are set of two or more layers that are called hidden layers. Hidden layers are the part of the architecture where the actual processing took place. Every layer has some neurons. Neurons are mathematical units that perform some mathematical operations on gathered information. Deep neural networks have many numbers of hidden layers. The number of hidden layers represents the depth of the model. These neurons are connected with neurons of their neighbor layers to transfer information with each other. Neurons of same layer are not connected to each other. Neuron of a layer extracts features from image and learns these features for prediction. Mathematical operations performed by neurons are called activation functions. Number of neurons on the final layers generates output of an input image. This output can be in form of an image or some information extracted from input image.

Figure 8. Deep neural network architecture

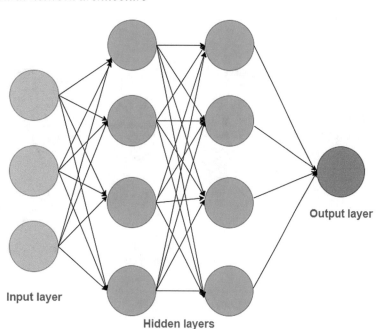

DEEP LEARNING IN MEDICAL SCIENCE

Deep neural networks are designed to imitate the working of the human brain. The high-performance level of deep neural networks makes them useful in various fields. Medical imaging techniques help doctors to present the internal view of body parts, deep learning models can assist doctors in decision making. By applying deep learning algorithms to medical imaging applications, the classification and detection of various diseases could be possible. Deep learning methods are neither imaging techniques dependent nor body part dependent. Deep learning itself is a huge area to work on. Various studies have been conducted to identify diseases of different-different body parts with the help of deep neural networks.

Convolutional neural networks (CNN) are deep neural networks that are used widely in the segmentation of medical images. CNN architecture shown in Figure 9 is a multilayered neural network that performs convolution operation on input images to extract features. These convolution operations are performed by the convolutional layer. Other layers in CNN architecture are the pooling layer, rectified linear unit layer, and fully connected layer. The fully connected layer is the last layer of this architecture that generates the output. A study by Wen (2015 conducted for liver tumor segmentation on CT scans used the CNN model. While authors (Roth et al., 2015) used the CNN model on CT scans for pancreas segmentation. CNN model has also used the by authors (Pereira, 2016) to perform brain tumor segmentation on MR images of the brain. The segmentation of the first-trimester placenta on 3D ultrasounds was presented in a study used CNN. Deep learning model CNN was applied on PET images to segment cervical tumors (Chen et al., 2019). Segmentation of ribs was performed on chest X-ray images with the help of a convolutional neural network (Wessel, 2019).

Figure 9. Architecture of CNN

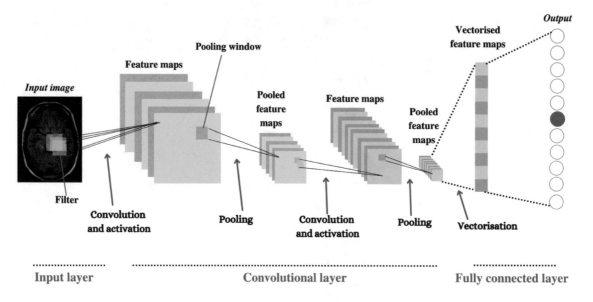

In year the 2015, authors Ronneberger et al., presented a deep model named "U-Net". The U-net architecture displayed in Figure 10 was specifically designed for segmentation on medical images. The fast and accurate segmentation quality of the U-Net model made this famous among researchers. U-Net model was used in the study by authors (Dalmış, 2017) to segment the breast and fibro-glandular tissue on MR images of the breast. While a modified U-Net model was used in the study by (Shreyas & Pankajakshan, 2017) to segment the brain region on MR images of the brain. To detect the organs-at-risk from CT scans of head and neck, the U-Net model was used by authors neck (HaN Zhu et al., 2019). In another study by authors (Blanc-Durand et al., 2018) the U-net model was used for detection and segmentation of gliomas tumor on PET images of the brain. U-net model was also applied on CT scans for the segmentation of lung parenchyma in the study by authors (Skourt et al., 2018) and for segmentation of whole heart by authors (Ye et al., 2019). Knee cartilage segmentation on knee MR images was conducted in the study by authors (Panfilov et al., 2019) using the U-Net model.

Figure 10. Architecture of U-Net model
(Ronneberger, 2015)

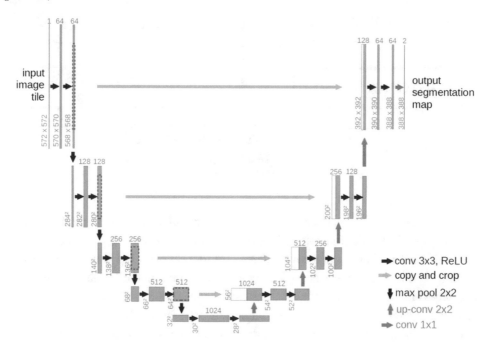

IMAGE SEGMENTATION

Segmentation is an important point of digital image processing. Separating the object present in the picture and placing the object with the same attribute in same category is part of the segmentation. The separated object is selected for further processing. At times, not all objects present in the image are required. Unnecessary objects are removed and necessary objects are kept for further processing. There are many different ways of doing segmentation.

Image segmentation is considered a very important part of image processing that divides the image into different segments mostly used for object recognition. Sometimes only a few parts of an image needed for processing and to get some kind of information, segmentation plays a vital role here. When an image is divided into parts then it becomes easy to select the required parts for further processing. Various image segmentation methods have been introduced by researchers depicted in Figure 11, and explained below in brief:

Figure 11. Image Segmentation Methods

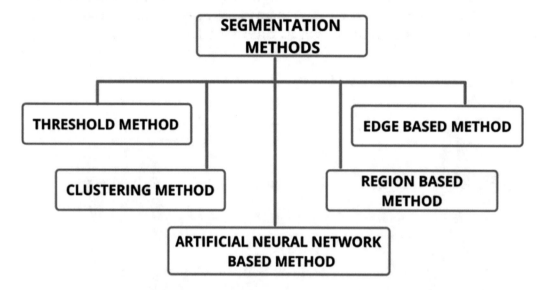

1. Threshold Segmentation Method: One of the simplest methods of segmentation is Threshold method. A threshold value T decides the color of the particular pixel according to its intensity value. If the intensity value is less than T, then color black is set for that pixel but if intensity value is equal or greater than T, then color white is set for pixel. Thus in this method, image is segmented on the basis of white and black colors only.
2. Edge Based Segmentation Method: As the name suggests, this method segments the objects on the basis of their edges. Edges are detected on the basis of intensity value. Pixels of similar intensity values are selected as edges of the same object while the change in intensity value disconnects edges.
3. Region-Based Segmentation Method: In this method image is segmented into regions and elements in a region have similar kind of characteristics. Two main region-based segmentation techniques are:
    a. Region Growing Technique: In this method, by manually or automatically an initial pixel is selected that is called seed. Segmentation performed on basis of seed's growth.
    b. Region Splitting & Merging Technique: In this method splitting is performed for segmenting the image into regions and merging is performed to combine regions with similar adjacent.
4. Clustering Based Segmentation Methods: Clusters of pixels that have characteristics are selected and grouped in same cluster. Thus objects are segmented in clustering way. Pixels of one cluster have characteristics different from pixels from other cluster.
5. Artificial Neural Network Based Segmentation Method: ANN-based algorithms try to simulate the human brain's learning process and make decisions as a human does. In medical imaging, ANN-based methods are currently the most popular methods. Important information is extracted and requisite objects are detached from the background. This process is achieved in two steps, first objects are extracted, and then neural network segment the image.

HOW DEEP LEARNING IS HELPFUL IN BRAIN MRI SEGMENTATION?

Various researches have shown the use of deep learning techniques in different areas like healthcare, Natural Language Processing (NLP), Visual Recognition, Image Processing. Neural networks can help with images for image classification, object detection, segmentation and image reconstruction, etc. In medical science, segmentation can help to segment ROI from the whole image captured through different imaging applications.

MRI technique gives a detailed inside picture of the brain. Recently, deep learning models are performing effectively for the segmentation of MRI scans of brain. That is why, this technology is attracting researchers to work on it and generate high performace models. Authors (Zhang et al., 2015) presented study of segmentation of brain tissues of isointense stage of infants in multimodality MR images, authors proposed a deep learning model. Multimodality MR Images were input to the model and output was segmented map. Multiple intermediate layers perform different operations between inputs and outputs so that nonlinear mapping can be captures. In another study, authors (Kleesiesk et al., 2016) developed a 3D CNN model that handles random number of MR image modalities including contrast-enhanced scans. Aim of the study was to establish a model with less or no parameter tuning and to develop a model that could perform better with single modality or with grouping of these modalities like T1, T2, T2-FLAIR. This study was to distinguish between brain tissues or non-brain tissues. Authors (Pereira et. al, 2016) presented a CNN based novel automatic segmentation model .MR images of brain tumor were collected for the study. The model has convolutional layers with 3X3 kernel size. The kernel size consents a deeper architecture. In pre-processing step, examination of Intensity normalization was performed. Authors also suggested that for the segmentation process, data augmentation plays an effective role. A comparative analysis between shallow and deep architectures in this study shows that performance of shallow architecture is low. Another comparative analysis between activation functions ReLU and LReLU shows that, LReLU performed well for training of CNN. Authors (Telrandhe et al., 2016) suggested system for detecting and identifying brain tumor from MR images. The system can find the tumor area and its type. Authors used k-means clustering with image pre-processing. Support Vector Machine technique was used to make system adaptive.

While authors (Akkus et al., 2017), presented a review of recent segmentation techniques for brain MRI. Study shows that deep learning based architectures has overtaken the traditional machine learning algorithms and supervised learning based deep learning algorithms needs cohort of manual ground truth labels that is not an easy task if applied on large scale of datasets; that is why deep learning models with few requirements on ground truth labels and unsupervised learning could make a highly robust model. Transfer learning could also make model very reliable. Authors (Havaei et al., 2017) proposed a DNN based segmentation method that is fully automatic to diagnose the brain tumor in brain region. Study is done to diagnose both high and low grade glioblastomas in MR images. Proposed CNN model feats with the local, and global contextual features. The last layer of network was convolutional execution of fully connected layer to increase the speed. A 2-phase training process holds the difficulties in inequity of tumor labels. A three cascaded CNN architecture is considered where once output is others input. Authors (Kamnitsas et al., 2017) presented a CNN based segmentation model that is a 3D architecture that automatically segments the brain lesion. The model also focuses on the intrinsic class imbalance of segmentation problems. Authors fined that small convolutional kernels are beneficial for developing a deeper network. For multi scale processing, parallel pathways were used for processing the image context of larger size. Proposed network was 11-layers deep. Input images were processed simultaneously at multiple scales by dual pathway architecture. MR Image data sets of brain injuries, stroke and tumors were used for segmentation and to evaluate the performance of the system. In a study by Kapoor and Thakur, 2017, authors examined several segmentation approaches and found that machine learning techniques are playing very important role in this area. Authors (Patil et al., 2017) presented different techniques for segmentation and finding of brain tumor on brain MR images. For segmentation and feature extraction techniques like k-mean clustering, curvelet transform, SOM clustering, fuzzy C-mean clustering was used.

Authors (Kong et al., 2018) used different methods on head MRI dataset for the extraction of precise shapes of different tissues of brain then CNN was applied with deep learning for automatic image segmentation. This process reduces the processing time. For increment in speed authors introduces parallel computing. Compared to manual segmentation or semi-automatic, parallel computing has great impact on reducing the processing time. Authors have shown that deep learning with image processing can perform automatic segmentation of tissues, and can play vital role in neurology. Authors (McClure et al., 2018) developed a Bayesian deep neural network. This model can predict FreeSurfer segmentations from MR images. The model was trained on large number of datasets. Model was trained by variational inference technique. Proposed method could be applied on any new deep network that performs segmentation. In another study by (Roy et al., 2018) authors proposed a framework for extraction of intracranial tissues based on deep learning. For study purposes, multi-contrast MR images were used in occurrence of TBI. This framework could be applied to unlike species also. Authors (Selvathi & Vanmathi, 2018) proposed a deep learning based model that is fully automated and segment brain region. The model not only segments the brain region but also defines the locations of brain image. Model segment the brain then detects tumor and affected area of brain, number of tumors present, and also detects the size and type of tumor. Thus the model presents the complete information about the disease. By resembling the skull boundaries the brain region is segmented. Morphological area constraints help in identifying the tumor region. Connected component labeling segments the tumor region. MR images are used for study. The proposed model generates output after completion of two phases. First is pre-processing stage in which MR image is input and with the help of Non Local Mean filter, rician noise was removed. In second phase, segmentation was done and skull portion is removed by CNN. Architecture of this model is three layered neural network. While authors (Sobhaninia et al., 2018), presented an automatic segmentation model for brain tumor segmentation. A new method was introduced for CNN in this model that does not required preprocessing steps. Results from the study presented that, to improve accuracy of segmentation, angles based separations of images can make this possible. Sagittal view image segmentation scored high in this study.

Authors (Mlynarski et al., 2019) proposed segmentation model based on CNN that can be trained equally on fully and weakly annotated training datasets. Idea behind the study was to add a new branch to segmentation model that perform classification on images. Model was trained in a way that it does not learn irrelevant features and can perform both classification and segmentation. Myronenko (2019) described a semantic segmentation architecture using 3D MR images. For this, an encoder and decoder based CNN architecture was implemented. Deep image features were extracted by encoder part while dense segmentation masks were reconstructed by decoder part. A variational-autoencoder branch was used for the reconstruction of input image. Authors (Wu et al., 2019) presented a novel CNN model that is Multi-cascaded architecture for segmenting brain tumor. Several components linked for transitional outcomes. Multi-scale features applied for the rough segmentation. Fake outputs were discarded by using CRFs. Resultant segmentation was obtained by combining three segmentation models.

Naser & Deen (2020) showed the potential of the use of both DL and transfer learning to diagnose the brain tumor on MRI scans of the brain. The architecture was based on U-Net model for the segmentation . Authors (Qamar et al., 2020) developed a novel mixed design on the groundwork of dense and residual connection and Inception module to segment the infant's brain MRI. The proposed model was based on UNet model that has encoder and decoder architecture. Authors (Ramzan et al., 2020) presented a deep neural network for the cortical and subcortical brain region segmentation. The proposed model performs the segmentation of multiple brain regions in approximately nine regions. The proposed model was based on 3D CNN.

Authors (Díaz-Pernas et al., 2021) proposed a segmentation and classification deep CNN model. The proposed model works on brain MRI and can diagnose glioma, pituitary, and meningioma tumor. Raja and Viswasa, (2021) used MR Images for segmentation using the technique of thresholding segmentation that diagnose brain tumor. In another study by authors (Khairandish et al., 2021) for the detection and classification of brain tumor, hybrid CNN and SVM methods were used on MR images of the brain. The presented study classifies the MR images of the brain as a malignant tumor or benign tumor. Authors (Zhang et al., 2021) suggested a cross-modality deep neural network to segment the brain tumor region. The multi-modality MR scans were used as input image dataset to the deep model. Figure 12 presents two MRI images of brain. Fig12.a is the input MRI image of brain and Figure 12.b is the brain region segmented in the input image through CNN model.

Figure 12. MRI scans of brain with segmented brain region: (a) MRI image of brain (b) Segmented brain region

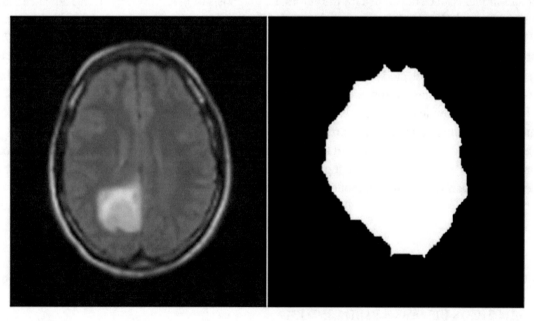

DISCUSSION

Brain is the most crucial body part that is also part of central nervous system. Any kind of abnormality inside the brain can make it's difficult to work. Abnormality could be due to tumor, damage in tissues, blood clotting, Alzheimer's disease, etc. MRI imaging technique has been considered as one of the important imaging technique that can show internal area of brain and doctors can diagnose the presence of abnormality through MR images. Images captured through MRI scanner are processed for clearer picture and to get detailed information. Deep learning technique comes in the category of machine learning where models are designed to perform automatic task. In the area of medical science, deep neural networks can be used to diagnose different disease on images captured through various imaging techniques. Researchers have used deep learning in the area of neuroimaging where these models can make brain disease detection task easy and automatic on brain MR images. Studies have suggested that deep models can assist medical team in decision making. Deep models require large amount of datasets for training. Deep models can perform segmentation on brain MR images to remove skull area, detect the size and location of tumor. Convolutional neural networks are deep models that are known as the favourite of researchers to develop the brain MR image segmentation models. U-Net architecture is particularly designed to perform the segmentation task on medical images. Various studies have used U-Net architecture as the backbone to develop a new model.

This chapter explores the interesting sub-area of artificial intelligence that is deep learning. Though, the deep learning technique has a wide area of applications. The motive of this chapter is to make focus on importance of deep learning in the medical line. With the help of deep learning technique, advance computer models can be developed for the automatic diagnosis of brain diseases. These advance models can help neurologist in their decision making to detect the problem area and design the treatment procedure. For this purpose, various studies have been included in literature review from year 2015 to year 2021. By studying various previous research works, it shows that CNN and U-Net are deep models that have been part of almost all selected studies for the segmentation of brain MRI. Researchers have developed deep models by updating these models and to get the required results. Thus, these studies suggest that CNN and U-Net deep learning models have performed well for the problem domain. Though accurate segmentation of the brain region is a critical task; deep learning techniques can help in make this task automatic and also can help the medical team in decision making. A lot of work has been conducted on the segmentation of brain MRI with deep learning models; experiments and updating on deep learning models can make more prominent models in the medical imaging area.

REFERENCES

Akkus, Z., Galimzianova, A., Hoogi, A., Rubin, D. L., & Erickson, B. J. (2017). Deep learning for brain MRI segmentation: State of the art and future directions. *Journal of Digital Imaging*, *30*(4), 449–459. doi:10.100710278-017-9983-4 PMID:28577131

Blanc-Durand, P., Van Der Gucht, A., Schaefer, N., Itti, E., & Prior, J. O. (2018). Automatic lesion detection and segmentation of 18F-FET PET in gliomas: A full 3D U-Net convolutional neural network study. *PLoS One*, *13*(4), e0195798. doi:10.1371/journal.pone.0195798 PMID:29652908

Chen, L., Shen, C., Zhou, Z., Maquilan, G., Albuquerque, K., Folkert, M. R., & Wang, J. (2019). Automatic PET cervical tumor segmentation by combining deep learning and anatomic prior. *Physics in Medicine and Biology*, *64*(8), 085019. doi:10.1088/1361-6560/ab0b64 PMID:30818303

Dalmış, M. U., Litjens, G., Holland, K., Setio, A., Mann, R., Karssemeijer, N., & Gubern-Mérida, A. (2017). Using deep learning to segment breast and fibroglandular tissue in MRI volumes. *Medical Physics*, *44*(2), 533–546. doi:10.1002/mp.12079 PMID:28035663

Díaz-Pernas, F. J., Martínez-Zarzuela, M., Antón-Rodríguez, M., & González-Ortega, D. (2021, February). A Deep Learning Approach for Brain Tumor Classification and Segmentation Using a Multiscale Convolutional Neural Network. *Health Care*, *9*(2), 153. PMID:33540873

Fonseca, L. M., & Costa, M. H. (1997, October). Automatic registration of satellite images. In *Proceedings X Brazilian Symposium on Computer Graphics and Image Processing* (pp. 219-226). IEEE. 10.1109/SIGRA.1997.625182

Havaei, M., Davy, A., Warde-Farley, D., Biard, A., Courville, A., Bengio, Y., Pal, C., Jodoin, P.-M., & Larochelle, H. (2017). Brain tumor segmentation with deep neural networks. *Medical Image Analysis*, *35*, 18–31. doi:10.1016/j.media.2016.05.004 PMID:27310171

Kamnitsas, K., Ledig, C., Newcombe, V. F., Simpson, J. P., Kane, A. D., Menon, D. K., Rueckert, D., & Glocker, B. (2017). Efficient multi-scale 3D CNN with fully connected CRF for accurate brain lesion segmentation. *Medical Image Analysis*, *36*, 61–78. doi:10.1016/j.media.2016.10.004 PMID:27865153

Kapoor, L., & Thakur, S. (2017, January). A survey on brain tumor detection using image processing techniques. In *2017 7th International Conference on Cloud Computing, Data Science & Engineering-Confluence* (pp. 582-585). IEEE. 10.1109/CONFLUENCE.2017.7943218

Khairandish, M. O., Sharma, M., Jain, V., Chatterjee, J. M., & Jhanjhi, N. Z. (2021). A Hybrid CNN-SVM Threshold Segmentation Approach for Tumor Detection and Classification of MRI Brain Images. *IRBM*. Advance online publication. doi:10.1016/j.irbm.2021.06.003

Kleesiek, J., Urban, G., Hubert, A., Schwarz, D., Maier-Hein, K., Bendszus, M., & Biller, A. (2016). Deep MRI brain extraction: A 3D convolutional neural network for skull stripping. *NeuroImage*, *129*, 460–469. doi:10.1016/j.neuroimage.2016.01.024 PMID:26808333

Kong, Z., Luo, J., Xu, S., & Li, T. (2018, February). Automatic tissue image segmentation based on image processing and deep learning. In *Neural Imaging and Sensing 2018* (Vol. 10481, p. 104811T). International Society for Optics and Photonics. doi:10.1117/12.2293481

Li, W., Jia, F., & Hu, Q. (2015). Automatic segmentation of liver tumor in CT images with deep convolutional neural networks. *Journal of Computer and Communications*, *3*(11), 146–151. doi:10.4236/jcc.2015.311023

McClure, P., Rho, N., Lee, J. A., Kaczmarzyk, J. R., Zheng, C., Ghosh, S. S., ... Pereira, F. (2018). *Knowing what you know in brain segmentation using deep neural networks*. arXiv preprint arXiv:1812.01719.

Mlynarski, P., Delingette, H., Criminisi, A., & Ayache, N. (2019). Deep learning with mixed supervision for brain tumor segmentation. *Journal of Medical Imaging (Bellingham, Wash.)*, *6*(3), 034002. doi:10.1117/1.JMI.6.3.034002 PMID:31423456

Myronenko, A. (2018, September). 3D MRI brain tumor segmentation using autoencoder regularization. In *International MICCAI Brainlesion Workshop* (pp. 311-320). Springer.

Nagel, S. (2019). *Towards a home-use BCI: fast asynchronous control and robust non-control state detection* (Doctoral dissertation). Eberhard Karls Universität Tübingen.

Naser, M. A., & Deen, M. J. (2020). Brain tumor segmentation and grading of lower-grade glioma using deep learning in MRI images. *Computers in Biology and Medicine*, *121*, 103758. doi:10.1016/j.compbiomed.2020.103758 PMID:32568668

Panfilov, E., Tiulpin, A., Klein, S., Nieminen, M. T., & Saarakkala, S. (2019). Improving robustness of deep learning based knee mri segmentation: Mixup and adversarial domain adaptation. *Proceedings of the IEEE/CVF International Conference on Computer Vision Workshops*. 10.1109/ICCVW.2019.00057

Patil, M., Pawar, M., Patil, M., & Nichal, A. (2017). A review paper on brain tumor segmentation and detection. *IJIREEICE*, *5*(1), 12–15. doi:10.17148/IJIREEICE.2017.5103

Pereira, S., Pinto, A., Alves, V., & Silva, C. A. (2016). Brain tumor segmentation using convolutional neural networks in MRI images. *IEEE Transactions on Medical Imaging*, *35*(5), 1240–1251. doi:10.1109/TMI.2016.2538465 PMID:26960222

Phelps, M. E. (2000). Positron emission tomography provides molecular imaging of biological processes. *Proceedings of the National Academy of Sciences of the United States of America*, *97*(16), 9226–9233. doi:10.1073/pnas.97.16.9226 PMID:10922074

Preston, D. C. (2006). Magnetic resonance imaging (mri) of the brain and spine: Basics. *MRI Basics, Case Med, 30*.

Qamar, S., Jin, H., Zheng, R., Ahmad, P., & Usama, M. (2020). A variant form of 3D-UNet for infant brain segmentation. *Future Generation Computer Systems*, *108*, 613–623. doi:10.1016/j.future.2019.11.021

Raja, P. M. S., & Viswasa, A. (2021). ScienceDirect Brain tumor classification using a hybrid deep autoencoder with Bayesian fuzzy clustering-based segmentation approach. *Integrative Medicine Research*, 1–14.

Ramzan, F., Khan, M. U. G., Iqbal, S., Saba, T., & Rehman, A. (2020). Volumetric segmentation of brain regions from MRI scans using 3D convolutional neural networks. *IEEE Access: Practical Innovations, Open Solutions*, *8*, 103697–103709. doi:10.1109/ACCESS.2020.2998901

Rani, S., Jindal, S., & Kaur, B. (2016). A brief review on image restoration techniques. *International Journal of Computers and Applications*, *150*(12), 30–33. doi:10.5120/ijca2016911623

Rao, C. H., Naganjaneyulu, P. V., & Prasad, K. S. (2017). Brain tumor detection and segmentation using conditional random field. In *2017 IEEE 7th International Advance Computing Conference (IACC)* (pp. 807-810). IEEE. 10.1109/IACC.2017.0166

Ronneberger, O., Fischer, P., & Brox, T. (2015, October). U-net: Convolutional networks for biomedical image segmentation. In *International Conference on Medical image computing and computer-assisted intervention* (pp. 234-241). Springer. 10.1007/978-3-319-24574-4_28

Roth, H. R., Lu, L., Farag, A., Shin, H. C., Liu, J., Turkbey, E. B., & Summers, R. M. (2015, October). Deeporgan: Multi-level deep convolutional networks for automated pancreas segmentation. In *International conference on medical image computing and computer-assisted intervention* (pp. 556-564). Springer.

Roy, S., Knutsen, A., Korotcov, A., Bosomtwi, A., Dardzinski, B., Butman, J. A., & Pham, D. L. (2018, April). A deep learning framework for brain extraction in humans and animals with traumatic brain injury. In *2018 IEEE 15th International Symposium on Biomedical Imaging (ISBI 2018)* (pp. 687-691). IEEE. 10.1109/ISBI.2018.8363667

Saxena, S., Kumari, N., & Pattnaik, S. (2021). Brain Tumour Segmentation in FLAIR MRI Using Sliding Window Texture Feature Extraction Followed by Fuzzy C-Means Clustering. *International Journal of Healthcare Information Systems and Informatics*, *16*(3), 1–20. doi:10.4018/IJHISI.20210701.oa1

Selvathi, D., & Vanmathi, T. (2018, February). Brain region segmentation using convolutional neural network. In *2018 4th International Conference on Electrical Energy Systems (ICEES)* (pp. 661-666). IEEE. 10.1109/ICEES.2018.8442394

Shreyas, V., & Pankajakshan, V. (2017, October). A deep learning architecture for brain tumor segmentation in MRI images. In *2017 IEEE 19th International Workshop on Multimedia Signal Processing (MMSP)* (pp. 1-6). IEEE. 10.1109/MMSP.2017.8122291

Skourt, B. A., El Hassani, A., & Majda, A. (2018). Lung CT image segmentation using deep neural networks. *Procedia Computer Science*, *127*, 109–113. doi:10.1016/j.procs.2018.01.104

Sobhaninia, Z., Rezaei, S., Noroozi, A., Ahmadi, M., Zarrabi, H., Karimi, N., . . . Samavi, S. (2018). Brain tumor segmentation using deep learning by type specific sorting of images. *arXiv preprint arXiv:1809.07786*.

Telrandhe, S. R., Pimpalkar, A., & Kendhe, A. (2016, February). Detection of brain tumor from MRI images by using segmentation & SVM. In *2016 World Conference on Futuristic Trends in Research and Innovation for Social Welfare (Startup Conclave)* (pp. 1-6). IEEE. 10.1109/STARTUP.2016.7583949

The Basics. (2011). *Learning Neuroradiology*. Retrieved from https://sites.google.com/a/wisc.edu/neuroradiology/image-acquisition/the-basics

Wessel, J., Heinrich, M. P., von Berg, J., Franz, A., & Saalbach, A. (2019). *Sequential rib labeling and segmentation in chest X-ray using Mask R-CNN*. arXiv preprint arXiv:1908.08329.

Wu, X., Jiang, G., Wang, X., Xie, P., & Li, X. (2019). A multi-level-denoising autoencoder approach for wind turbine fault detection. *IEEE Access: Practical Innovations, Open Solutions*, *7*, 59376–59387. doi:10.1109/ACCESS.2019.2914731

Ye, C., Wang, W., Zhang, S., & Wang, K. (2019). Multi-depth fusion network for whole-heart CT image segmentation. *IEEE Access: Practical Innovations, Open Solutions*, *7*, 23421–23429. doi:10.1109/ACCESS.2019.2899635

Zhang, D., Huang, G., Zhang, Q., Han, J., Han, J., & Yu, Y. (2021). Cross-modality deep feature learning for brain tumor segmentation. *Pattern Recognition*, *110*, 107562. doi:10.1016/j.patcog.2020.107562

Zhu, W., Huang, Y., Zeng, L., Chen, X., Liu, Y., Qian, Z., Du, N., Fan, W., & Xie, X. (2019). AnatomyNet: Deep learning for fast and fully automated whole-volume segmentation of head and neck anatomy. *Medical Physics*, *46*(2), 576–589. doi:10.1002/mp.13300 PMID:30480818

ADDITIONAL READING

Bhatt, D. P., Bhatnagar, V., & Sharma, P. (2021). Meta-analysis of predictions of COVID-19 disease based on CT-scan and X-ray images. *Journal of Interdisciplinary Mathematics*, *24*(2), 381–409. doi:10.1080/09720502.2021.1884385

Bhatt, D. P., & Srimal, G. (2020). Lung Cancer Detection through CT scan images using Convolution Neural Networks. *International Journal of Advanced Science and Technology*, *29*(3), 11125–11131. http://sersc.org/journals/index.php/IJAST/article/view/28007

Dougherty, G. (2009). *Digital image processing for medical applications*. Cambridge University Press. doi:10.1017/CBO9780511609657

Gaur, L., Bhatia, U., Jhanjhi, N. Z., Muhammad, G., & Masud, M. (2021). Medical image-based detection of COVID-19 using Deep Convolution Neural Networks. *Multimedia Systems*, 1–10. doi:10.100700530-021-00794-6 PMID:33935377

Gaur, L., Solanki, A., Wamba, S. F., & Jhanjhi, N. Z. (Eds.). (2021). *Advanced AI Techniques and Applications in Bioinformatics*. CRC Press. doi:10.1201/9781003126164

Hsu, C. Y., Schneller, B., Ghaffari, M., Alaraj, A., & Linninger, A. (2015). Medical image processing for fully integrated subject specific whole brain mesh generation. *Technologies*, *3*(2), 126–141. doi:10.3390/technologies3020126

Hussein, S., Kandel, P., Bolan, C. W., Wallace, M. B., & Bagci, U. (2019). Lung and pancreatic tumor characterization in the deep learning era: Novel supervised and unsupervised learning approaches. *IEEE Transactions on Medical Imaging*, *38*(8), 1777–1787. doi:10.1109/TMI.2019.2894349 PMID:30676950

Kaswan, K. S., Gaur, L., Dhatterwal, J. S., & Kumar, R. (2021). AI-Based Natural Language Processing for the Generation of Meaningful Information Electronic Health Record (EHR) Data. In Advanced AI Techniques and Applications in Bioinformatics (pp. 41-86). CRC Press.

Latif, J., Xiao, C., Imran, A., & Tu, S. (2019, January). Medical imaging using machine learning and deep learning algorithms: a review. In *2019 2nd International Conference on Computing, Mathematics and Engineering Technologies (iCoMET)* (pp. 1-5). IEEE. 10.1109/ICOMET.2019.8673502

Modi, A. S. (2018, June). Review article on deep learning approaches. In *2018 Second International Conference on Intelligent Computing and Control Systems (ICICCS)* (pp. 1635-1639). IEEE. 10.1109/ICCONS.2018.8663057

Niyaz, U., & Sambyal, A. S. (2018, December). Advances in deep learning techniques for medical image analysis. In *2018 Fifth International Conference on Parallel, Distributed and Grid Computing (PDGC)* (pp. 271-277). IEEE. 10.1109/PDGC.2018.8745790

Somasundaram, S., & Gobinath, R. (2019, February). Current trends on deep learning models for brain tumor segmentation and detection–a review. In *2019 International Conference on Machine Learning, Big Data, Cloud and Parallel Computing (COMITCon)* (pp. 217-221). IEEE.

KEY TERMS AND DEFINITIONS

Deep Learning: A self-learning technique of machines that is inspired by the working of human brain.

Digital Image Processing: Computerized processing of digital images to make images clearer and to get information from the image.

Image Segmentation: Partitioning image into different clusters.

Machine Learning: A technique which makes machines self-learner.

Medical Imaging: Techniques that are used to get inside details of the human body.

Neuroscience: It is the study of how the sensory system creates, its construction, and what it does.

Tumor: Abnormal growth of cell inside the human body.

Chapter 2
Optimized Breast Cancer Premature Detection Method With Computational Segmentation:
A Systematic Review Mapping

Soobia Saeed

Taylor's University, Malaysia

Noor Zaman Jhanjhi

ⓘ https://orcid.org/0000-0001-8116-4733

Taylor's University, Malaysia

Mehmood Naqvi

Mohawk College, Canada

Mamoona Humyun

ⓘ https://orcid.org/0000-0001-6339-2257

Jouf University, Saudi Arabia

Muneer Ahmad

School of Electrical Engineering and Computer Science (SEECS), National University of Science and Technology, Pakistan

Loveleen Gaur

Amity University, Noida, India

ABSTRACT

Breast cancer is the most common cancer in women aged 59 to 69 years old. Studies have shown that early detection and treatment of breast cancer increases the chances of survival significantly. They also demonstrated that detecting small lesions early improves forecasting and results in a significant reduction in death cases. The most effective screening diagnostic technique in this case is mammography. However, interpretation of mammograms is difficult due to small differences in tissue densities within mammographic images. This is especially true for dense breasts, and this study suggests that screening mammography is more effective in fatty breast tissue than in dense breast tissue. This study focuses on breast cancer diagnosis as well as identifying risk factors and their assessments of breast cancer as well as premature detection of breast cancer by analyzing 3D MRI mammography methods and segmentation of mammographic images using machine learning.

DOI: 10.4018/978-1-7998-8929-8.ch002

INTRODUCTION

When the healthy cells grow abnormally in the breast and continue to accumulate resulting in a mass or lumps called tumor. The tumor is categorizing as benign and malignant. A benign tumor cannot spread in the other part of the body but possibly grow but the malignant tumor can quickly grow and spread throughout the body. Breast cancer can expand in other parts of the body through arteries or lymph vessels known as metastasis. The study covers both non-invasive and invasive cancers, as well as Premature stages of breast cancer to localize cancer in the breast, which include I, II, and III.These stages describe how cancer has progressed, including how much it has grown and where it has spread. Despite the fact that breast cancer spreads prematurely to lymph nodes, it can also migrate to other parts of the body such as the bones, lungs, liver, and brain, which is known as metastatic or stage IV breast cancer.While it depends on the condition of breast cancer, normally it is not often considered the relationship of lymph nodes comes to stage IV breast cancer. It depends on different types of breast cancer which are based on the cells that exist in the breast to become cancerous. Breast cancer can have started in any area of the breast, a breast consists of three major parts including (1) lobules, (2) ducts, and (3) connective tissue. The lobules indicate the glands which produce milk, ducts are the tube that brings milk to the nipples and associated with tissues containing fibrous and fatty tissues surround and holds everything together. Normally breast cancer starts in the lobules or ducts. Breast cancer can metastasis, or spread outside of the breast, through lymphatic and blood channels to other regions of the body. Table 1 depicts the various kinds of breast cancer and their associated breast diseases.

Table 1. Breast malignant tumors

Types of Breast Cancer	Ratio of growth
In Situ Carcinoma	15-30%
Ductal Carcinoma in Situ	80%
Lobular Carcinoma in Situ	20%
Invasive Carcinoma	70-85%
Ductal Carcinoma(General Type)	79%
Lobular Carcinoma	10%
Tubular Cribriform Carcinoma	6%
Mucinous Carcinoma	2%
Medullary Carcinoma	2%
Papillary Carcinoma	1%

Invasive and non-invasive breast cancers are also possible. Non-invasive breast cancer does not expand beyond the milk ducts or lobules in the breast, whereas invasive breast cancer spreads to distant organs and tissues. Ductal carcinoma and lobular carcinoma are cancers that begin in the ducts or lobes. Other types of breast cancer, such as invasive ductal carcinoma, can spread outside the ducts and into other regions of the breast tissue. The other type of breast cancer is invasive lobular carcinoma, which can migrate from the lobules to the adjacent breast tissues, allowing the cancer cells to migrate to other parts of the body. Ductal carcinoma is frequently developing cancer in the breast from the beginning of the cell that contour the milk ducts. In the end, ductal carcinoma in situ (DCIS) cannot spread to another part of the body but it affects only the duct due to non-invasive cancer

Multi-Grading and Staging of Breast Cancer

The irregular shape of cancer cells and tissues is depicted in the breast cancer classification. Breast cancer is classified in this stage based on the types, grades, and stages of the disease. Table 1 defines and categorizes various types, grades, and stages of cancer, as well as various ranges:

- Grade I (Low-grade):Normal cells and tissues are similar to cancer cells and tissues. These cancers are well-differentiated, according to research.
- Grade II (Low-grade):Cells and tissues are irregular and slightly different, but they are considered low grade.
- Grade III (High-grade):Cancer cells and tissues are frequently abnormal. These cracks are well-known for being difficult to distinguish because they no longer have an architectural shape or theme.
- Grade IV (High-grade):These undifferentiated tumors produce the rarest cells. They are of the highest grade and generally develop and spread faster than lower grade cancers.
- Stage 0:None-growth cancer.
- Stages 1 to 3:Primary cancer spread only to surrounding tissues.
- Stage 4:Cancer has extent to distant parts of the body.

The stages of breast cancer are described in table.2 to demonstrate the various subtypes and stages of breast cancer. It displays the survival rates' mortalities.

Table 2. Stages of breast cancer

Stages	Grades	Types of Breast Cancer	Survival Rate
0	Low Grade-I	Ductal Carcinoma or Lobular Carcinoma in Situ	92%
I	Low Grade-I	Invasive Carcinoma 2cm or less in size without nodal involvement and no distance metastasis	87%
II	Low Grade-II	Invasive Carcinoma less than 5cm without nodal involvement but movable axillary nodes and no distance metastasis	75%
III	High Grade-I	Invasive Carcinoma less than 5cm with nodal involvement and fixed axillary nodes	46%
IV	High Grade-II	Any form of breast cancer with distance metastasis	13%

Premature Detection of Breast Cancer

As breast cancer is one of the most frequent cancers, there are a variety of screening tests available to detect it Premature. Mammography, MRI, ultrasound, and clinical breast examinations are all used to detect breast cancer. Medical science has recently developed an advanced screening procedure to improve the options for breast cancer screening and Premature diagnosis. The development of a 3D mammography screening procedure known as breast tomosynthesis is one of the new technologies. This method combines images of the breast from various angles to create 3D approximation images. This cutting-edge technology is widely available in clinics and breast screening centres, and it is considered superior to 2D mammography (Local mammography technology) in terms of detecting cancer at an earlier stage. However, the Premature detection of breast cancer is easy to treat with fewer risk chances and can reduce the mortality rate to 25%. Mostly, this Premature detection reduced the risk factor of breast cancer diagnosing in female's breasts such as postmenopausal female to mammography of every two years later because it enhances after 5 years later to breast tumor to spread 1mm for a year, < 2 years longer than 5mm spread, and 1 or 2 years measure this tumor around 2cm which is diagnosing by palpation (Dupont & Page, 1985; Fakhro et al., 1999; Fattah et al., 2000; Hamid et al., 2001; Harirchi et al., 2000; Key et al., 2001).In this study, we describe how to use the most up-to-date mammography technology to detect breast cancer Premature and the many types of breast cancer. The literature review is discussed in detail in Section 2. Section 3 discusses the experimental work and screening method implementation criteria, as well as how breast density might be considered a risk factor. Section 4 show the results and discussion and section 6 mention the conclusion with future work.

LITERATURE REVIEW

Breast cancer is common cancer in females globally for the cause of death. The mortality rate varies about fivefold around the world, but they are rapidly increasing the region that until had a low rate of diseases currently. Numerous of the recognized risk factors are associated with oestrogens. Risk can be increase by obesity in postmenopausal females, late menopause and initial menarche, and high concentrations of endogenous oestradiol are linked to an increase in risk which is declared by potential studies. In addition, childbearing may reduce risk with superior protection of Premature birth and a greater number of births; according to the research, breastfeeding has a protective effect on females. Menopause has a lesser chance of breast cancer risk in females depends on both hormonal therapy and oral contraceptives which seems to reduce once usage stops. However, alcohol increase the risk of breast cancer but probably physical activity is creating the protective zone of females. In addition, we consider the Mutations in minority cases of breast cancer that increase the risk in certain genes significantly (Siegel et al., 2017).We know that breast cancer is one of the most dangerous diseases who is the second leading cancer in the world that causes the death ratio is high in females. The cure of breast cancer is one of the challenging faces in the world as the growth of cancer including different types of cells are an uncontrollable way in the breast. The best approach to the prevention of breast cancer is Premature diagnosing to reduce the death ratio of breast cancer. For an instant, few modern countries follow-up and increase the survival rate of breast cancer is above 80% in 5 years due to the prevention of the Premature detection process.

In the current era, the development of preventive methods has great progress made in the understanding of breast cancer. Breast cancer stem cells have been discovered the numerous genes associated with breast cancer and mechanism of tumor drug-resistant and also pathogenesis have been disclosed. To improve the patient's quality of life through biological prevention, which is recently developed and more pharmacological options are now available for chemoprevention of breast cancer. In this research review, we summarize the major components of breast cancer pathogenesis, risk factor, preventive strategies and associated breast cancer genes have been published in the last years. These collections represent the significant development in the ongoing battle against the breast cancer

Breast cancer is one of the most regular malignancies in females worldwide, with 570,000 mortalities reported in 2015. Every year at least 1.5 million women face breast abnormalities globally (25% of all females are cancer patients) are diagnosed with breast cancer (DeSantis et al., 2016; Siegel et al., 2017). In 2017, the ratio has been increased and around 30% of new cases reported for breast cancer in females all over the world (Drukteinis et al., 2013). We know that breast cancer is one of common cancer to easily transfer to the other part of the body such as bone, liver, lung and brain due to the reason of incurability and only Premature diagnose of breast cancer is the best leading approach to reduce the death cases of this diseases (Majeed et al., 2014). From now Mammography is the best solution for detecting breast cancer which is widely used to diagnose Premature detection and help to reduce mortality efficiently. On the other hand, Magnetic Resonance Imaging (MRI) is also available for the screening process of breast cancer diagnosing which is more sensitive compare to mammography that has been implemented in the previous decades. There are different types of risk factors that increase the chance of growing breast cancer such as sex, ageing, estrogen, gene mutation, prior family history, unhealthy lifestyle etc. (Sun et al., 2014). Mostly, breast cancer occurs in females compared to men and the number of death cases are 100 times more than a man (DeSantis et al., 2016)However, the incident rate increases last year but the mortality rate is decreased due to the reason of screening process of Premature diagnoses of breast cancer and modern medical therapies (Hegan et al., 2010).

A mammogram is a machine of advanced level of an X-ray to diagnose tumour or nodules in the breast which is particularly located in the breast to show the presence may specify the existence of breast cancer (Makarem et al., 2013). Remember that one thing mammography is not shown always tumor and cancer in the breast, it allows the doctor to check the abnormalities in the breast. The radiologist or doctor conduct the physical examination of the female breast in the appearance of skin and nipples through a mammogram.To confirm the diagnosis, additional tests will be required (breast ultrasound, breast MRI and sampling). CAD improves mammography interpretation accuracy, early detection of potential tumors, and differentiation between benign and malignant tumors. (Blot & Zwiggelaar, 2014; Catsburg et al., 2015; Hela et al., 2013). Clusters of microcalcifications (3 or more per cm2) on mammography, for example, are aPremature indicator of breast cancer. However, due to their small size and similarity to breast tissue, they are difficult to identify.

Breast tissue can be affected by a variety of abnormalities. The opacities, micro-calcifications, and architectural distortions are the three most common types of abnormalities:

Masses

As shown in fig.1, there are two effects seen on lesions that consume space, and they are classified by their shape, for example, round, oval, lobulated, irregular, their curve, for example, circumscribed, micro-lobulated, obscured, indistinct, speculated, and density like high, medium, and low fat. Breast cancer never delivers fats that are radiotransparent, permitting fat to be caught. Oil growths, lipomas, galactocele, and mixed lesions (hamartoma) are generally instances of fat-containing lesions, and fat-containing masses are consistently benign (Bouyahia et al., 2009).

Figure 1. Examples of masses

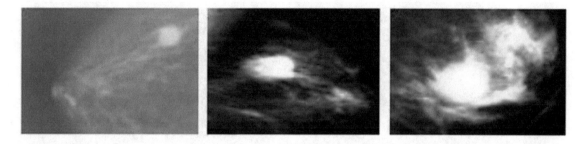

Micro-Calcifications

Micro-calcifications are divided into three categories benign such as cutaneous, vascular, staghorn, sticks, apprehensive condition namely dusty amorphous or heterogeneous, and malignancy with high probability like polymorphic linear spreading, triangular or diverged. Fig.2 show some experimental results of micro-calcifications is given in Figure 2.

Figure 2. (a) annular or arcuate (b) regular full round (c) Linear, stick (d) rail (vascular) (e) vermicular, connected (f) Irregular, blocky (g) powder of microcalcifications

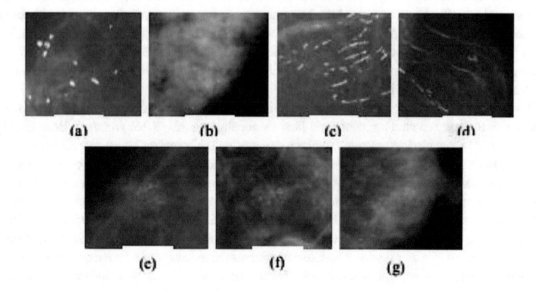

Architectural Distortions

Architectural distortions are representing the out of the normal architecture of breast tissue without visibility of mass. They can show the central opacity and can show the dense centre or clear centre depend upon the situation as shown in fig.3.

Figure 3. Architectural bias (a) with dense centre (b) with a clear centre

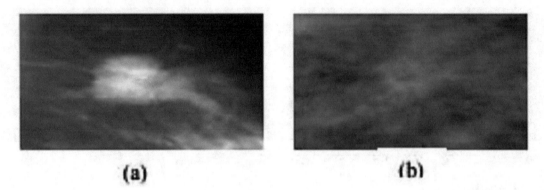

(a)   **(b)**

Asymmetric tubular structure, intra-mammary lymph node (clear centre in oval shape or ground spherical), asymmetry breast tissue, and focal asymmetric density are all examples of breast abnormalities. Breast cancer can be diagnosed using symptoms such as Skin retraction, nipple retraction, skin clots, and skin scratches are all frequently associated with a variety of abnormalities (Bouyahia et al., 2009).According to the literature, datasets that were used for mammography assessment belong to those anomalies that generate the larger CAD outcomes of a breast cancer situation. However, few of the researches were utilized their developed databases with the mutual understanding of trained radiologists (Beucher & Lenteuejoul, 1979; Davies & Dance, 1990; Dheeba & Jiji, 2010; Eddaoudi et al., 2011; Jasmine et al., 2010), the other is used the Mammographic Image Analysis Society (MIAS) database to generates the results of CAD which is belongs to UK research groups (Bovis & Singh, 2002). The rest of the other databases such as the Nijmegen database (Kestener, 2003) and digital database for the screening process of mammography(DDSM) (Muhimmah & Zwiggelaar, 2006) have been evaluated over than MIAS database and compare both results.

Tissue density has a big impact on mammogram reading. There is a difference between two types of tissues in the breast including: dense and fatty (Mandelblatt et al., 2016; Woods & Bowyer, 1994). All fatty tissues show black on mammography it depends on the breast architecture varies from female to female, few are very small tissues (dense breasts) which may be difficult tumor because cancer has different contrast same as that type of tissue. Wolfe (Oeffinger et al., 2015), was the first to identify the relationship between both breast cancer risk and density of the breast tissues. Based on connective distribution tissues and density, this study was able to classify mammographic images into four different types of groups: N1 represents fat with less dense tissues, P1 represents dense components that occupy less than a quarter of the breast area, P2 dense components that occupy more than a quarter of the breast area, and DY dense elements that occupy more than a quarter of the breast area, indicating that the area is fat with some dense tissues. According to Wolfe's research, only P2 and DY have a high sensitivity to illness (Bouyahia et al., 2009).

According to the research investigation, the most recent United States Preventive Services Task Force (USPSTF) study, females with average risk should begin screening mammography at the age of 50 and have it done every two years until the age of 74. They suggested that women between the ages of 40 and 50 take a customized approach, evaluating the benefits and hazards of false positives. The American cancer society also recommended beneficial information about mammography for females with average risk. They refer to the screening mammography starting at the age of 45 and continue this process on yearly basis between the age of 45-54. They refer to endure biennial screening for females who are the age 55. They also suggest the breast screening process continues to life expectancy till longer or at least 10 years. Furthermore, the American cancer society recommended the breast screening process at the beginning age of 40 who are asymptomatic and has a chance of risk of breast cancer. They follow the decision approaching implement in the U.S for females when she has the age of 40s, the care providers provide care services about the breast cancer screening process to maintain their health routine. The goal of this research is to develop the criteria of female's breast assessment with average, higher and prior history of breast cancer. In addition, this research also supports those females who are facing breast cancer genetically and their chance of risk is increased with untested first-degree families. This research also recommended these females and calculate their lifetime's risk of 20% or more, and another history of chest or mantle radiation therapy at a young age. They recommend magnetic resonance imaging (MRI) with enhancing the contract breast supplemental screening process. Normally, Breast MRIs are always recommending those females who have a previous family history of breast cancer who have dense tissues and diagnose the breast cancer before the age of 50. The researcher also discussed the surveillance with MRI of those females who need a biopsy confirmed atypia especially if there is any other risk factor chance. They refer to the screening of whole breast ultrasound to be considered if females need to do a biopsy (Monticciolo et al., 2018).

Risk Assessment

To determine the risk assessment by using the screening approach. This research refers to the following instruction to identify the risk factor of breast cancer of females with their ages (Kuhl et al., 2005).

1. Check the family history of malignancies and genetic testing of the unaffected results
2. Check the women prior histories of atypical hyperplasia or lobular carcinoma in situ (LCIS)
3. Check if the females have a prior history of chest or mantle radiation therapy at the age of 10-30.
4. Check if the females have a history or finding genetic proneness relate to prior atypia or history of mantle radiation then females considered higher risk of breast cancer
5. Follow the risk assessment at regular intervals

Breast Cancer Risk

The absolute possibility is utilized to clarify an individual's probability of developing breast cancer. In view of the number of individuals who will get breast cancer within a specific period. The absolute possibility can likewise be communicated as a percentage. Presently, 1 in every 8 females in the world, or 12%, will foster breast cancer growth over their lifetime. The absolute risk of securing breast cancer sooner or later during a specific decade of life is less than one of every eight The lower the risk, the younger you are. For instance, a 30-year-elderly person with no other breast cancer risk factors faces like 1 of every 228 chance at creating breast cancer in the following ten years or 0.44 percent. On the other hand, a female who is 60 years of age and has no additional breast cancer risk factors has a one-in-29 chance of creating breast cancer in the next g ten years or 3.49 percent. In the examination, a relative risk is a number or rate that actions the danger of breast cancer spreading starting with one institution then onto the next. Females with moderate risk are considered to have an absolute risk comparable to the general populace at a specific age for the motivations behind the current recommendations. Besides, a

20% last lifetime risk threshold was picked to coordinate with the different thresholds utilized in global MRI screening preliminaries where the attention was on more young females with higher risk. In any case, for females, as they age, the utilization of remaining lifetime risk is characteristically dangerous because fast time-frame occurrence growing at the same time that final lifetime. Therefore, females who were qualified for screening MRI when they were younger may fall underneath the 20% rule while as yet experiencing peak short-term disease occurrence. Notwithstanding the way that no association in the United States suggests MRI screening, short-term risk assessments (5 or 10-year chances) ought to be remembered for future exploration, preferably related to breast density (Sung et al., 2011).

Supplemental Screening Modalities

In high-risk groups, contrast-enhanced breast magnetic resonance imaging (MRI) is more sensitive than mammography or ultrasound (Berg et al., 2008; Tieu et al., 2014). MRI is indicated as an additional screening technique for Breast Cancer genes and other germline mutation carriers beginning at the age of 25(with mammography starting at age 30). The incremental rate of cancer detection including MRI is 4% under the age of 30 who have a prior history of chest and mantle radiation therapy (Berg et al., 2008). Breast cancer has increased in females day by day since the last eight years after the accomplishment of radiation therapy. Thus, MRI surveillance should start that time at the age of 25. The other screening modalities are also considering if females decline the avail the facility of MRI or are contraindicated (Brem et al., 2015).

Ultrasound

Multiple research confirms the incremental most cancers detection abilities of complete-breast ultrasound in teenagers with higher risk. This research conducts the huge potential multicenter have a look at comparing women with better chance and verified a supplemental cancer detection charge of 4.3 in step with 1,000 (Ohuchi et al., 2016). However, this supplemental detection is counterbalanced by using growth in fake-nice findings and lower effective predictive value as compared to mammography and MRI (World Health Organization, 2006). Some of these limitations may be mitigated when supplemental ultrasound screening evolves and automated generation improves. Females were randomized to screening mammography alone as opposed to screening mammography and additional screening ultrasound in the Japan Strategic Anti-Cancer Randomized Trial (J-START). Females who received supplemental screening ultrasound had a bigger number of tumors diagnose than the individuals who had standard mammography [184 (0.50%) versus 117 (0.32%), p=0.0003], and the malignancies were all the more frequently Stage 0 and Stage I. (Lyon, 2002).

Computed Tomography (CT)

The benefits of investigative computed tomography seem to be minor, given its high cost and the probable for high radiation exposure. As a result, it has very few threatening signs (Baxter, 2001).

Magnetic Resonance Imaging (MRI)

The benefit of MRI is that it has a high sensitivity (approximately 95 percent) for breast analysis but a low specificity (approximately 53-70 percent). This study uses a false positive strategy to diagnose proliferative fibrocystic diseases, adenomatous fibroadenomas, radial scars, fat, necrosis, intramammary lymph nodes, and breast parenchyma after surgery and shows the outcomes of breast cancer. Microcalcifications are also imperceptible on MRI scans, and dynamic differentiation upgraded MRIs can help rule out excursion malignancy in non-palpable lesions. The most compelling reason for a breast MRI is the fear of recurrence of breast cancer in patients who have received conservative treatment (recurrence versus fibrosis).MRI was found to have a 98% specificity for these patients. (Baxter, 2001).

Figure 4. MRI breast cancer

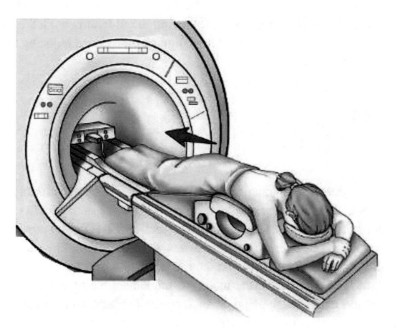

Molecular Breast Imaging (MBI).

There are currently no big trials to validate MBI's screening efficacy. However, when utilized as a supplement to mammography, some studies have shown considerable increases in cancer detection rates (Shitara et al., 2021).MBI is not too effective as mammography for sensitivity and specificity to identify breast density. At present time, more advances in detector technology are being made to allow for lower doses, and prospective trials are required before MBI may be recommended as a screening tool for females at high risk of breast cancer.

Contrast-Enhanced Mammography (CEM)

CEM is a new breast imaging approach that uses contrast-enhanced recombined images to assess neovascularityin the same way as MRI does (Barton et al., 1999). To date, this technique has not been widely adopted. Additional ionizing radiation is less beneficial than alternative options. Furthermore, no commercially available techniques to biopsy suspected augmentation zones under CEM direction are currently available. However, as this modality's technology advances, CEM's use as a second imaging modality may become more common.

Positron Emission Tomographic Screening (PET)

Breast tumors are thought to have increased metabolic activity, which can be detected using fluorine 18-labelled glucose, according to Premature research. PET imaging could be used to stage breast tumors and determine the likelihood of recurrence following initial treatment.PET is still being studied as a diagnostic tool for distinguishing benign from malignant tumors and reducing the need for needle aspiration biopsies (Baxter, 2001).

METHODOLOGIES

Overview

This article presents the systematic literature review for analysis of Premature detection of breast cancer and clinical examination of the female for risk assessment. This research consists of multiple phases containing Premature cancer detection, Care/disease intervention, Screening approaches, Clinical breast examination, and mammography approaches. This review describes the clinical techniques in different sections, along with the overall approaches and their examination process for detecting breast cancer with different age groups of females. Furthermore, we implement multiple computational techniques for detecting breast cancer using image preprocessing, contrast enhancement of the images, image segmentation, SVM-k-NN classification of abnormal masses of Breast cancer and Evaluation Metricsto identifying the stages with grades of breast cancer in the images. In addition, we use mammograms analysis techniquesaiming to detect abnormalities, and the various techniques developed for that purpose. This research is based on two components including qualitative and quantitative research. The first component relates to quantitative systematic review research and the second component is relating to qualitative research of breast cancer to calculate the sensitivity, specificity and accuracy of the breast cancer through mammographic images after taking the MRI mammogram. Below figure 6 show the strategy of a systematic literature review of breast cancer.

Figure 5. Flowchart of the qualitative analysis of breast cancer

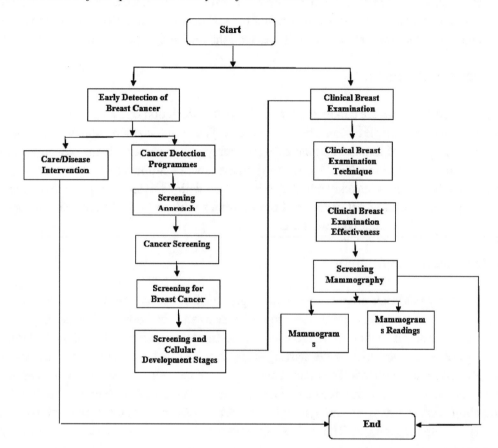

Methods and Materials

Premature Detection

The premature detection process is one of the great achievements of prevention (screening) of breast cancer which is reduce the mortality and morbidity rates in females all over the world. The breast cancer screening process can be accomplished in many ways such as:

1. Cancer groups and authorities all over the world have authorized and widely promoted breast self-examination. Its effectiveness, on the other hand, is contingent on women's education and outreach, as well as conscientious and regular self-examination.
2. Clinical assessment of a breast is one of the common screening processes that can analyse and diagnose the breast condition with the help of health care workers and provide the facilities of the females. The health care worker guides you properly and gives beneficial knowledge about the breast cancer examination

3. Mammography has been reducing the death ratio of females in breast cancer but it's dependent on the number of factors that have been utilizing the technician's skills, the way of the use of mammography machine, and radiologist ability to read the mammogram readings.

Care/Disease Intervention

The cancer care programmes are conducted for the Premature detection of cancer at the beginning stage of breast cancer that can cure the diseases by the treatment. The Premature detection of diagnosing cancer reduce the mortality rate of females and increase the therapy of cancer that is the reason for low cases of females overall the world. In addition to surgery, breast cancer treatment should involve drug therapy and radiation methods. Breast cancer should also be treated with adjuvant therapy to avoid recurrence. Finally, giving women with breast cancer and their families with additional psychosocial support and palliative care can improve their quality of life.

Cancer Detection Programmes

The motive of early detection programmes is to diagnose cancer when the cancer is still localized to the specific part of the breast and not migrate to the other part of the body or surrounding tissues. The technique involves early detection for diagnosing the asymptomatic neoplastic lesions and understand the knowledge of cancer detection at the starting stage of cancer that can they suggest the therapy and other cost-effective measurements. The importance of public education and professional continuing education in an early detection programme cannot be overstated. The goal of public education is to inform the public about cancer's dangers and symptoms to encourage early detection and improve access to diagnostic and treatment facilities. The subject of professional continuing the education program in the healthcare system is the initial point of contact between the cancer patient in this continuing program.

These specialists must be aware of cancer's Premature signs and symptoms in order to assist in the disease's discovery.Continuing education programmes, meanwhile, increase disease burden knowledge among government officials and policymakers in charge of formulating and executing national health care agendas and programmes. Premature detection programmes enhance patients' prognoses, provide additional and less toxic treatment alternatives, and enable more cost-effective delivery of services. It's worth noting that a large proportion of malignancies detected in the Premature stages in rich countries are nevertheless diagnosed at later, and frequently deadly, stages in poor countries, hence increasing the disease burdenIt's worth mentioning that a considerable proportion of cancers recognized in the Premature stages in developed countries are diagnosed at later, and often fatal, stages in developing countries, hence increasing the disease burden. This is especially true in nations where healthcare resources are scarce.

Cancer Screening

The motive of cancer screening programmes is to diagnose breast cancer in females during the asymptomatic stages that have probably the chance of cancer detection. the screening programmes permit the females to check up regularly that can easy for the physician to diagnose an earlier stage and possibly treat cancer that has a greater chance of success to reduce the deaths cases. Three factors should be considered when developing and implementing screening programmes.

Screening for Breast Cancer

When breast cancer is diagnosed as Premature, it is most simply and efficiently treated. When women present with advanced cases, their survival chances drop drastically, regardless of setting; hence, enhancing the number of cases diagnosed Premature in the disease is a fundamental strategy for lowering breast cancer mortality. Unfortunately, women in resource-limited countries present at a later stage of disease than women in other countries, owing to a lack of mass screening programmes in many of these countries. Regular screening of all women over the age of 50 has the potential to significantly increase the proportion of cancer cases discovered in their early stages (Miller et al., 2000). The screening guidelines have two objectives.

1.   To guide the proper use of screening tools for the detection of breast cancer;
2.   To help doctors and patients make informed decisions about breast cancer screening in asymptomatic women of all ages.

Screening Approach

A screening program's main conceptual framework is to design a process that will reduce breast cancer mortality rates while improving the target population's quality and longevity of life. This process should be carried out in a well-defined high-risk population in a cost-effective manner. The primary strategy should be a mechanism capable of detecting malignant disorders at their earliest stages of development. This process's outcome will be determined by two distinct conditions.

Screening and Cellular Development Stages

There is a period throughout the screening process when there is no recognizable disease, even though Premature cancer changes have effectively started. The sojourn time or detectable preclinical stage is the point at which a tumor is first identified through the screening. It is the result of the lesions just as the screening test. The lead-time is the time when a threat is located by screening and whilst medical signs and symptoms appearances. The frequency of screening may influence it. Neither the sojourn time nor the lead-time is straightforwardly detectable for a person till a screening take a look at is repeated at regular intervals(Barton et al., 1999; Miller et al., 2000).Breast cancer development should be considered when deciding screening recurrence spans. Premenopausalhas a shorter sojourn time for all malignancy types.

Clinical Breast Examination

A clinical breast examination is conducted by a health care proficient, like a doctor, nurse, attendant, or physician's assistant. It involves both a visual assessment and palpation of the breasts (feeling). The whole breasts /chest region is checked (including lymph nodes), as well as the area above and underneath the collarbone and under each arm. Clinical breast examination combined with mammography is regarded to be significant in decreasing breast cancer mortality. Clinical breast examination is believed to be a decent beginning step in distinguishing whether a female has the condition. Be that as it may, without the data offered by indicative mammography and fine-needle aspiration, it can't be utilized in detachment. The feasibility of a medical breast exam is determined by several parameters, consisting of good enough patient positioning, thoroughness of the search, use of a vertical strip technique, right finger positioning and movement, and an examination time of a minimum of five minutes in step with breast (Lyon, 2000).

Clinical Breast Examination Technique

At each palpation point, three levels of pressure (superficial, medium, and deep) must be applied. Palpation is completed using the finger pads of the 3 middle hands, and the pressing factor is brought in circular motions at each side. For the lateral half of the breast, the body is turned medially; for the average portion of the breast, the torso is turned around along the side to spread out the breast tissue (Figure 7). At the point whilst an abnormality is located, the opposing breast's nearly similar region is examined. If the finding isn't always reciprocal, similarly examining is required (Lyon, 2000). A female's regular check-up has to contain a clinical breast exam. Starting at twenty years 'old, females must undergo a medical examination for each 2-3 years later, increasing to once every 12 months above the age of 40.

Figure 6. Clinical breast examination techniques
(Lyon, 2000)

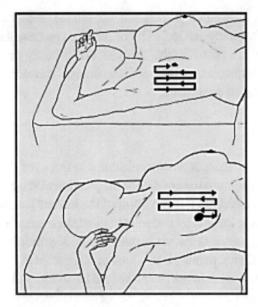

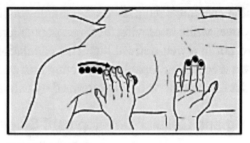

Palpation technique
Pads of the index, third and fourth fingers
(inset) make small circular motions.

**Position of patient and direction of palpation
for clinical breast examination**
The top shows the lateral portion of the breast
and the bottom shows the medial portion of the
breast. Arrows indicate vertical strip pattern of
examination.

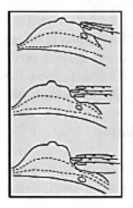

Pressure levels
Superficial, medium and
deep levels of pressure for
palpation of breast tissue
shown in a cross-sectional
view of the right breast.

Clinical Breast Examination Effectiveness

Clinical breast examination has been studied extensively and in conjunction with other screening procedures. In trials, clinical breast examination alone has been proven to detect 3–5% of breast cancers missed by screening mammography in women over 50, and 10% or more in women aged 40–49. The vast majority of breast tumors with a diameter of 2 cm or more, as well as many with a diameter of 1–2 cm, are detected by clinical breast examination. The results of two randomized trials comparing clinical breast examination vs no screening have yet to be published. Clinical breast examination plus annual mammography screening was compared in one randomized experiment to clinical breast examination alone.Mammography did not affect breast cancer mortality when used to detect tiny impalpable tumors (Zheng et al., 2015). Breast screening with clinical breast assessment alone or in the mix with screening mammography doesn't seem to diminish breast malignancy mortality, as per a functioning gathering of the International Agency for Research on Cancer (Shitara et al., 2021). However, a clinical breast assessment doesn't prevent the occurrence of incurable illness, it is suggested that it be utilized as a screening tool for identifying certain irregularities that can progress to breast cancer.

Screening Mammography

Another screening approach for Premature-stage breast cancer is mammography. A typical two-view mammogram conducted on an asymptomatic woman to detect breast cancer Premature is known as screening mammography. The motivation behind population-based mammography screening is to decreasebreast cancer mortality and morbidity by recognizing and treating malignancies almost immediately. According to a variety of well-documented sources, Premature or two-Premature mammography helps lowerbreast cancer mortality in females aged 50–69 years (Barton et al., 1999). females under 50 with no family background of breast cancer or a previous malignancy diagnosis are viewed as low risk, however, they might be benefited from normal mammograms at their doctor's discretion. females more than 50 years old, those with a first-degree relative with premenopausal breast cancer, and those with a background marked by breast or gynaecological malignant growth are viewed as high risk and should have to screen mammography each 1–3 years in industrialized countries.

Despite all of the advantages indicated, mammography alone is not a useful screening method, with a false-negative rate of 12 percent. False-negative outcomes are more common in younger patients. The effectiveness of breast screening was examined by a working group of the International Agency for Research on Cancer. They came to the following conclusion:

1. Mammography as the sole screening method for women aged 50–69 years has enough data to suggest its efficacy in lowering breast cancer mortality. In women aged 50–69 years, there is evidence of a 25% drop.
2. The women aged 40-49 years is controversial in mortality of breast cancer reducing due to the single screening technique of mammography. There was evidence of reduced breast cancer around 11% in the women aged 40-49 when all studies are eligible after evaluation.
3. No clear conclusion was reached regarding the efficacy of mammography in women under the age of 40 or over the age of 69.

Figure 7. The mammography screening process shows that both breasts compressed horizontally then obliquely and x-rays are taken of each position

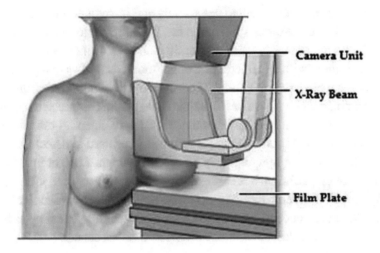

Mammograms

Mammography is a type of X-ray that is used to look for abnormalities in the breast. Various forms of breast tissue, such as fat, fibro glandular tissue, cysts, tumors, and calcifications, absorb different amounts of X-rays, which is utilized to diagnose, assess, and determine the outcomes. The imaging system must be tuned during the processes to deliver the needed radiation dose with the least quantity of radiation. Radiation levels should be harmonized according to national and international guidelines. The mean absorbed dosage in the breast gland per mammographic film for the average breast evaluated with modern equipment is in the region of 1.0–1.5 mGy. When it comes to mammographic density, there are a few aspects to keep in mind:

1. The sensitivity of mammography is determined by breast parenchymal density as seen on a mammogram.
2. with age, the density of the breast parenchyma decreases;
3. combination hormone replacement therapy may result in increased breast density;
4. Tamoxifen has been shown to reduce breast density

Mostly author proposes a double reading of mammographic images which increase the sensitivity of the reading at 10-15% compare to single readings. In the modern era, digital mammography has been replacing by traditional mammography. The image receptor has been utilized by the traditional mammography which is replaced by the digital receptor.In every other way, the imaging procedures, on the other hand, remain the same. According to the point of view of the female being checked, a Digital mammogram is indistinguishable from a traditional mammogram because the compression and positioning are something very similar. Digital mammography, rather than screen-film mammography, can deliver images with decreased radiation exposures. Moreover, computer-aided detection can be coordinated into the workstation, with the aftereffects of the computer investigation being added to the image, supporting the radiologist in recognizing problematic lesions. Several studies have looked at computer-assisted detection and found that it has an incremental value in terms of sensitivity, however evidence on specificity is mixed. Many women who have been advised to get this form of screening have expressed worries about the potential for radiation exposure through mammography. The average dose per examination (single view per breast) is around 2 mGy, according to research, with the dose varying based on breast thickness and exposure factors. Radiation risk builds up over time, increasing with age and reducing with adolescent exposure.In people above the age of 50, the probability of cancer induction during a single view examination is about 1 in 100 000 (Li et al., 2017). The radiographers perform mammograms who are an expert for the use of mammography as well as an expert in the procedures and techniques of use.

Mammography Reading

Two views of each breast are obtained during a mammogram: one from the top and the other from the side. The breast must be compressed to a uniform thickness to acquire reliable images, reducing radiation exposure while permitting precise imaging of potential abnormalities. To detect breast cancer is to distinguish between the abnormality or masses of normal breast tissues, whereas, the greater quantity of fats available in the breast the easier it is to find cancer. When the breast is dense, the anomaly may be hidden in the tissue, needing further testing, such as an ultrasound if a cystic mass is detected or a tiny needle aspirate for cytologic evaluation. Figure.8 (a) shows a low-density mass with a hollow sign surrounding it. Most likely, it's a fibro-adenoma.

Figure 8. Mammography interpretations

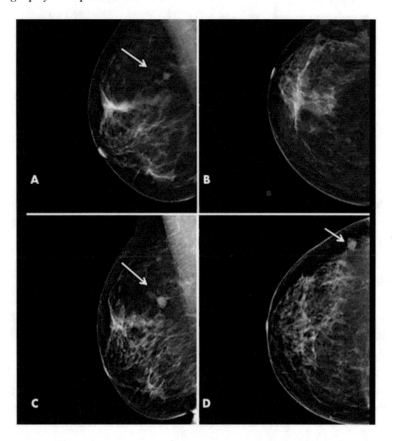

Microcalcifications aren't frequently linked to cancer in general. Figures 8(b) and (b) depict a low density, benign-appearing, well-defined mass surrounded by a hollow sign atop benign-appearing macro calcifications. Microcalcifications, on the other hand, necessitate further examination and analysis of the mass to differentiate benign from malignant microcalcifications. Figure 8 depicts a malignant tumor with a lobulated margin, high density, microcalcifications, and nipple retraction 8(c). Figure 8(d) shows three masses of varied sizes that, due to their high density, irregularspeculated edge, and the bigger one having micro-calcifications, raise the likelihood of malignancy. According to studies, the size of tumors detected by clinical breast examination differs significantly from those detected by mammography, indicating that both are efficient Premature detection techniques for breast cancer.

Figure 9. Flowchart of the proposed mammogram technique

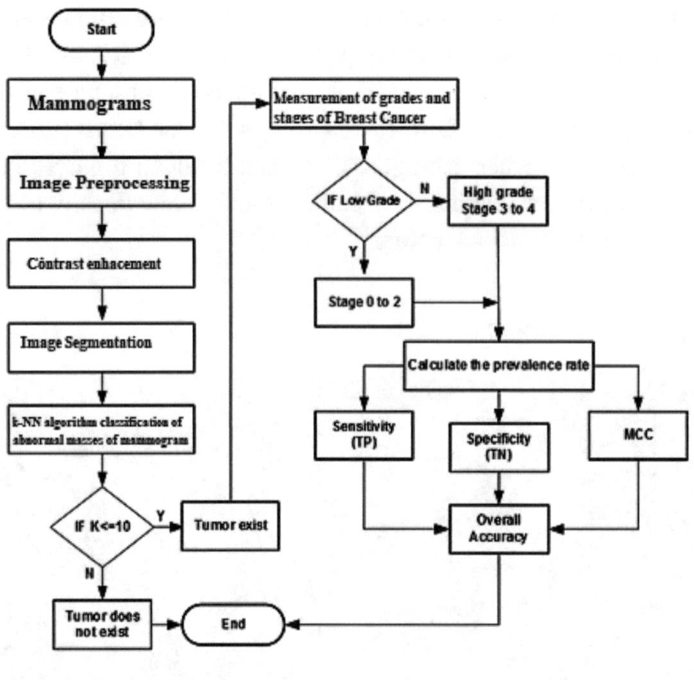

The figure. 9 show the quantitative research-based implementation process of mammographic images. This research conducts multiple techniques to identify the accuracy of digital mammography and calculate the survival ratio of all stages and grades of breast cancer in females.

Image Preprocessing

Pre-processing is the first step in classifying mammogram images. Each mammogram image will be pre-processed first to achieve a much higher image quality. The pre-processing step aimed to improve image quality by removing any irrelevant data, resulting in more accurate and reliable results. Pre-processing steps are essential for detecting cancer masses in the background of mammograms. During this study, we used 3000 mammogram images. Cropping and resizing each mammogram image to 129 x 129 pixels is another step in this study's pre-processing. Image The first images are different in size and direction because they are being pre-processed for the automated mammogram analysis system. Furthermore, some mammograms may contain artefacts and noise, resulting in incorrect or poor analysis results. As a result, several mammogram preprocessing steps were implemented to regularize image appearance and remove unnecessary artefacts and noise. The following actions were taken during this project:

Figure 10. (a)-(c) MLO view mammogram from Right and Left side of the breast and the image afterward orientation corresponding of MLO mammogram.

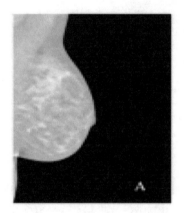 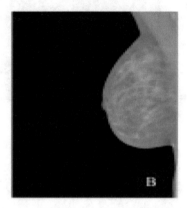 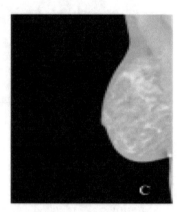

This research is only concerned with the presentation of MLO mammograms. In those, the proper right and left breasts factor to the other aspects of the mammogram image. As a result, flipping one of the breasts in the opposite direction ensures that every image is pointed in the identical direction, preventing modifications within the wavelet transform coefficients because of simplest the directionality exchange among the right and left images. The sharp edge among the tissue and accordingly the dark background can also be an extensive feature that influences this change. The depth of right breast images decreases from left to proper across this side, as shown in Fig. 10, whereas it increases in left breast pictures. This is frequently used to modify the sign of the calculated wavelet coefficient. The orientation matching consequences of the MLO view mammogram are proven in Fig. 10. Figures 10A and B depict the right and left breast images of a patient who has tiny microcalcifications in her breast tissue. The contemplated images of proper breast orientation matching are shown in Fig. 10 C.

Contrast Enhancement

Image enhancement in this context refers to the processing of images to increase contrast and suppress noise, thereby supporting radiologists in detecting abnormalities. There are several image enhancement strategies, considered one of that's the image contrast enhancement method (ICEM). The image contrast enhancement method technique can enhance neighbourhood assessment and bring out additional information in images. It is a great approach for enhancing contrast in each natural and medical image. The contrast-confined histogram equalization approach (CLHEM), a form of ICEM, was used in this paper to enhance photograph assessment. An improved image of the usage of CLHEM is proven in Figure 11.

Figure 11. Enhanced image using contrast-limited histogram equalization method (CLHEM).

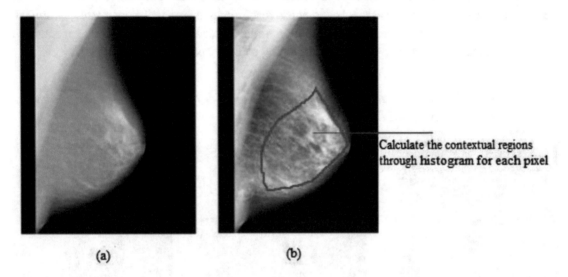

The CLHEM algorithm is frequently summed up as follows: (1) Section of the first image into contextual regions. (2) Generate an area histogram for each pixel. (3) The clip level was used to limit this histogram. (4) Use binary search to redistribute the histogram. (5) Using histogram integration, obtain the improved pixel value.

Image Segmentation

Image segmentation is the system of dividing an image into parts that have similar capabilities and properties. The aim of segmentation is a simplification or representing the image in a simple analyzable manner. The region of interest (ROI) turned into extracted from the primary mammogram image all through this have a look at through suppressing the whole breast, except the pectoral and as a consequence the other artefacts. Pectoral muscle mass is a Triangulum- shaped area located on one side of the mammogram's MLO view, both on the left or right pinnacle corner. Because of the dense tissues within the mammogram image, the pectoral muscle mass appears roughly with a uniform density. As a result, getting rid of the pectoral plays a critical position in exactly detecting the tumor cellular.

The steps for ROI segmentation are regularly summarized as follows: (1) Align all mammogram samples within a similar direction. This step is completed to keep away from using distinct techniques for left and right-oriented MLO mammograms. As an instance, flip all the RMLO perspectives to appear to be the LMLO view samples. (2) Remove any radiopaque artefacts, which include labels, from the mammogram picture. This is frequently performed through the usage of thresholding and morphological operations (Cover & Hart, 1967). An international threshold of 18 become discovered to be the maximum appropriate threshold for converting grayscale photographs into binary (0,1) layout (Cover & Hart, 1967). Figure 3 depicts a mammogram photo with artefacts removed. (3) Remove the pectoral through photo segmentation based totally on a cluster of points (Kumar & Balakrishnan, 2013).

SVM-k-NN Classification of Abnormal Masses of Breast Cancer

This experiment employs SVM: the first is trained to classify normal and peculiar training data, and the second one is trained to classify benign and malignant tumors, which can be used all through the testing phase of the segment. If the input is completely particular, the first SVM will determine whether it's normal or abnormal. If the input is abnormal, the second SVM will automatically classify the data as benign or malignant breast. The k-Nearest Neighbor (k-NN) algorithm is the most basic of the machine learning algorithms (Harefa et al., 2017). The k-NN classifier is used to categories an object-based item of its neighbour supported "k" similar vectors in the feature space, in which k can also be a positive integer and is commonly small. The following formula becomes used to discover the maximum similar vector the use of Euclidian Distance between points:

$$d\left(X,Y\right) = \sqrt{\sum_{i=1}^{n}\left(x_i - y_i\right)^2}$$

where X = (x1, x2..., xn) and Y = (x1, x2..., xn) (y1, y2..., yn). Here's a simple illustration of k-nearest neighbour.

We can see that if k-NN is primarily based on 1 Nearest Neighbor, the circle (unknown object) may be labelled as a plus (primarily based at the closest point). If the closest neighbour count is 2, the k-NN might be not able to categories the circle's result due to the fact the second one closest point can be a minus. If the number of nearest neighbours is increased to five, the ability of k-NN's is to classify the circle can be a minus (3 minus and more than one plus). Confusion Matrix is used to evaluate the accuracy rateof SVM and ok-NN classifiers (Harefa et al., 2017).

Evaluation Metrics

Two parameters may be used to assess the overall performance of a mammography screening system: sensitivity and specificity. The proportion of cases deemed abnormal whilst breast cancers is referred to as sensitivity (true positive rate). Sensitivity may be affected by a variety of factors, along with lesion size, breast tissue density, and standard image quality. Because failure to diagnose breast cancer can bring about serious fitness effects, sensitivity is deemed more vital than specificity in most cancers screening protocols. Premature half of all scientific malpractice instances involve "false-negative mammograms". The proportion of cases considered normal when breast cancer is absent is referred to as specificity (true negative fraction). Although the consequences of a false positive (diagnosing a healthy patient as having breast cancers) are less life-threatening than the effects of missing a positive cancer diagnosis, specificity ought to be as high as feasible. False-positive outcomes can lead to unnecessary follow-up checks and approaches, as well as significant anxiety and issue for the affected person. For the proposed method, overall accuracy can be categorized as True Positive (TP), False Negative (FN), False Positive (FP), and True Negative (TN).We used the Sensitivity/Recovery (Se) ratio, Specific (Sp) ratio, Accuracy (ACC) ratio, and F score to measure classification performance in terms of recall and accuracy. All metrics are defined by Equations 4, 5, 6, and 7, in that order.

$$Accuracy = \frac{TP + TN}{TP + FP + TN + FN} \times 100 \qquad (1)$$

$$Sensitivity = \frac{TP}{TP + FN} \times 100 \qquad (2)$$

$$Specificity = \frac{TP}{FP + TN} \times 100 \qquad (3)$$

Table 3. Overall result of breast cancer

Screening Interval	Type	Age	Grade	Tumor Size	Stage	Survival Rate (%)	Sensitivity (%)	Specificity (%)	Overall Accuracy (%)
1 year	Ductal Carcinoma or Lobular Carcinoma in Situ	50–54	Low-Grade (I)	625	0	92	75.9	98.3	88.32
>1 year		55–59		720	1	87	82.7	98.5	88.77
2 year	Invasive Carcinoma less than 5cm in size, no nodal involvement, movable axillary nodes, and no distant metastasis	60–64	Low-Grade (II)	110	2	75	85.6	99.03	89.02
>2 years	Invasive Carcinoma less than 5cm with nodal involvement and fixed axillary nodes	60–64	High-Grade (III)	209	3	46	86.7	99.05	89.57
All intervals	Breast Cancer with distance metastasis	65–69	High-Grade (IV)	834	4	13	88.9	99.08	90.03
Total							**83.96**	**98.79**	**89.14**

Moreover, the proposed method is compared with the existing methods. In 3D MRI mammographic images is used based on a digital mammographic method to create a predictive radiation signature with 93.57% accuracy. However, Table 2 shows the overall result of the proposed method which includes the types, grades, and stages based on the size of breast cancer with 89.14% accuracy, sensitivity 83.96% and specificity of 98.79%.

CONCLUSION

In this paper, we studied both qualitative and quantitative analysis of the breast cancer risk factors with Premature detection as well as discuss the 3D digital mammography follow up and aged female cases analysis that identifies and assesses the severity factor of breast cancer to enhance the entire identification and classification results of the digital mammography. For this purpose, we examined the 3D MRI digital mammography results that categorized breast cancer with different aged female and their condition as per different types, grades, and stages respectively. Consequently, the experimental results determine the effectiveness of this research to make accurate details of breast cancer analysis in different ages of females and their history regarding the four grades with stages of breast cancer. The simulation results verified that the review of the detection method of 3D MRI digital mammography achieved improved results in terms of collecting data confirmed that digital mammography is a highly accurate tool for breast cancer detection, to have to find the evaluation of metrics through the prevalence of diseases of sensitivity 83.96% sensitivity, 98.79% specificity, and 89.14% with diagnostic accuracy, respectively. Digital mammography has a few more advantages over traditional film-screen mammography and is rapidly replacing the older technique around the world. However, special care should be taken when selecting equipment because not much data is available publicly, but in the future, this will change. we aim to extend our current work for the detailed classification of each grade by investigating the digital 3D mammography using the KNN algorithm to achieve a balance between efficiency and accuracy.

REFERENCES

Barton, M., Harris, R., & Fletcher, S. W. (1999). Does this patient have breast cancer? The screening clinical breast examination: Should it be done? *Journal of the American Medical Association, 282*(13), 1270–1280. doi:10.1001/jama.282.13.1270 PMID:10517431

Baxter, N. (2001). Preventive health care. update: Should women be routinely taught breast self-examination to screen for breast cancer? *Canadian Medical Association Journal, 164*, 1837–1846. PMID:11450279

Berg, W. A., Blume, J. D., & Cormack, J. B. (2008). Combined screening with ultrasound and mammography versus mammography alone in women at elevated risk of breast cancer. *Journal of the American Medical Association, 299*(18), 2151–2163. doi:10.1001/jama.299.18.2151 PMID:18477782

Beucher, S. S., & Lenteuejoul, C. (1979). Use of watersheds in contour detection. *Proceedings of the International Workshop on Image Processing: Real-Time Edge and Motion Detection/Estimation*, 1–12.

Blot, L., & Zwiggelaar, R. (2014). Background Texture Extraction for the Classification of Mammographic Parenchymal Patterns. *Medical Image Understanding and Analysis*, 1-5.

Bouyahia, S., Mbainaibeye, J., & Ellouze, N. (2009). Wavelet based microcalcifications detection in digitized mammograms. *Graphics. Vision and Image Processing Journal, 8*, 1–12.

Bovis, K., & Singh, S. (2002). Classification of mammographic breast density using a combined classifier paradigm. *4th International Workshop on Digital Mammography*, 177–180.

Brem, R. F., Tabar, L., & Duggy, S. W. (2015). Assessing improvement in detection of breast cancer with three-dimensional automated breast US in women with dense breast tissue: The SonoSight Study. *Radiology*, *274*(3), 663–673. doi:10.1148/radiol.14132832 PMID:25329763

Catsburg, C., Miller, A. B., & Rohan, T. E. (2015). Active cigarette smoking and risk of breast cancer. *International Journal of Cancer*, *136*(9), 2204–2209. doi:10.1002/ijc.29266 PMID:25307527

Cover, T., & Hart, P. (1967). Nearest neighbor pattern classification. IEEE Transactions on Information Theory, 1-12.

Davies, D. H., & Dance, D. R. (1990). Automatic computer detection of clustered calcifications in digital mammograms. *Physics in Medicine and Biology*, *35*(8), 1111–1118. doi:10.1088/0031-9155/35/8/007 PMID:2217536

DeSantis, C.E., Fedewa, S.A., Sauer, A.G., Kramer, J.L., Smith, R.A., & Jemal, A. (2016). Breast cancer statistics, 2015: Convergence of incidence rates between black and white women. *A Cancer Journal for Clinicians*, *66*, 31-42.

Dheeba, J., & Jiji, G. C. (2010). Detection of Microcalcification Clusters in Mammograms using Neural Network. *International Journal of Advanced Science and Technology*, *130*, 31–45.

Drukteinis, J. S., Mooney, B. P., Flowers, C. I., & Gatenby, R. A. (2013). Beyond mammography: New frontiers in breast cancer screening. *The American Journal of Medicine*, *126*(6), 472–479. doi:10.1016/j.amjmed.2012.11.025 PMID:23561631

Dupont, W. D., & Page, D. L. (1985). Risk factors for breast cancer in women with proliferative disease. *The New England Journal of Medicine*, *312*(3), 146–151. doi:10.1056/NEJM198501173120303 PMID:3965932

Eddaoudi, F., Regragui, F., Mahmoudi, A., & Lamouri, N. (2011). Masses Detection Using SVM Classifier Based on Textures Analysis. *Applied Mathematical Sciences*, *5*, 367–379.

Fakhro, A. E., Fateha, B. E., al-Asheeri, N., & al-Ekri, S. A. (1999). Breast cancer: Patient characteristics and survival analysis at Salmaniya Medical Complex, Bahrain. *Eastern Mediterranean Health Journal*, *5*(3), 430–439. doi:10.26719/1999.5.3.430 PMID:10793821

Fattah, M. A., Zaki, A., Bassili, A., Shazly, M., & Tognoni, G. (2000). Breast self-examination practice and its impact on breast cancer diagnosis in Alexandria, Egypt. *Eastern Mediterranean Health Journal*, *6*(1), 34–40. doi:10.26719/2000.6.1.34 PMID:11370338

Hamid, A., Tayeb, M. S., & Bawazir, A. A. (2001). Breast cancer in south-east Republic of Yemen. *Eastern Mediterranean Health Journal*, *7*(06), 1012–1016. doi:10.26719/2001.7.6.1012 PMID:15332743

Harefa, J., Alexander, A., & Pratiwi, M. (2017). Comparison classifier: Support vector machine (SVM) and K-nearest neighbor (K-NN) in digital mammogram images. *Journal InformatikadanSistemInformasi*, *2*, 35–40.

Harirchi, I., Ebrahimi, M., Zamani, N., Jarvandi, S., & Montazeri, A. (2000). Breast cancer in Iran: A review of 903 case records. *Public Health. National Library of Medicine*, *114*, 143–145. PMID:10800155

Hegan, D. C., Lu, Y., Stachelek, G. C., Crosby, M. E., Bindra, R. S., & Glazer, P. M. (2010). Inhibition of poly(ADP-ribose) polymerase down-regulates BRCA1 and RAD51 in a pathway mediated by E2F4 and p130. *Proceedings of the National Academy of Sciences of the United States of America, 107*(5), 2201–2206. doi:10.1073/pnas.0904783107 PMID:20133863

Hela, B., Hela, M., Kamel, H., Sana, B., & Najla, M. (2013). *Breast cancer detection: A review on mammograms analysis techniques. In 10th International Multi-Conferences on Systems.* Signals & Devices.

Jasmine, J. S., Govardhan, A., & Baskaran, S. (2010). Classification of Microcalcification in Mammograms using NonsubsampledContourlet Transform and Neural Network. *European Journal of Scientific Research*, 531–539.

Kestener, P. (2003). *Analysemultifractale 2D et 3D à l'aide de la transformation enondelettes: application enmammographie et en turbulence développée.* Université Bordeaux I, Ecoledoctorale de sciences physiques et de l'ingénieur, No d'ordre 2729.

Key, T. J., Verkasalo, P. K., & Banks, E. (2001). Epidemiology of breast cancer. *The Lancet. Oncology, 2*(3), 133–140. doi:10.1016/S1470-2045(00)00254-0 PMID:11902563

Kuhl, C. K., Schrading, S., Leutner, C. C., Morakkabati-Spitz, N., Wardelmann, E., Fimmers, R., Kuhn, W., & Schild, H. H. (2005). Mammography, breast ultrasound, and magnetic resonance imaging for surveillance of women at high familial risk for breast cancer. *Journal of Clinical Oncology, 23*(33), 8469–8476. doi:10.1200/JCO.2004.00.4960 PMID:16293877

Kumar, S. M., & Balakrishnan, G. (2013). Classification of Microcalcification in Digital Mammogram using Stochastic Neighbor Embedding and KNN Classifier. International *Conference on Emerging Technology Trends on Advanced Engineering Research (ICETT'12)*, 1-9.

Li, H., Meng, X., Wang, T., Tang, Y., & Yin, Y. (2017). Breast masses in mammography classification with local contour features. *Biomedical Engineering Online, 16*(1), 1–12. doi:10.118612938-017-0332-0 PMID:28410616

Lyon. (2000). *International Agency for Research on Cancer.* Monographs on the evaluation of carcinogenic risks to humans, International Agency for Research on Cancer Press.

Lyon. (2002). IARC handbooks of cancer prevention. *International Agency for Research on Cancer, 7*, 9-12.

Maffini, M. V., Soto, A. M., Calabro, J. M., Ucci, A. A., & Sonnenschein, C. (2004). The stroma as a crucial target in rat mammary gland carcinogenesis. *Journal of Cell Science, 117*(8), 1495–1502. doi:10.1242/jcs.01000 PMID:14996910

Majeed, W., Aslam, B., Javed, I., Khaliq, T., Muhammad, F., Ali, A., & Raza, A. (2014). Breast cancer: Major risk factors and recent developments in treatment. *APJCP, 15*(8), 3353–3358. doi:10.7314/APJCP.2014.15.8.3353 PMID:24870721

Makarem, N., Chandran, U., Bandera, E. V., & Parekh, N. (2013). Dietary fat in breast cancer survival. *Annual Review of Nutrition, 33*(1), 319–348. doi:10.1146/annurev-nutr-112912-095300 PMID:23701588

Mandelblatt, J. S., Stout, N. K., Schechter, C. B., Broek, J. J. D., Miglioretti, D. L., Krapcho, M., Dietz, A. T., Munoz, D., Lee, S. J., Berry, D. A., Ravesteyn, N. T., Alagoz, O., Kerlikowske, K., Tosteson, A. N., Near, A. M., Hoeffken, A., Chang, Y., Heijnsdijk, E. A., Chisholm, G., ... Cronin, K. A. (2016). Collaborative modeling of the benefits and harms associated with different U.S. breast cancer screening strategies. *Annals of Internal Medicine*, *16*(4), 164. doi:10.7326/M15-1536 PMID:26756606

Miller, T. T., Baines, C. J., & Wall, C. (2000). Canadian National Breast Screening Study-2: 13–year results of a randomized trial in women age 50–59 years. *Journal of the National Cancer Institute*, *92*(18), 1490–1499. doi:10.1093/jnci/92.18.1490 PMID:10995804

Monticciolo, D. L., Newell, M. S., Moy, L., Niell, B., Monsees, B., & Sickle, E. A. (2018). Breast cancer screening in women at higher-than-average risk: Recommendations from the ACR. *Journal of the American College of Radiology*, *15*(3), 408–414. doi:10.1016/j.jacr.2017.11.034 PMID:29371086

Muhimmah, I., & Zwiggelaar, R. (2006). Mammographic Density Classification using Multiresolution Histogram Informatio. *Proceedings of the ITAB 2006*, 1-6.

Oeffinger, K. C., Fontham, E. T. H., Etzioni, R., Herzig, A., Michaelson, J. S., Shih, Y.-C. T., Walter, L. C., Church, T. R., Flowers, C. R., LaMonte, S. J., Wolf, A. M. D., DeSantis, C., Lortet-Tieulent, J., Andrews, K., Manassaram-Baptiste, D., Saslow, D., Smith, R. A., Brawley, O. W., & Wender, R. (2015). Breast cancer screening for women at average risk: 2015 Guideline Update from the American Cancer Society. *Journal of the American Medical Association*, *314*(15), 1599–1614. doi:10.1001/jama.2015.12783 PMID:26501536

Ohuchi, N., Suzuki, A., Sobue, T., Kawai, M., Yamamoto, S., Zheng, Y.-F., Shiono, Y. N., Saito, H., Kuriyama, S., Tohno, E., Endo, T., Fukao, A., Tsuji, I., Yamaguchi, T., Ohashi, Y., Fukuda, M., & Ishida, T. (2016). Sensitivity and specificity of mammography and adjunctive ultrasonography to screen for breast cancer in the Japan Strategic Anti-Cancer Randomized Trial (JSTART): A randomized controlled trial. *Lancet*, *387*(10016), 341–348. doi:10.1016/S0140-6736(15)00774-6 PMID:26547101

Shitara, K., Özgüroğlu, M., Bang, Y. J., Bartolomeo, M. D., Mandalà, M., Ryu, M. H., Caglevic, C., Chung, H. C., Muro, K., Cutsem, E. V., Kobie, J., Cristescu, R., Garg, A. A., Lu, J., Shih, C. S., Adelberg, D., Cao, Z. A., & Fuchs, C. S. (2021). National breast screening programme: Organization and results. *Bulletin EpidemiologiqueHebdomadaire*, *32*(10), 39–40.

Siegel, R.L., Miller, K.D., & Jemal, A. (2017). Cancer Statistics. *A Cancer Journal for Clinicians*, *67*, 7-30.

Stewart, B. W., & Wild, C. P. (2014). *World Cancer Report*. International Agency for Research on Cancer.

Sun, Y. S., Zhao, Z., Yang, Z. N., Xu, F., Lu, H. J., Zhu, Z. Y., & Zhu, H. P. (2014). Risk factors and pre-ventions of breast cancer. *International Journal of Biological Sciences*, *13*(11), 1387–1397. doi:10.7150/ijbs.21635 PMID:29209143

Sung, J. S., Lee, C. H., Morris, E. A., Oeffinger, K. C., & Dershaw, D. D. (2011). Screening breast MRI imaging in women with a history of chest irradiation. *Radiology*, *259*(1), 65–71. doi:10.1148/radiol.10100991 PMID:21325032

Tieu, M. T., Cigsar, C., Ahmed, S., Ng, A., Diller, L., Millar, B. A., Crystal, P., & Hodgson, D. C. (2014). Crysta Pl, Hodgson DC. Breast cancer detection among young survivors of pediatric Hodgkin lymphoma with screening magnetic resonance imaging. *Cancer*, *120*(16), 2507–2513. doi:10.1002/cncr.28747 PMID:24888639

Woods, K. S., & Bowyer, K. W. (1994). Computer detection of stellate lesions. *International Workshop on Digital Mammography*, 221–229.

World Health Organization. (2006). Guidelines for the early detection and screening of breast cancer. *EMRO Technical Publications Series*, 55.

Zheng, Y., Keller, B. M., Ray, S., Wang, Y., Conant, E. F., Gee, J. C., & Kontos, D. (2015). Parenchymal texture analysis in digital mammography: A fully automated pipeline for breast cancer risk assessment. *Medical Physics*, *42*(7), 4149–4160. doi:10.1118/1.4921996 PMID:26133615

Chapter 3
Overview and Analysis of Present–Day Diabetic Retinopathy (DR) Detection Techniques

Smita Das
MBB College, India

Swanirbhar Majumder
ⓘ https://orcid.org/0000-0002-1046-1682
Tripura University, India

ABSTRACT

Diabetic retinopathy (DR) detection techniques is a biometric modality that deserves systematic review and analysis of the connected algorithms for further improvement. The ophthalmologist uses retinal fundus images for the early detection of DR by segmenting the images. There are several segmentation algorithms reported as earlier. This chapter presents a comprehensive review of the methodology associated with retinal blood vessel extraction presented to date. The vessel segmentation techniques are divided into four main categories depending on their underlying methodology as pattern recognition, vessel tracking, model based, and hybrid approaches. A few of these methods are further classified into subsections. Finally, a comparative analysis of a few of the DR detection techniques will be presented here based on their merits, demerits, and other parameters like sensitivity, specificity, and accuracy and provide detailed information about its significance, present status, limitations, and future scope.

INTRODUCTION

Diabetic Retinopathy (DR) is a dynamic microvascular incurable disorder of diabetes mellitus which includes blurred vision, difficulty seeing colors, floaters, and sometimes causes permanent loss of vision. So, DR detection needs systematic discussion and review of the connected methods and findings.

DOI: 10.4018/978-1-7998-8929-8.ch003

These studies assist ophthalmologists to analyze the early stages of DR. The features of retinal vessels, such as width, length, and branching structures, are very important in the detection of such diseases. The uneven illumination of blood vessels and irregular retinal image contrast during the acquisition process are some of the influencing factors that confuse the extraction process. Moreover, the features of blood vessels (grey level, shape, and size) may be puzzled by some background effects with similar characteristics. Other challenges like image intensity, signal noise, and lack of image contrast affect the extraction of retinal blood vessels. Therefore, the exact extraction of blood vessels is a crucial job which plays a very significant role in the diagnosis of retinal vascular complaints. Segmentation is the main step to analyze retinal blood vessels for the detection of DR by extracting vessels from the background which can minimize the issues of the fundus image. In automatic vessel segmentation, the system processes the fundus image and produces the output directly. Preprocessing is the primary step of segmentation. Preprocessing improves the intensity of inhomogeneity and enhances vessels for further processing. Then segmentation does the main task of analyzing each pixel of images. Finally, post processing is applied for quality improvement of segmented images. Due to the fast improvement of such techniques, extensive study is needed. Segmentation plays a great role in retinal image analysis for early detection of ophthalmologic diseases such as arteriosclerosis, glaucoma, hypertension, DR, and choroidal neovascularization by Ophthalmologists. So, this chapter will give a comprehensive review of the problems associated with retinal vessel segmentation, analyzing different extraction methods and giving a short illustration of quantitative performance measures for retinal vessel segmentation like sensitivity, specificity and accuracy. Finally, a comparative study of a few DR detection approaches is presented on the basis of their features and other parameters like Sensitivity, Specificity and Accuracy. The analysis shows that most of the techniques that have been proposed for DR detection perform well to extract wide and normal vessels from retinal images. However, few techniques can't extract the tiny, thin and abnormal vessels. As a result, performance degradation occurs and only a few of the proposed DR detection methods appear to be able to support performance improvement.

DIABETIC RETINOPATHY DETECTION TECHNIQUE ANALYSIS

The automatic extraction process of the retinal blood vessel is a necessary step before the decision of the ophthalmologist to perform early screening and accomplish the treatment of DR disease. Different Researchers use different methods to extract blood vessels from fundus images. These vessel extraction techniques are divided into four main categories depending on their underlying methodology as pattern recognition, vessel tracking, model based and hybrid approaches. Few of these classifications are further classified into subsections.

Figure 1. Categorization of retinal vessel extraction technique

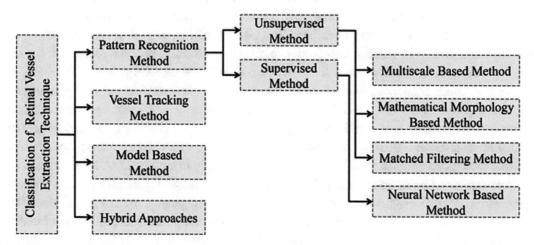

Pattern Recognition Based Method

Pattern recognition (PR) is the identification of data or patterns based on the information collected from their patterns or representation by applying a machine learning approach. PR can also be defined as the categorization of data on the basis of knowledge already acquired or on statistical facts extracted from their representation or patterns. PR helps in the clustering and classification of various patterns. In classification, a suitable class label is assigned to a pattern on the basis of an abstractiveness which is produced by applying a set of domain knowledge. In Clustering, the whole data is partitioned to help in decision making. Supervised learning uses the Classification process whereas, Clustering is used by Unsupervised learning. For example, in 2016, Khan et al. (2016) proposed a Pattern Recognition based unsupervised automated technique for retinal vessel segmentation. In Preprocessing, image enhancement is done by Contrast Limited Adaptive Histogram Equalization (CLAHE) followed by morphological filters. Then Hessian matrix with Eigenvalues transformation is used to extract thin and wide vessel images from enhanced images. Then Otsu thresholding is applied in the classification of non-vessel and vessel pixels from all enhanced images. Lastly, Pixel Count based thresholding is used for the elimination of the unwanted noise, segment/region, disease abnormalities and non-vessel pixels, to get the required output image.

Figure 2. Step-wise illustration of the method.

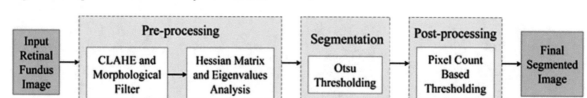

This technique was examined on the publicly accessible STARE (STructured Analysis of the Retina) and DRIVE (Digital Retinal Images for Vessel Extraction) databases. Due to robustness and computational efficiency, the method extracts thin vessels and performs accurately against noise. The PR based approaches can be categorized into two groups: Unsupervised and Supervised approaches.

Unsupervised Method

The Unsupervised method is performed the vessel extraction without any prior labeling information means without any trained dataset. The main aim of this method is to search the patterns/structures from the input data without any training/supervision. It provides the input data to the model and permits the model to search the hidden structures/patterns from the input dataset. It does not take any feedback. So, it is suitable for those cases where there is only input datasets without any corresponding output datasets. Depending on the underlying methodology, this method is mainly categorized into three methods: Multiscale, Mathematical Morphology and matched filtering based algorithms.

Multiscale Based Method

The multi-scale method represents the image at multiple levels/scales. It performs the segmentation of the retinal image on the basis of the variation of the image resolution. This process produced a scale space for the extraction of various structures from the input retinal images. Multi-scale approaches outperform readily at the alternate resolution of an image with an escalated processing speed, where the large retinal vessels are bifurcated from very low resolution and fine retinal vessels from high resolution. Robustness and increased execution speed are the main features of this approach. For example, Yu et al.(2012) in 2012 use morphological pre-processing operations followed by a vessel probability map to generate the Hessian matrix Eigenvalues. A Second order local entropy based thresholding is used for segmentation. Lastly, a rule-based approach is applied to reduce false detection. The method is examined on the STARE and DRIVE datasets and images from Friedrich-Alexander University Erlangen-Nuremberg (Germany). This algorithm faces over-segmentation issues in some retinal structures and under-segmentation issues in some blood vessel segments. Again, detection of thin vessels of low contrast images is difficult. Otherwise, the algorithm needs less time for segmentation. Then in 2014, Ravichandran et al (2014). Use histogram matching and CLAHE techniques for image enhancement and Wiener filtering to remove the background noise. Then 2D Gabor Filtering is used for the vessel enhancement. A local entropy based thresholding technique is then applied to extract blood vessels from the 2D Gabor filter response of the CLAHE'd image. Finally, Post Processing is done by Length Filtering. The method was evaluated on STARE and DRIVE databases which shows that the sensitivity of the technique is a little bit lower. Moreover, the method detects retinal blood vessels in real time, which is useful in high resolution image detection.

The second-order entropy used for vessel segmentation proposed by Yu et al.(2012) in 2012 and Ravichandran et al (2014)in 2014 is defined as:

$$H_2 = -\frac{1}{2}\sum_{x=0}^{a-1}\sum_{y=0}^{a-1} S_{xy} \log_2 S_{xy}$$

Where, S_{xy} is the probability of co-occurrence of the gray level x and y, and a is the total intensity level of image.

In 2018, Gharaibeh et al. (2018)was conducted Pre-processing by three stages: HSI (Hue, Saturation and Intensity) conversion, DE noising by Non-Linear Wiener Filter (NLWF), and then CLAHE for image enhancement. Therefore, Circular Hough Transform (CHT) is used for the detection of the Optic disc (OD). Then, Blood vessel segmentation by applying Spatially Constrained Possibilistic Fuzzy CMeans algorithm (SCPFCM) followed by contour detection, Edge detection and fovea elimination. For effective features extraction, features are categorized into three types: Micro-aneurysms, retinal hemorrhage and exudates. The selection of relevant features is done by Deep Belief Network (DBN). Then, the Support vector machine genetic algorithm (SVMGA) is applied as a classification algorithm. So, SVM is used for the separation of the feature vectors and lastly, classification of DR diseases using a genetic algorithm.

Figure 3. Step-wise illustration of the method.

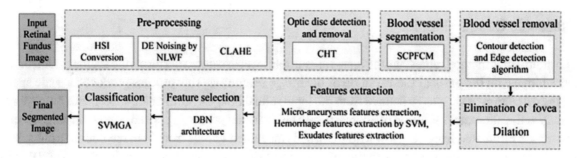

Finally, a simulation using the DIARETDB1 dataset is conducted, which shows that the algorithm is effective and efficient in specificity, sensitivity and accuracy. So, this method is a good option to efficiently segment the vessels to detect DR with high accuracy. In 2019, Mallick et al.(2019) proposes the white top-hat transform and CLAHE for enhancement of images in preprocessing stage. Then enhanced image is segmented by multiple filters, which is obtained by the modified Matched Filter with the First Derivative of Gaussian (MF-FDOG).

Figure 4. Step-wise illustration of the method.

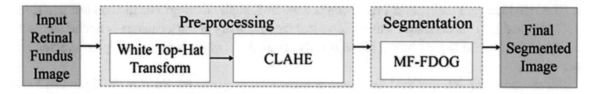

Finally, a simulation using the DRIVE dataset is conducted which provides that the method achieves higher accuracy. Moreover, the false detection rate is lower by the proposed filter than its other variants. Few pixels belong to the background but are wrongly identified as vessel pixels and few vessel pixels are wrongly assigned as background pixels. Further, the applied filter parameters increase the response of the MF-FDOG filter. The method is efficient in identifying thin and thick vessels in the presence of optic disc, exudates, and fovea. Furthermore, the method significantly decreases the false detection and increases the true positive detection. In 2020, Kushol et al. (2020)conducted preprocessing by Central light reflex diminution by using morphological opening, CLAHE and then border extension. Retinal vessel enhancement by Bottom-hat and Top-hat transformation and Measuring Edge Content-based contrast matrix, then feature extraction by applying the new multiscale directional transforms methodology named Bendlets. The output of Bendlet transform is used to construct a 4-D feature vector which is used to collect directional information. Afterward, a set of ensemble classifiers is employed for classification. Finally, postprocessing is done by a multiscale line detection algorithm, removing small noise/objects with the help of morphological area open operation.

Figure 5. Step-wise illustration of the method

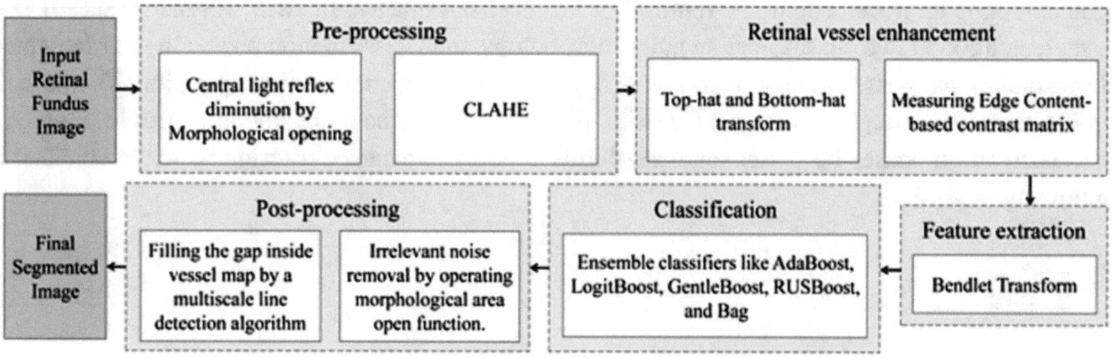

The method was examined on STARE and DRIVE datasets. Due to the multiscale line detection algorithm, some broken vessel segments can be observed which reduces the accuracy of the outcome. The method faces an over-fitting problem in a specific portion of the data. To reduce the problem of overfitting as well as variance the Bagging or Bootstrap aggregation of sample data can be used primarily but it can't remove the problem. Moreover, the major advantage of an ensemble classifier is having the ability to avoid the mistakes of a single classification model. Bendlets can successfully solve a lot of complex clinical applications. Moreover, this methodology uses only a limited number of filters that could run in any lightweight system.

Mathematical Morphology Based Method

Morphological processing technique is basically combined with other vessel properties, to obtain vessel-like patterns from retinal fundus images. Objective image and Structuring Element (SE) are the main two parts of this technique. This technique offers the identification and segmentation of images by processing and analyzing SE in a binary image. It does shape and region based features extraction like convex hulls, skeletons, boundaries etc by using SE of the images. Morphological operations are a strong tool for extraction and Morphology based filters are well suited at reducing both nonlinear and linear noise forms. Imani et al. (2014) do the segmentation in three steps: preprocessing, by green channel selection and removal of useless parts of retinal images by applying morphological opening and closing operations, and a median filter for image enhancement. Then retinal image cleaning by Morphological Component Analysis (MCA) algorithm with Shearlet transforms and Non-Subsampled Contourlet Transform (NSCT) for separation of lesions and vessels and finally, vessel segmentation by Morlet Wavelet Transform followed by Adaptive thresholding to obtain the final vessel map. The Morlet Wavelet Transform at time t can be expressed as:

$$\psi_M\left(t\right) = \exp\left(ik_0 t\right)\exp\left(-\frac{1}{2}\left|Pt\right|^2\right)$$

Where, i $= \sqrt{-1}$ and P is a diagonal matrix. The nonzero parameter $\mathbf{k}_0$ is the wave vector of the plane wave. This technique is examined on STARE and DRIVE databases, which shows that the method has less false positive rate and can gain a higher detection rate in abnormal images. The result of vessel segmentation is improved due to the removal of lesions from images. In 2015, Hassan et al.(2015) do the segmentation in two phases, mathematics morphology and Classification phase. In the Mathematical Morphological phase opening operation is applied and then reconstruction operation. Then use the Top-Hat transformation followed by a Gaussian filter to generate the more smoothed image. Finally, in the Classification phase, the vessel segmentation is done by K-means clustering which is obtained by minimizing

$$V = \sum_{n-1}^{m}\sum_{x_j \in S_n}\left(X_j - \mu_n\right)^2$$

Where, m is the number of clusters to be founded S_n, n = 1, 2,...., m and μ_n is mean point of all the points $X_j \in S_n$ or centroid. The algorithm is examined on the DRIVE database. The technique gives better outputs, which proves that it is more effective than others. Again, the method achieves high accuracy with lower misclassification. In 2018, Setiawan et al.(2018) use green channel extraction, overlap masking and opening operation followed by the top-hat morphology in the preprocessing phase. A morphological operation (Dilation and Erosion) was carried out to improve the image. Then Top-Hat Transformation operation is applied to obtain details and small elements of the image. Then Segmentation is done using Global Thresholding. Finally, in postprocessing, hole filling and pixel removal are added to improve the segmented image. The algorithm used the DRIVE image database for the experiment. The small part of the artery and vessel could not be well segmented using this process. In 2019, Kumar et al.(2019) uses white top-hat transformation and CLAHE for image enhancement followed by removal of the local intensity change due to fovea, OD and exudates from the background. Then, preprocessed images are segmented by multiscale 2-D Gabor wavelet filters to obtain a better results. Finally, Global Otsu thresholding is applied to obtain the segmented image.

Figure 6. Step-wise illustration of the method

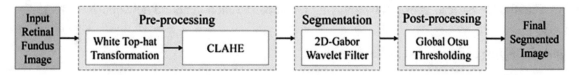

The method is tested on DRIVE dataset. The method is efficient in blood vessel identification even under illuminance conditions and uneven pigmentation in the presence of fovea, and exudates. The non vessel pixels are suppressed in the preprocessing step whereas, 2D Gabor wavelets illustrate the thin and thick retinal vessels effectively and accurately even under unequal pigmentation. In 2020, Adidja et al (2020) conducted the segmentation in 3 steps: Firstly, Pre-processing for conversion of retinal color images to grayscale image and enhancement by using CLAHE, Secondly, Feature extraction is done by using different techniques of mathematical morphological operations, partial contrast stretching and Kirsch's template for retinal vessels network extraction. Kirsch's template is one of the discrete versions of first order derivative used for retinal blood vessels edge enhancement and detection. Finally, Post processing for unwanted regions and noise removal by using a 2D median filter.

Figure 7. Step-wise illustration of the method

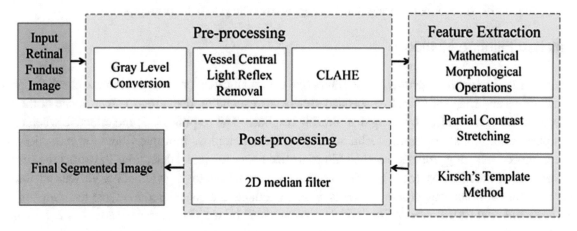

The method was analyzed on the DRIVE dataset. Kirsch's templates have the drawback of creating small holes within the blood vessels and the unwanted small objects going through the detected blood vessels. To minimize this tradeoff and eliminate the unwanted species, the morphological closing operation, with disk shaped structuring element is applied for closing the small holes in the image and preventing the shapes and size of the object image. The algorithm achieves high accuracy and takes less execution time. In 2020, Kumar et al.(2020) proposed Morphological Operations and CLAHE for preprocessing and detection of blood vessels. Then, Watershed transform (WT) is applied for OD segmentation. This Watershed transform contains several steps namely, morphological gradient (MG), marker-controlled watershed segmentation (MCWS), erosion-based and dilation-based gray-scale image reconstruction.

Then MM is used for fovea localization followed by feature extraction of hemorrhages and microaneurysm. Finally, Classification of DR by applying radial basis function neural network (RBFNN).

Figure 8. Step-wise illustration of the method

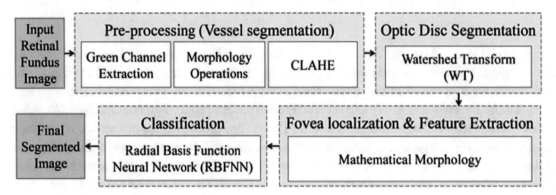

The algorithm is tested on Diaretdb0 v 1 1 and the DIABET DB1 dataset. MCWS algorithm is efficient in reducing the grayscale image over segmentation. RBFNN is very much effective in classification and its parameters are trained by the features of hemorrhages and microaneurysm. The algorithm is very much effective for hemorrhages as well as microaneurysm detection.

Matched Filtering Method

Matched filtering methods primarily use filters like Gaussian filters or their variation to check the gray distributions and shape of retinal vessels and collect corresponding responses. The presence of the required feature is recognized by using this filtering response. The response is found effective when used as a part of additional processing techniques. The method employs multiple filters for extraction, so designing and selecting properly matched filters are necessary for vessel detection. To extract the vascular network of the retina Matched Filtering convolves a retinal photograph template. Various attributes like bifurcation, branching, crossover points, vessel width etc are considered to create the template. In 2015, Zhang et al.(2015) used a filter which is constructed by the Gaussian derivatives (left-invariant second-order) in the orientation score domain. With proper parameter settings and scale selection, the method matches the vessel profile and maximizes the filter response. By applying an anisotropic wavelet transform, 2D images are lifted to 3D orientation scores. Then set a rotation and translation Gaussian derivatives (left-invariant second-order) in the domain. Finally, the method extract vessel-like patterns from different orientation scores by matching the Gaussian derivatives (left-invariant second-order) filters response with orientation score data. The method is evaluated on STARE and DRIVE datasets. The proposed filter can preserve both tiny vessels and crossings. The testing shows that the proposed filter is able to deal with generally difficult vessel patterns and gives fruitful results on large data sets. In 2015, Chakraborti (2015) uses Eigen-analysis of Hessian Matrix of each image pixel at different scales followed by the vesselness filter for the analysis of retinal images. The vesselness value for each pixel of the image is obtained and then finds Grayscale output where intensity corresponds to vesselness. Orientation Histogram of the above grayscale output where histogram contains five minimally overlapping Gaussians is used to design a self-adaptive matched filter. The Kernel of the filter is designed as a linear combination of these Gaussians. Finally, the matched filter is used to detect the retinal vessels from the response of the vesselness filter.

The modified MF kernel for each pixel at (p,q) is expressed as:

$$K\left(p,q\right) = \sum_{n=1}^{5} A_n e^{-\frac{\left(p - \mu_n\right)^2}{2\sigma_n^{\,2}}} \, for \, |q| \leq \frac{L}{2}$$

Where, A_n, σ_n (n = 1–5) and μ_n are the gains, standard deviations and means of the Gaussian kernels. L denotes the length for fixed orientation of vessels. The method is evaluated on CHASE, DRIVE and STARE datasets. This process detects vessels with very high accuracy but needs improvement in sensitivity. In 2016, Kar et al.(2016) proposes Curvelet transform for retinal vasculature enhancement. Then MF is applied to the retinal blood vessels. The MF response is used by fuzzy c-means algorithm (kernel based) for extraction of the vessel contour from the background by non-linear mapping. Laplacian of Gaussian filter is applied with MF when the test is done on pathological images. To test the ability of this approach, the algorithm is examined by additive Gaussian noise where image denoising is done by curvelet transform.

Figure 9. Step-wise illustration of the method

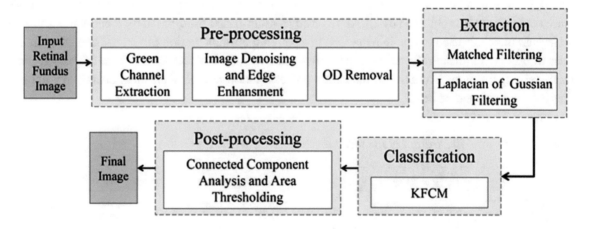

The method is evaluated on STARE, DRIVE and DIARETB1 databases. The result shows that the above mentioned method is very effective in the detection of the thick and the long as well as the thin and the short vessels. In 2020 Gao et al. (2020) proposed random walk algorithms on the basis of the centerlines for segmentation of retinal vessels. Firstly, grayscale images are extracted from retinal fundus images and then extraction of Field of View (FOV) mask. Secondly, blood vessel Enhancement Filtering is done by applying a multiscale vessel enhancement filter on the basis of the eigenvalues of the Hessian matrix. Thirdly, locating the centerlines based on the normalized gradient vector field (GVF) divergence value and bottom-hat operators. Then, the random walker algorithm (RWA) is used for blood vessel segmentation where Seed groups of the RWA are labeled by using the centerlines.

Figure 10. Step-wise illustration of the method

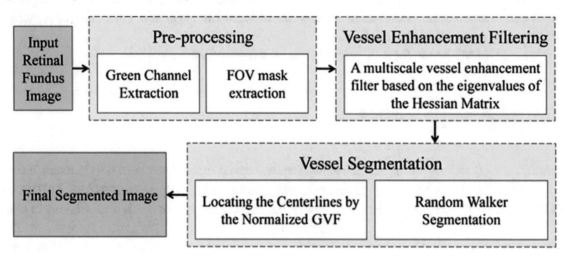

The method is implemented on STARE Dataset. The method achieves higher sensitivity and less misclassification of the nonvessel objects. Only Consideration of the intersection ratio between the skeletons and the candidate centerlines may lose some details of the vessel structure. However, the real-time performance of the method needs to be improved. Low-contrast areas of blood vessels are well detected by using this process, which is more effective for both healthy and pathological images. In 2020, Dash et al. (2020) applied a 2D Gabor filter in the spatial domain for the extraction of vessel features from the image obtained by CLAHE. Then Hessian-based filter based on eigen-value study of the Hessian matrix is used to obtain enhanced images. In the segmentation phase, the enhanced image passes through the k-means clustering step for the extraction of the blood vessels from the background. After receiving the output from the segmentation process, a morphological cleaning operation is applied to get the final segmented image.

Figure 11. Step-wise illustration of the method

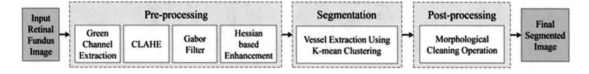

The algorithm is evaluated on Child heart and health studies in England (CHASE_DB1) and DRIVE datasets. This algorithm overcomes few existing problems of extraction techniques like false detection of vessels, connectivity issues among pixels, inaccurate detection of thin vessels etc. The main merit of the proposed algorithm is that it is easier and simple to implement and does not need any training.

Supervised Method

Supervised method is a machine learning method where vessel extraction is performed by trained labeling data. In this method, trained data is given to the model with the output. So, it is mandatory to train the model first for each input data, and then it can compute the accurate output. The model always collects feedback to confirm whether the output is correct or not. This learning model gives accurate output then the unsupervised method. The Neural Network method is one of the important supervised methods used for the extraction of blood vessels.

Neural Network Based Method

Neural network consists of interconnected nodes which work like neurons of the human brain. Basically, it is a set of the algorithm, which is constructed to identify hidden patterns. It interprets data by using machine perception or labeling raw input. The patterns it identifies are numerically contained in vectors, where all real-world data, like sound, images, time series or text must be translated. There are several kinds of neural networks – and each has its merits and demerits. Examples include artificial neural network(ANN), convolutional neural network (CNN) etc. Neural network based methods decrease the computational cost by parallel processing. In 2016, Ceylan et al. (2016) proposed a Complex ripplet-I (CRI) transform to extract the features of retinal fundus images. These features are used by a complex valued ANN to obtain a blood vessel network. The coefficients are collected from the output of the ANN which, was resized by applying inverse transforms. Then binary thresholding is applied and finally gets desired extracted vessels.

The output A_k of neuron k is defined as:

$$A_k = F\left(\sum W_{k,i} \cdot x_i + \theta_k\right)$$

Where, $W_{k,i}$ is the complex weight from an input. x_i is the unit and θ_k is the complex valued threshold. The output function is defined by F.

The STARE and DRIVE datasets were used to evaluate the method. The main advantage of this method is that the complex valued ANN directly process features. The proposed method achieved better accuracy. CRI transforms shows better results than other multiresolution analysis. The ANN gives improved performance than SVM. The proposed ANN considers the input image as a whole which makes to co-operate vessels with one another. The proposed system achieved a good response even in small vein structures. The results obtained from the CRI transform are better than the curvelet transform. In 2017, Nivetha et al.(2017) proposes a new method where green channel images are processed by applying Daubechies wavelet transform (DWT) to obtain the features of grey level cooccurrence matrix (GLCM). These features are extracted by

$$Energy, E = \sum_x \sum_y p(x,y)^2$$

$$Entropy, S = -\sum_{x}\sum_{y} p(x,y) \, X \log p(x,y)$$

$$Contrast, I = \sum\sum (x - y)^2 \, p(x,y)$$

$$Homogenity = \sum\sum \left[\frac{p(x,y)}{1 + (x,y)} \right]$$

Where, $p(x,y)$ is pixel of the grey level co-occurrence matrix (GLCM) Entropy.

Then these features are analyzed by applying a probabilistic neural network (PNN) and input images are compared with the dataset image for the classification of images as abnormal or normal. To extract the retinal blood vessels Morphological operations are used on the abnormal images. Then exudates are detected by applying fuzzy cmeans(FCM) clustering in the extracted blood vessels. FCM clustering improves the accuracy under noise. The publicly available fundus image databases are used for the evaluation. The method is applied successfully and the exudates and blood vessels are effectively detected. In 2018, Khojasteh et al. (2018)applied a method using the probabilistic output of Convolution neural network (CNN) to detect microaneurysms, exudates and hemorrhages. First, the image enhancement is done by CLAHE and then train the CNN by manually annotated segmented patches. The trained CNN was utilized to explore the other images and a probability map is created to identify the location of the pathological signs. Then the isolated signs are removed by the probability map. Then comparison takes place between the output images and the manually annotated images to the determination of the accuracy of this approach.

Figure 12. Step-wise illustration of the method

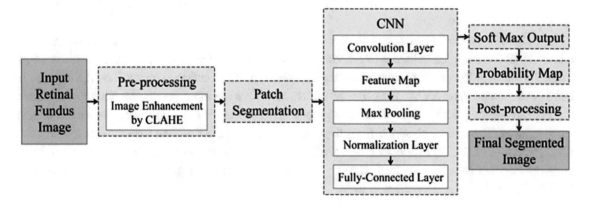

The technique was evaluated by two methods: patch based and image-based analysis on two datasets: e-Ophtha and DIARETDB1. The proposed technique analyzed the images by using probability maps instead of binary output. A demerit of this method is that it is not able to differentiate between microaneurysms and hemorrhages when there is an overlapping between these. The network was trained using single database and evaluated on two databases, which shows the universality of the method. The technique performs well without requiring a large database. In 2019, Li et al. (2019) presents an algorithm using Deep Convolutional Neural network (DCNN), SVM, and teaching-learning-based optimization (TLBO). DCNN consists of multiple convolution layer, Fractional max-pooling and Softmax classifier. Then combined features from DCNNs and metadata of the image for classification by SVM classifier. Finally, optimizing the parameters of SVM with TLBO to get final image.

Figure 13. Step-wise illustration of the method

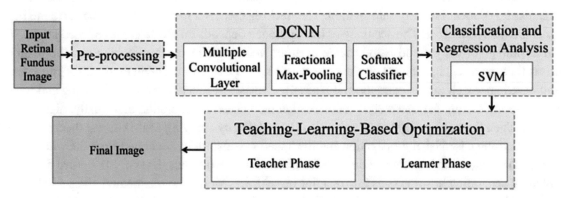

The algorithm was evaluated on a dataset collected from Kaggle. Images labeled with lesion numbers are used by the approach instead of labeling the location of symptoms. The dataset preprocessing step requires less time for processing. Overall the method is time-efficient compared to other machine learning methods used for DR detection. In 2020, Mateen et al. (2020) proposed pretrained CNN architecture for exudates detection. After data preprocessing, localization of region of interest (ROI) is done by Gaussian mixture model (GMM) and adaptive learning rate (ALR). Then feature extraction is achieved by the DCNN model. Then transfer learning is applied and then, the fused features are fed into the softmax classifier for exudate classification.

Figure 14. Step-wise illustration of the method

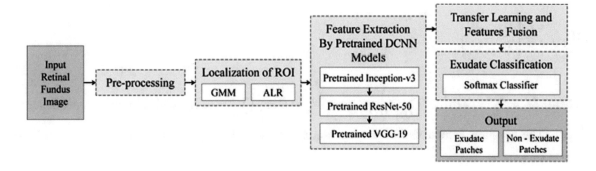

The algorithm was evaluated on two datasets DIARETDB1 and e-Ophtha. The accuracy of the transfer learning method outperforms in feature extraction. The proposed method may be reconstituted in the future to discriminate between soft and hard exudates. Moreover, the method can also be applied to diagnose microaneurysms and hemorrhages for DR.

Vessel Tracking Method

Vessel tracking methods are used to segment the retinal vessels by tracking the vessels. The algorithms usually work with a set of reliable seed points and use them to track the retinal vasculature on the basis of the texture of local intensity information. The tracking creates a tree-like pattern because the blood vessels are interconnected. The accuracy of this approach depends on the selection of seed points. The main advantage of the method is to provide accurate vessel widths during tracking and the main demerit is that the tracking depends on the pre-processing step. In 2014, Cheng et al. (2014) proposed a graph based approach for the extraction. It basically consists of two phases: preprocessing and tracing step. In preprocessing, the first step is segmentation then skeleton extraction and finally, digraph construction. Then the tracing step to trace vessels is completed by applying Matrix-forest theorem (MFT) in directed graph based label propagation and the traced vessels finally separated from the whole vessel network. This algorithm is examined on the STARE and DRIVE datasets. Uses of MFT solve the tracing problem of separating blood vessels into disjoint vessel trees. Moreover, the method gives reliable tracing results. In future, the approach may be applied for neurite tracing. In 2014, Chen et al. (2014) proposed Optimally Oriented Flux and Metric construction, Anisotropic Fast Marching using Basis Reduction, Curve Length calculation and Geodesic Extraction for vessel extraction. The oriented flux of an image I, of dimension d, is defined by the amount of the image gradient projected along the orientation $\vec{p}$ flowing out from a 2D circle (or 3D local sphere) at point $\tilde{x}$ with radius r:

$$f\left(\tilde{x}; r, \vec{p}\right) = \int_{\partial S_r} \left(\nabla\left(G_\sigma * I\right)\left(\tilde{x} + r\vec{n}\right) \cdot \vec{p}\right)\left(\vec{p} \cdot \vec{n}\right) dA,$$

Where, G_σ is a Gaussian function with variance σ and $\vec{n}$ is the outward unit normal vector along ∂Sr. dA is the infinitesimal length (area) on ∂S_r.

The metric used for vessel extraction is…

$$M\left(\tilde{x}, r\right) = \begin{pmatrix} M_s & 0 \\ 0 & M_r \end{pmatrix}$$

Where, $M_s = \sum_{i=1}^{d} \exp\left(\propto \sum_{j \neq i} \lambda_j\right) v_i v_i^T$ and $M_r = \beta \exp\left(\sum_{i=1}^{d} \propto \lambda_i\right)$, which implicit dependence on $\left(\tilde{x}, r\right)$. The constant β controls FM propagation speed along the radius direction, and α controls the metric anisotropy.

Anisotropic Fast Marching with path score helps to find key points separated by small curve lengths in vessel tree extraction. Curve length threshold (CLT) is most useful for a tree like structure extraction. CLT can find small structures. Evaluation results show that this approach can extract vessel tree structures at a very finer scale, with increased accuracy. In 2016, Singh et al. (2016) proposes principal component analysis (PCA) followed by CLAHE for enhancement of retinal fundus image in preprocessing stage. Then a new MF based on the Gumbel probability density function (PDF) is designed with an appropriate parameter value for segmentation of the vessels. MF response image is generated by Gumbel PDF based MF. The final phase includes the entropy based optimal thresholding, then length filtering and removing outer artifacts to get the segmented image.

Figure 15. Step-wise illustration of the method

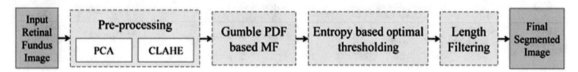

The approach is tested on STARE and DRIVE databases. The method achieves the highest accuracy due to the presence of a Gumbel PDF based kernel. Comparison of this filter with the Cauchy PDF based MF and Gaussian distribution function shows that the proposed filter achieved better performance. In 2019, Luo et al. (2019) proposes an active contour tracking for OD segmentation. Firstly, denoising and image enhancement is done in preprocessing. Then, the center of OD was collected by applying the least squares method. The ROI was calculated on the basis of the features and center of OD. Finally, segmentation was obtained by active contour tracking.

Figure 16. Step-wise illustration of the method

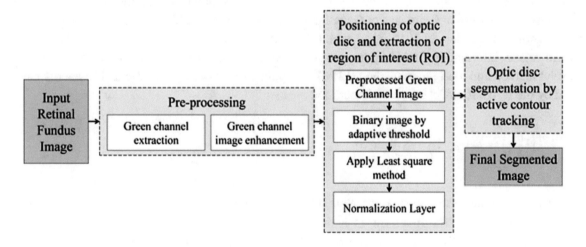

The method was evaluated on STARE, DRIVE, Messidor and Drishti-GS1 datasets. The least square method uses by the proposed method identifies the center of OD effectively. The technique works well with mild or low contrast images and achieves lower computing complexity and higher segmentation accuracy. In the future, the method will improve the accuracy with severe lesions of images. In 2020,

Jainish et al. (2020) proposed method consists of preprocessing and extraction of vessels. Preprocessing follows firstly, image acquisition secondly, grey scale conversion then bias correction and finally adaptive histogram equalization for enhancement of the blood vessels. Then region segmentation of images is achieved by Probabilistic modeling. Finally, a maximum entropy based expectation maximization (MEEM) algorithm is applied for the extraction of the retinal blood vessels.

Figure 17. Step-wise illustration of the method

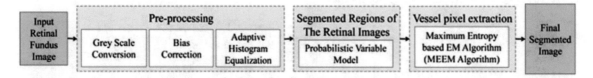

The algorithm is evaluated on STARE and DRIVE datasets. This experiment shows that the proposed approach is robust and achieves accurate segmentation results in abnormal and normal images. In addition, the approach outperforms with good sensitivity. In the future, the method will apply to the detection of lesions in retinal vessel images.

Model Based Method

In model-based methods, the explicit vessel models are used to extract the retinal vessel map. The method mainly consists of vector fields, the Hermite model, region growing, active contour, level set, and other methods. The method is classified into two types: (i) deformable models and (ii) vessel profile models. Deformable models can be classified into geometric and parametric approaches. In vessel profile models, a mixture of Gaussians or Gaussian curves is used for the blood vessel cross-sectional intensity profile projection. In 2015, Zhao et al. (2015) applied an infinite perimeter active contour with hybrid region information (IPACHI) for automated vessel segmentation. Eigenvalue-based method, wavelet method and local phase method (LPM) are applied for vessel enhancement. The energy calculated by the IPACHI model in γ neighbourhood area is:

$$F^{IPACHI}\left(\Gamma,r_n\right) = \mathcal{L}^2\left(\gamma - \Gamma\right) + \sum_{n=1}^{N}\lambda_n R_n,$$

where $\mathcal{L}^2$ is the 2D Lebesgue measure, R_n is the nth region information, and N is the total number of different region terms. The first term $\mathcal{L}^2$ is the area of the γ-neighborhood of the edge set Γ. The experiment is done in DRIVE, STARE and VAMPIRE datasets. The LPM preserves vessel edges. The phase map gives a more accurate and reliable vesselness map. Infinite perimeter regularization is well suited for the detection of vasculature structures than other traditional approaches. The method can be used for other evaluations like corneal neovascularization. The method can also be used for the segmentation of other images like MRI, CT, and X-ray. In 2016, Oliveira et al. uses three combined filters namely, MF, Frangi's filter (FF) and GWF for retinal vessel segmentation. The Gaussian filters are obtained using the following function:

$$K_i\left(x,y\right) = e^{-\frac{u^2}{2\sigma^2}} \forall \overline{p} \in Z$$

Where, $\overline{p}$ =(x, y) be a discrete point in the kernel, Z is a neighborhood such that Z = {(u, v), |u| ≤ 3σ, |v| ≤ δ/2} and σ is the parameter that controls the scale, δ is the length of the filter and the direction of the blood vessel is aligned along the y-axis. In preprocessing enhanced images by using intensity normalization, then combined MF, FF and GWF by median ranking and weighted mean. The threshold criterion is used to segment the images enhanced by using median ranking. Deformable models and the FCM clustering method are used to segment the images enhanced by weighted mean. Then post processing to remove noise and finally get the segmented image. The method is evaluated using two datasets, STARE and DRIVE. The combined filter gives a better results than a single filter. The median ranking is far better than the weighted mean method. But the areas close to the borders and thin vessels are not well segmented. In 2016, Rad et al. (2016) used the Morphological Region-Based Initial Contour (MRBIC) model for vessel segmentation. At first Binarization algorithm (Histogram based image thresholding) is applied on input images for binarization. The morphologically open binary image technique is used to remove unwanted objects. Then a region-based map function is used to collect the best IC of images to perform by level set function. Finally, segmentation is completed by using the MRBIC method.

Figure 18. Step-wise illustration of the method

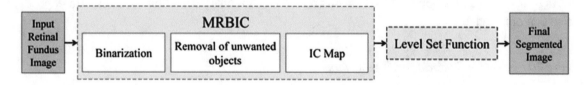

The method is evaluated on the STARE and DRIVE datasets. The method shows appropriate segmentation of noisy images by selecting accurate IC. Moreover, the method is robust and easy to implement. In 2018, Karn et al. (2018) applied a hybrid active contour model for segmentation. Preprocessing includes vessel enhancement by CLAHE and removal of central vessel reflex by Contour driven black top-hat transformation algorithm (CDBTHTA). Then, phase-based binarisation is implemented by Phase congruency-centred feature map and main binarisation to get the final preprocessed image. Finally, vessel Segmentation is accomplished by a Hybrid active contour model where the Gradient vector flow (GVF)-based snake and balloon method are combined to carry out the final segmentation. The GVF based snake and balloon method efficiently do the detection of blood vessels.

Figure 19. Step-wise illustration of the method

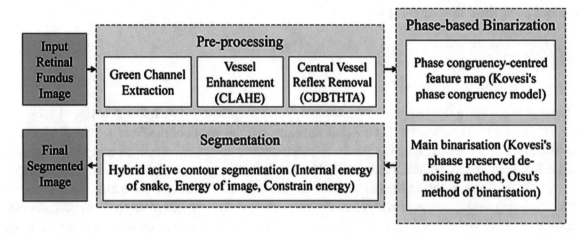

The method is evaluated by DRIVE, STARE, VAMPIRE and CHASE datasets. The uses of phase based binarization increase the performance metrics of the method. Ballon algorithm minimizes few demerits of the snake model. This method can also be utilized to detect Islands or coastlines during satellite image processing. In 2019, Naqvi et al. (2019) presents a method consists of Optic Disk (OD) Localization, OD homogenization and OD contour estimation for OD detection and segmentation. OD localization does Haze-removal and Iterative normalization by the difference of Gaussian (DoG) filter for image enhancement. Edge-aware Image smoothing is applied for OD homogenization. Finally, OD contour estimation employed the Ellipse Fitting approach and Variational Active contour model for effective detection and segmentation of OD. However, most vascular patterns are detected by Laplacian filtering-based inpainting approach and unconstrained OD boundary detection by gradient-independent active contour model.

Figure 20. Step-wise illustration of the method

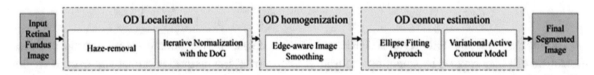

MESSIDOR, DRIONS-DB and ONHSD datasets are used here for the evaluation of the method. Vascular structure inpainting before contour estimation improved the performance of this method by the most accurate extraction of OD boundary. The approach omits unnecessary information and concentrates on true contours. Its real time application result will be fruitful in all aspects.

Hybrid Approaches

Hybrid techniques are a combination of two or more computational techniques which provide more advantage to detect components than any other individual technique. It helps to improve data analysis.

The hybrid technique helps qualitative research to be effective. It can collect and correlate more tangible solutions more quickly. So, Hybrid Machine Learning approaches are a technique to Improve Expected Output from any raw data. Here, Hybrid approaches used multiple classifiers for the extraction of retinal fundus images. Hence, Different researchers combine different individual approaches for agile and effective extraction. Gaussian mixture model (GMM) method with Gray-voting process is used by Dai et al. (2015) for segmentation of the vessels. GMM parameters are updated by

$$\omega_i^{t+1} = \frac{1}{N} \sum_{j=1}^{N} p_i\left(x_j \mid \mu_i^t, \sigma_i^t\right)$$

$$\mu_i^{t+1} = \frac{\sum_{j=1}^{N} p_i\left(x_j \mid \mu_i^t, \sigma_i^t\right) x_j}{\sum_{j=1}^{N} p_i\left(x_j \mid \mu_i^t, \sigma_i^t\right)},$$

$$\sigma_i^{t+1} = \frac{\sum_{j=1}^{N} p_i\left(x_j \mid \mu_i^t, \sigma_i^t\right)\left(x_j - \mu_i^{t+1}\right)^2}{\sum_{j=1}^{N} p_i\left(x_j \mid \mu_i^t, \sigma_i^t\right)}$$

where N is the number of pixels to be classified and t denotes the tth iteration. The grey value of the center point in the window is denoted as (x,y).

Preprocessing is accomplished by 2D-Gabor filter, Gray-vote algorithm and Image fusion whereas, Postprocessing is done by vessel complement and elimination of fragments to get the segmented image. The result of this approach contains small vessel details, which proves that the proposed method achieved a higher sensitivity whereas; over-segmentation rate is high, which lowers the specificity and accuracy of the proposed approach. Jiang et al. (2015) use a combination of isotropic undecimated wavelet transforms(IUWT), Texture Entropy, and Fuzzy C-mean Clustering (FCM) classifier, which has some limitations such as easy local minimum results during FCM calculating, and the discontinuous segmented vessels after skeleton processing, which need further optimum processing and refinement. In IUWT original signal was reconstructed from wavelet coefficient by

$$f = c_n + \sum_{j=1}^{n} w_j$$

Where, at each iteration j, scaling coefficients c_j are computed by lowpass filtering, and wavelet coefficients w_j by subtraction.

Texture Features Extracted Based on Gray Value Entropy obtained by:

$$H = -\sum_{i=0}^{255} p_{ij} \log 2 p_{ij}$$

$$p_{ij} = f(i,j) / N^2$$

Where, i ($0 \leq i \leq 255$) represents the detected center pixel, j ($0 \leq j \leq 255$) represents the mean gray value of i's neighborhood pixels, $f(i,j)$ was the frequency of (i,j), N was defined as the scale of image.

Panchal et al. (2016) proposed a hybrid method which combines morphological operation and knowledge of Scanning Window Analysis (SWA) for obtaining the reliable result from the fundus image of the retina. Basically, segmentation includes thresholding, erosion and dilation morphological operations, morphological opening and closing and finally SWA. This method works well even with the retinal images with complex disorder patterns. Sundaram et al. (2019) hybridized the method with morphological operations, bottom hat transform, multi-scale vessel enhancement (MSVE) algorithm, and image fusion.

Figure 21. Step-wise illustration of the method

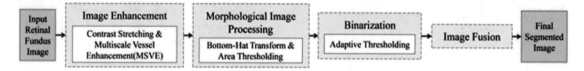

The proposed approach is tested on HRF, CHASE, and DRIVE datasets. Due to the varying aspect ratio and low-resolution images, the algorithm achieves lower sensitivity but efficiency is better given classification parameters. If this algorithm can be added to artifacts removal approaches then it will achieve better segmentation outputs. Diaz et al. (2019) combined two different approaches: Lateral Inhibition (LI) and Differential Evolution (DE). The LI method creates a new image with enhanced contrast between retinal vessels and the background. After that, a proper threshold value by decreasing the cross entropy function from the enhanced retinal image is achieved by the DE algorithm.

Figure 22. Step-wise illustration of the method

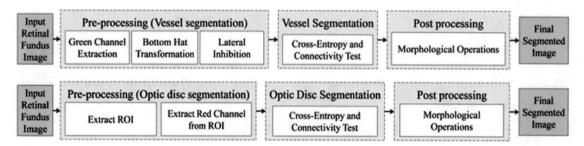

The performance of the algorithm is tested using DRIVE, STARE, and DRISHTI-GS datasets. The proposed algorithm is an accurate method for retinal vessel segmentation as well as OD segmentation. Tamin et al. (2020) done the Feature extraction of green channel image by Local Intensity Feature, Morphological White Top-Hat Transformation, Morphological Black Bottom-Hat Transformation, The Principal Moments of Phase Congruency, Multi-Scale Second-Order of Local Image Structure (Hessian matrix)and Difference of Gaussian (DoG).

Figure 23. Step-wise illustration of the method

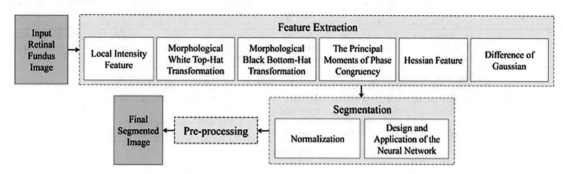

The performance of the algorithm is tested using DRIVE, STARE, and CHASED_DB1 datasets. The method outperforms with DRIVE and STARE database but, shows poor performance for CHASE_DB1. Due to the nonuniform background illumination and poor contrast between vessels and the background, performance degradation occurs.

COMPARATIVE ANALYSIS

Different researchers use different techniques for the extraction of blood vessels from different fundus images. It is noticed that the STARE and DRIVE public databases are commonly used for the verification of retinal blood vessel extraction approaches. Merits and Demerits of different retinal blood vessel extraction techniques are presented here. Then, a comparative analysis of a few of the DR detection techniques is presented on the basis of parameters like Sensitivity, Specificity and Accuracy. Table 2 shows the performance comparison based on Sensitivity, Specificity and Accuracy of retinal blood vessel extraction methodologies whereas table 1 shows the merits and demerits of different techniques.

Table 1. Merits and Demerits of different retinal blood vessel extraction technique

Extraction Technique	Merits	Demerits
Multiscale Based	• It works well on healthy retinal images. • The main advantages of multiscale methods include dramatic reductions in the necessary sample size to achieve these results. • At lower resolutions, most of the slide is visible, and a person can investigate bigger features. At high resolutions, very small features are captured in a small space within the sample.	• Sometimes does false detection in overlapping areas. • Segmentation criteria may be arbitrarily complex and can consider local as well as global criteria. • A common necessity is that each region must be linked in some sense.
Mathematical Morphological Based	• Binary images may contain numerous imperfections. The Morphological method removes these imperfections by considering the structure and form of the image. • This method uses a set of tools for feature extraction. Dilation and erosion operations used in this method are primitive.	• Cannot properly segment the smaller part of the retinal vessel, which is smaller than the vein. • For effective lesion detection, it is important to enhance only the target lesions without surrounding tissue whereas, the method usually enhances full structures of images without any discrimination.
Matched Filtering Based	• Very much effective in the detection of thick and long retinal vessels as well as the thin and the short vessels. • The Filter maximizes the signal to noise ratio (SNR). • Optimal detection performance and low computational cost. • Requires fewer signal samples to achieve good detection. • The probability of false alarm or missing detection is low.	• The filter does not preserve the input signal shape. • Requires prior knowledge of the primary user. • High Complexity. • Requires a large amount of power consumption.
Neural Network (NN) Based	• Focuses mainly on the abnormal retinal images and gives a better result. • It can model difficult functions. • A NN can complete tasks which a linear program can't. • It can be imposed in any application and without any problem. • A NN learns and never needs to be programmed again.	• Large Complexity in network architecture. • The NN needs proper training to operate. • Large NN needs high execution time. • As the number of neurons increases the network becomes complex.
Vessel Tracking Based	• For images with noise and poor contrast, vessel tracking is reliable, but it may unable to track blood vessels which have the substantial central reflex. • Vessel tracking is computationally effective but the segmentation depends on the neighborhood pixels, for which some of the vessel pixels are left unnoticed during segmentation. • It didn't use any edge information to locate the vessel so, the noise effect is reduced in vessel tracking.	• The main demerit of this process is the full dependency on the pre-processing steps of segmentation. • The method has a complex intensity profile at branching or crossover positions. • Boundary locations and vessel bifurcation are not well modeled and sometimes lead to incompletion in the extraction.
Model Based	• The model provides a more accurate and reliable vessel map and the intensity information helps in excluding few potential outliers in the fundus image. • The Model-based Design is a convenient graphical representation of systems, continuous validation at all stages as well as it has robustness against coding errors.	• Cannot follow topological changes of objects. • Need suitable parameters, and long runtime. • It is not capable to segment the nearest objects. • When image size is too large, this method works slowly.
Hybrid Approaches	• The main advantage of hybrid based segmentation is that it employs multiple approaches for accurate and effective output. • Higher accuracy, performance than Filter. Less computational complexity. • More flexible and robust upon high resolution data.	• It is a classifier specific method. • Dependent on the combination of different feature selection method. • The low-resolution images and varying aspect ratio does a huge drop in sensitivity during segmentation.

Table 2. Performance comparison based on Sensitivity, Specificity and Accuracy of the retinal blood vessel extraction technique

Authors	Year	Extraction Technique	Dataset	Sensitivity	Specificity	Accuracy
Gharaibeh et. al.	2018	Support Vector machine Genetic Algorithm (SVMGA)	DIARETDB1	99%	96%	98.4%
Mallick et. al	2019	Matched filter with first-order derivative of Gaussian (MF-FDOG)	DRIVE	0.7193	0.9764	0.9434
Kushol et. al.	2020	Bendlet transform	DRIVE STARE	0.7588 0.7798	0.9748 0.9746	0.9456 0.9528
Kumar et. al.	2019	2D-Gabor Wavelet Filter	DRIVE	0.7503	0.9717	0.9432
Adidja et. al.	2020	Kirsch's Template Method	DRIVE	96.49	74.91	94.60
Kumar et. al.	2020	Watershed transform	DIABET DB1 and Diaretdb0 v 1 1	87%	93%	Not Available
Karv et. al.	2016	Curvelet Transform and Kernel Fuzzy c-means	DRIVE STARE	0.7548 0.7549	0.9792 0.9699	0.9616 0.9741
Gao et. al.	2020	Random Walk Algorithm	STARE	0.7581	0.9550	0.9401
Dash et. al.	2020	K-Mean Clustering	DRIVE CHASE_DB1	0.756 0.774	0.981 0.974	0.952 0.951
Khojasteh et. al.	2018	Convolution neural network-based analysis(CNN)	DIARETDB1 and e-Ophtha	0.98	0.96	0.98
Li et. al.	2019	Deep Convolutional Neural Network (DCNN)	Kaggle	0.8930	0.9089	91.05%
Mateen et. al.	**2020**	**Pretrained Convolutional Neural Network**	**e-Ophtha and DIARETDB1**	**Not Available**	**Not Available**	**98.43% 98.91%**
Singh et. al.	2016	Gumbel Probability Distribution Function based matched filter	DRIVE STARE	Not Available	Not Available	0.9522 0.9270
Luo et. al.	**2019**	**Active contour tracking**	**DRIVE, STARE, Drishti-GS1 and Messidor**	**Not Available**	**Not Available**	**100 92.6 99 95.7**
Jainish et. al.	2020	Maximum entropy based EM algorithm	DRIVE STARE	98.9% 99%	79% 85%	96.57 97.03
Rad et. al.	2016	Morphological Region-Based Initial Contour Algorithm	DRIVE STARE	69.65 73.42	97.22 96.08	96.08 92.89
Karn et. al.	2018	Hybrid Active Contour Model	DRIVE, STARE CHASE, VAMPIRE	0.78 0.80 0.78 0.79	0.98 0.96 0.97 0.97	0.97 0.96 0.97 0.96
Naqvi et. al.	**2019**	**Variational active contour model**	**DRIONS-DB, MESSIDOR and ONHSD**	**0.9130 0.9486 0.9364**	**0.9800 0.9896 0.9885**	**0.9672 0.9860 0.9851**
Sundaram et. al.	2019	Combination of BHT, Area based filtering, Binarization using Adaptive thresholding and image fusion	DRIVE, CHASE, HRF	0.69 0.71 78.32%	0.94 0.96 96.79%	0.93 0.95 95.82%
Diaz et. al.	2019	Combination of LI and DE	DRIVE, STARE, DRISHTI-GS	0.8464 0.8331 --	0.9701 0.9619 --	0.9619 0.9559 --
Tamin et. al.	2020	Local intensity, Top and Bottom hat transform, Hessian features, Moment of phase congruency and difference of Gaussian	DRIVE, STARE, CHASED_DB1	0.7542 0.7806 0.7585	0.9843 0.9825 0.9846	0.9607 0.9632 0.9577

From the comparison, it is clear that Neural Network based method and Active Contour model perform well in segmentation.

CONCLUSION

DR detection is an emerging biometric modality which deserves a discussion and systematic review of the connected methods and findings. The chapter presents a few of the retinal blood vessel extraction methods which play a vital role in the detection of DR. It is realized from the analysis that no unique extraction technique is suitable for images of various eye-related diseases and the deterioration of the vessels varies from patient to patient. The Hybrid approach focuses mainly on the abnormal retinal images. The future work will focus on Hybrid based approaches which eliminate the demerits of existing retinal vessel extraction technique. An optimal method based on hybrid approaches will be proposed to minimize issues of existing methods to obtain a more accurate output with the addition of soft computing approaches. Keeping these factors in mind, in future work the feature extraction will be done by using transform domain with dynamic neural network and finally, image resizing by inverse transform and thresholding. These approaches will be tested on publicly available databases like DRIVE, STARE databases, as well as on local retinal image databases. The performance of the proposed method is evaluated based on different performance parameters like Sensitivity, Specificity and Accuracy etc. Finally, the proposed approach is compared with alternative approaches. The proposed method will be a more efficient and fast process for the detection of blood vessels from fundus images. Other than the quantitative performance measures, the receiver operating characteristic (ROC) curve will be used to justify the effectiveness of the segmentation approach.

REFERENCES

Adidja, M., & Robleh, H. A. (2020). Automated Blood Vessels Segmentation Method for Retinal Fundus Image Based on Mathematical Morphology Operations and Kirsch's Template. *International Journal of Computer Science and Network*, 9(3), 114–122.

Agarwal, G., Gaur, L., & Bist, A. S. (2021). COVID-19 Real Time Impact Analysis India vs USA. In Futuristic Trends in Network and Communication Technologies. Springer. doi:10.1007/978-981-16-1480-4_29

Ceylan, M., & Yasar, H. (2016). A novel approach for automatic blood vessel extraction in retinal images: Complex ripplet-I transform and complex valued artificial neural network. *Turkish Journal of Electrical Engineering and Computer Sciences*, 2016(24), 3212–3227.

Chakraborty, T., Jha, D. K., Chowdhury, A. S., & Jiang, X. (2015). A Self-Adaptive matched filter for retinal blood vessel detection. *Machine Vision and Applications*, 2015(26), 55–68.

Chen, D., Cohen, L. D., & Mirebeau, J. M. (2014). *Vessel Exraction using anisotropic minimal paths and path score.* https://projet.liris.cnrs.fr/imagine/pub/proceedings/ICIP-2014/Papers/1569899543.pdf

Cheng, L., De, J., Zhang, X., Lin, F., & Li, H. (2014). *Tracing Retinal blood vessels by Matrix-Forest theorem of Directed Graphs.* Doi:10.1007/978-3-319-10404-1_78

Dai, P., Luo, H., Sheng, H., Zhao, Y., Li, L., & Wu, J. (2015). A New Approach to Segment Both Main and Peripheral Retinal Vessels Based on GrayVoting and Gaussian Mixture Model. *PLoS ONE, 10*(6). doi:10.1371/journal.pone.0127748

Das, S., & Majumder, S. (2021). A Review on Pattern Recognition based Retinal blood vessels extraction technique to detect Diabetic Retinopathy (DR). *2nd International Conference on Data Science and Applications (ICDSA 2021).*

Dash, J., Parida, P., & Bhoi, N. (2020). Retinal Blood Vessel Extraction from Fundus Images using Enhancement Filtering and Clustering. *ELCVIA. Electronic Letters on Computer Vision and Image Analysis, 19*(1), 38–52.

Diaz, P., Rodriguez, A., Cuevas, E., Valdivia, A., Chavolla, E., Pérez-Cisneros, M., & Zaldívar, D. (2019). A hybrid method for blood vessel segmentation in images. *Biocybernetics and Biomedical Engineering, 39*(1-2). doi:10.1016/j.bbe.2019.06.009

Gao, J., Chen, G., & Lin, W. (2020). *An Effective Retinal Blood Vessel Segmentation by Using Automatic Random Walks Based on Centerline Extraction.* Hindawi BioMed Research International.

Gaur, L., Bhatia, U., & Jhanjhi, N. Z. (2021). Medical image-based detection of COVID-19 using Deep Convolution Neural Networks. *Multimedia Systems.* Advance online publication. doi:10.100700530-021-00794-6 PMID:33935377

Gaur, L., Singh, G., & Agarwal, V. (2021). Leveraging Artificial Intelligence Tools to Combat the COVID-19 Crisis. In Futuristic Trends in Network and Communication Technologies. Springer. doi:10.1007/978-981-16-1480-4_28

Gaur, L., Solanki, A., Wamba, S. F., & Jhanjhi, N. Z. (2021). *Advanced AI Techniques and Applications in Bioinformatics.* CRC Press. doi:10.1201/9781003126164

Gharaibeh, N., Al-Hazaimeh, O. M., Al-Naami, B., & Nahar, K. M. O. (2018). An effective image processing method for detection of diabetic retinopathy diseases from retinal fundus images. *International Journal of Signal and Imaging Systems Engineering, 11*(4), 206–216.

Hassan, G., Bendary, N. E., Hassanien, A. E., Fahmy, A., Shoeb, A. M., & Snasel, V. (2015). Retinal blood vessel segmentation approach based on mathematical morphology. *Procedia Computer Science, 65*, 612–622.

Imani, E., Javidi, M., & Pourreza, H. R. (2015). Improvement of retinal blood vessel detection using morphological component analysis. *Computer Methods and Programs in Biomedicine, 118*(3), 263–279. PMID:25697986

Jainish, G. R., Jiji, G. W., & Infant, P. A. (2020). A novel automatic retinal vessel extraction using maximum entropy based EM algorithm. Multimedia Tools and Applications, 79, 22337–22353. doi:10.100711042-020-08958-8

Jiang, K., Zhou, Z., Geng, X., Tang, L., Wu, H., & Dong, J. (2015). Isotropic Undecimated Wavelet Transform Fuzzy Algorithm for Retinal Blood Vessel Segmentation. *Journal of Medical Imaging and Health Informatics, 5*(7), 1524–1527. doi:10.1166/jmihi.2015.1561

Kar, S. S., & Maity, S. P. (2016). Blood vessel extraction and optic disc removal using Curvelet Transform and Kernel Fuzzy C-means. Computers in Biology and Medicine, 1-16. doi:10.1016/j.compbiomed.2015.12.018

Karn, P. K., Biswal, B., & Samantaray, S. R. (2018). Robust retinal blood vessel segmentation using hybrid active contour model. *IET Image Processing*, 1–12. doi:10.1049/iet-ipr.2018.5413

Kaswan, K. S., Gaur, L., Dhatterwal, J. S., & Kumar, R. (2021). AI-Based Natural Language Processing for the Generation of Meaningful Information Electronic Health Record (EHR) Data. In Advanced AI Techniques and Applications in Bioinformatics. CRC Press. doi:10.1201/9781003126164

Khan, B.K., Khaliq, A.A., & Shahid, M. (2016). A Morphological Hessian Based Approach for Retinal Blood Vessels Segmentation and Denoising Using Region Based Otsu Thresholding. *PLOS ONE, 11*(7), 1-19.

Khojasteh, P., Aliahmad, B., & Kumar, D. K. (2018). Fundus images analysis using deep features for detection of exudates, hemorrhages and microaneurysms. *BMC Ophthalmology, 18*, 288. doi:10.1186/s12886-018-0954-4

Kumar, K., & Samal, D. (2019). Automated retinal vessel segmentation based on morphological preprocessing and 2D-Gabor wavelets. *Proceedings of ICACIE 2018*, 1. arXiv:1908.04123v1[eess.IV]

Kumar, S., Adarsh, A., Kumar, B., & Singh, A. K. (2020). An automated early diabetic retinopathy detection through improved blood vessel and optic disc segmentation. *Journal of Optics and Laser Technology, 121*, 1-11.

Kushol, R., Kabir, M. H., Abdullah-Al-Wadud, M., & Islam, M. S. (2020). Retinal blood vessel segmentation from fundus image using an efficient multiscale directional representation technique Bendlets. *Mathematical Biosciences and Engineering, 17*(6), 7751–7771. PMID:33378918

Li, Y. H., Yeh, N. N., Chen, S. J., & Chung, Y. C. (2019). *Computer-Assisted Diagnosis for Diabetic Retinopathy Based on Fundus Images Using Deep Convolutional Neural Network.* doi:10.1155/2019/6142839

Luo, Z., Jia, Y., & He, J. (2019). An Optic Disc Segmentation Method Based on Active Contour Tracking. International Information and Engineering Technology Association. *Traitement du Signal., 36*(3), 265–271. doi:10.18280/ts.360310

Mallick, D., Kumar, K., & Agarwal, S. (2019). *Blood Vessel Detection using Modified Multiscale MF-FDOG Filters for Diabetic Retinopathy.* arXiv:1910.12028v1 [eess.IV]

Mateen, M., Wen, J., Nasrullah, N., Sun, S., & Hayat, S. (2020). *Exudate Detection for Diabetic Retinopathy Using Pretrained Convolutional Neural Networks.* doi:10.1155/2020/5801870

Naqvi, S. S., Fatima, N., Khan, T. M., Rehman, Z. U., & Khan, M. A. (2019). Automatic optic disk detection and segmentation by variational active contour estimation in retinal fundus images. Springer. doi:10.100711760-019-01463-y

Nivetha, C., Sumathi, S., & Chandrasekaran, M. (2017). Retinal Blood Vessels Extraction and Detection of Exudates Using Wavelet Transform and PNN Approach for the Assessment of Diabetic Retinopathy. *IEEE International Conference on Communication and Signal Processing*, 1962-1966.

Oliveira, W.S., Teixeira, J.V., Ren, T.I., & Cavalcanti, G.D.C. (2016). Unsupervised Retinal Vessel Segmentation Using Combined Filters. *PLoS ONE, 11*(2). doi:10.1371/journal.pone.0149943

Panchal, P., Bhojani, R., & Panchal, T. (2016). An Algorithm for Retinal Feature Extraction using Hybrid Approach. *Procedia Computer Science, 79*, 61–68. doi:10.1016/j.procs.2016.03.009

Rad, A. E. R., Safry, M., Rahim, M., Kolivand, H., & Amin, I. B. M. (2016). Morphological Region-Based Initial Contour Algorithm for Level Set Methods in Image Segmentation. *Multimedia Tools and Applications*, 1–16.

Ravichandran, C., & Raja, J. B. (2014). A Fast Enhancement/Thresholding Based Blood Vessel Segmentation for Retinal Image Using Contrast Limited Adaptive Histogram Equalization. *Journal of Medical Imaging and Health Informatics, 4*(4), 567–575.

Setiawan, W., Utoyo, M. I., & Rulaningtyas, R. (2018). Retinal Vessel Segmentation using a Modified Morphology Process and Global Thresholding. *The 8th Annual Basic Science International Conference. AIP Conference Proceedings 2021*. 10.1063/1.5062795

Singh, N. P., & Srivastava, R. (2016). Retinal blood vessels segmentation by using Gumbel Probability Distribution Function based matched filter. *Computer Methods and Programs in Biomedicine*, 1–15. doi:10.1016/j.cmpb.2016.03.001 PMID:27084319

Sundaram, R. (2019). Extraction of Blood Vessels in Fundus Images of Retina through Hybrid Segmentation Approach. *Mathematics, 7*(169), 1–17. doi:10.3390/math7020169

Tamim, N., Elshrkawey, M., Azim, G.A., & Nassar, H. (2020). Retinal Blood Vessel Segmentation Using Hybrid Features and Multi-Layer Perceptron Neural Networks. *Symmetry 2020, 12*, 894. doi:10.3390/sym12060894

Yu, H., Barriga, S., Agurto, S., Zamora, G., Bauman, W., & Soliz, P. (2012). Fast Vessel Segmentation in Retinal Images Using Multiscale Enhancement and Second-order Local Entropy. *Medical Imaging 2012: Computer-Aided Diagnosis, Proc. of SPIE*, 8315, 1-12.

Zhang, J., Bekkers, E., Abbasi, S., & Dashtbozorg, R. B. H. (2015). *Robust and Fast Vessel Segmentation via Gaussian Derivatives in Orientation Scores*. Springer International Publishing.

Zhao, Y., Rada, L., Chen, K., Harding, S. P., & Zheng, Y. (2015). Automated Vessel Segmentation Using Infinite Perimeter Active Contour Model with Hybrid Region Information with Application to Retinal Images. *IEEE Transactions on Medical Imaging*, 1–11. doi:10.1109/TMI.2015.2409024 PMID:25769147

KEY TERMS AND DEFINITIONS

Hybrid Approaches: Hybrid techniques are a combination of two or more computational techniques which provide more advantage to detect components than any other individual technique. It helps to improve data analysis. The hybrid technique helps qualitative research to be effective.

Matched Filtering Method: Matched filtering methods primarily use filters like Gaussian filters or their variation to check the gray distributions and shape of retinal vessels and collect corresponding responses. The presence of the required feature is recognized by using this filtering response.

Mathematical Morphology-Based Method: Morphological processing technique is basically combined with other vessel properties, to obtain vessel-like patterns from retinal fundus images. Objective image and Structuring Element (SE) are the main two parts of this technique. This technique offers the identification and segmentation of images by processing and analyzing SE in a binary image.

Model-Based Method: In model-based methods, the explicit vessel models are used to extract the retinal vessel map. The method mainly consists of vector fields, the Hermite model, region growing, active contour, level set, and other methods. The method is classified into two types: (1) deformable models and (2) vessel profile models.

Multiscale-Based Method: The multi-scale method represents the image at multiple levels/scales. It performs the segmentation of the retinal image on the basis of the variation of the image resolution. This process produced a scale space for the extraction of various structures from the input retinal images.

Neural Network-Based Method: Neural network consists of interconnected nodes which work like neurons of the human brain. Basically, it is a set of the algorithm, which is constructed to identify hidden patterns. It interprets data by using machine perception or labeling raw input.

Vessel Tracking Method: Vessel tracking methods are used to segment the retinal vessels by tracking the vessels. The algorithms usually work with a set of reliable seed points and use them to track the retinal vasculature on the basis of the texture of local intensity information.

Chapter 4

Application of Deep Learning in Epilepsy:
A Catalyst in Better Diagnosis of Epileptic Seizures and Prevention

Gauri Sharma

Manipal University, Jaipur, India

ABSTRACT

Over the past few decades, chronic illnesses have been on a continuous rise of which epilepsy has been the most common neurological disorder. However, due to the recent progress that has been made by medical science, epilepsy can be controlled for about 70% of the cases. To diagnose epilepsy, EEG, CT scan, MRI, etc. are some of the most common ways, but in this chapter, diagnosis using EEG shall be most focused upon. Although EEG can be considered a good way to decide upon the results of epilepsy proving whether a person is epileptic or not, it is not a completely reliable method. Hence, for its accurate detection we must use sophisticated techniques like CNN and LSTM that will provide a timely and correct diagnosis, reducing the chances of frequent epileptic seizures and SUDEP. Using anti-epileptic drugs cannot guarantee epilepsy prevention, and even if they do, these drugs come with some serious side effects, so people must look back to yoga for a probable permanent treatment.

INTRODUCTION

Epilepsy is one of the most common chronic illness and people suffering from it have been on a continuous rise. There are many ways to detect Epilepsy caused by different factors however EEG remains the most common one, and this a major cause of concern for the results shown by EEG are not always correct and accurate. Hence this chapter focuses on bridging the gap between the lack of correct and timely diagnosis using deep learning so that memory impairment, mental decline and various other mental disorders caused by Epilepsy could be prevented in early stages. Also, prevention of Epilepsy has been discussed in this chapter following the ancient practice of Yoga.

DOI: 10.4018/978-1-7998-8929-8.ch004

BACKGROUND

Epilepsy is a group of neurological diseases characterised by recurrent seizures (Choi et al.,2016). Seizures happen as a result of a sudden surge in the brain's electrical activities. Depending on which part of the brain is affected a seizure may manifest as loss of awareness, unusual behaviours, uncontrollable movements and loss of consciousness (Acharya et al., 2013).

Brain is a complex network of billions of neurons and they can be excitatory or inhibitory. Excitatory neurons stimulate others to fire action potentials and transmit electrical messages while inhibitory neurons suppress this process, preventing excessive firing. A balance between the excitation and inhibition neuron is essential for normal brain functioning. In epilepsy there is an up regulation of excitation and /or down regulation of inhibition causing lots of neurons to fire synchronously at the same time. If this abnormal electric surge happens within a limited area of the brain, it causes partial or focal seizures. If the entire brain is involved generalised seizures will result. Partial seizures further subdivide to: Simple Partial Seizures and Complex Partial Seizures while Generalised seizures subdivide further into Absence Seizures, Tonic Seizures, Atonic Seizures, Clonic Seizures, Myoclonic Seizures and Convulsive Seizures.(Smith, 2005) The symptoms of the various types of seizures indicated above are as given below: Partial seizures subdivide further into:

- Simple Partial Seizures -People experience unusual feelings, strange sensations, uncontrollable jerky movements but remain conscious and aware of the surroundings.
- Complex Partial Seizures -Involve loss or change in consciousness awareness and responsiveness.

Generalised seizures subdivide further into:

- Absence Seizures-This type occurs most often in children and is characterised by a very brief loss of awareness, commonly manifested as a blank stare with or without subtle body movements such as lip smacking or eye blinking. People with absence seizures may not be aware that something is wrong with them for years. Kids who start having absence seizures stand a good chance to outgrow them without treatment.
- Tonic Seizures -They are often associated with stiffening of muscles or increased muscle tone that may cause a person to fall, often backwards.
- Atonic Seizures-They are also known as drop attacks; they may cause a person to collapse or drop down due to sudden loss of muscle tone.
- Clonic Seizures -They are associated with rhythmic jerking muscle movements most commonly affected are the muscles of the neck, arm, face and legs.
- Myoclonic Seizures- They are sudden brief jerks or twitches of muscles. When myoclonic seizure occurs patients typically react as if hit by a jolt of electricity.
- Convulsive Seizures-They are most dramatic Tonic-Clonic seizures involving muscle stiffening and jerking. This type is what most people relate to when they think of a seizure. It also involves sudden loss of consciousness and sometimes loss of bladder control. If this seizure lasts more than five minutes an immediate medical treatment will be required by the person.

Although there is no concrete evidence regarding the cause of Epilepsy but some of the common causes of these Epileptic seizures are injury, tumours, stroke, previous infection or birth defect however Generalised Seizures that start in childhood are likely to involve genetic factors.(Joseph et al., 2014)

Diagnosis is based on observation of symptoms, medical history and an electroencephalogram (EEG). An EEG may also help in differentiating between partial and generalised seizures. Also, Genetic Testing may be helpful when genetic factors are suspected. There is no cure for Epilepsy but various treatments are available that help to control seizures. There are various Anti-Epileptic drugs (AEDs) available that target sodium channels, GABA receptors and other components involved in neural transmission. Different types of medicines help with different type of seizures. Patients may need to try several drugs to find the most suitable. Also, Dietary therapy has been shown to reduce or prevent seizures in many children. Ketogenic diet has shown to reduce or prevent seizures in many children who do not respond to any medication. It is a high fat low carbohydrate diet that must be prescribed and followed strictly. With this diet, the body uses fat as a major source of energy instead of carbohydrates. However, the reason why this diet helps in control of Epilepsy is still unclear. Nerve stimulation therapy such as vagus nerve stimulation in which a device placed under skin is programmed to stimulate the vagus nerve at a certain rate. The device acts as a pacemaker for the brain. The underlying mechanism has been poorly understood but it has shown to reduce seizures significantly. Finally, a surgery(Mao et al.,2020) may be performed to remove part of brain that causes seizure. This is usually done when tests show that seizures are originated from small area that does not have any vital function.

WHY EEG IS NOT AN ACCURATE WAY OF TESTING EPILEPSY?

Electroencephalogram(EEG) records activity in brain. During the test, some small electrodes (Holmes, 2008)are placed on scalp using a special paste glue that records signals picked up from brain. EEG does not cause any pain nor does it interfere with the normal activity of the brain. EEG tests are done for various purposes like testing Epilepsy, checking the intensity or severity of Epilepsy so that it can be determined whether it can be controlled using medicines or surgery is a requirement. Also, it may be an interesting fact to know that there are many types of EEG tests like:

- Sleep EEG tests -In this test the patient might be given medicine to sleep in the hospital and then the brain wave patterns are recorded because when asleep some of the brain wave patterns may change and showcase an unusual electrical activity. This test is majorly useful for young children and older people for their seizures mainly happen in sleep.
- Sleep deprived EEG tests -This test is done when patient has had less sleep than usual. This test is done when a patient is tired because there is more chance of unusual activity in brain when the patient is tired.
- Ambulatory EEG tests -These tests record the everyday brain activity. The word ambulatory itself implies meant for walking. It is designed in such a way that it can record activity in brain over few hours, days or weeks. Hence this test significantly increases chances of recording unusual activities or seizures in brain. This test also uses electrodes similar to that used in standard EEG test, however the electrodes attached to the patients are plugged in small machine that records the results. The device can be easily carried out . It is just that a doctor asks the patient to maintain

the record of activities that are being done like sleeping and eating whenever wearing ambulatory EEG device.

- Video telemetry tests -Video telemetry is the term used to describe the procedure involving an EEG and a Video Recording. This is done if more information about the seizures of a patient is needed. This video telemetry test may be done in hospital or in home and are classified accordingly into hospital video-telemetry and home video-telemetry. Hospital video telemetry is done involving instrument similar to ambulatory EEG and at the same time all the activity is recorded into the camera. Also, sometimes the Epilepsy medicine is reduced or withdrawn in order to increase the chances of the patient having a seizure so that it can be recorded. While procedure of Home video telemetry is done similarly as hospital video telemetry but home video telemetry is advised in cases when the doctor needs to check the type of seizures a patient experiences, when Epilepsy medicine is not working well or when the patient is being accessed for Epilepsy Surgery.

- Invasive EEG-telemetry-Some people who are being considered for Epilepsy Surgery need to experience invasive EEG -telemetry (iEEG).It is a less common type of EEG usually done with people experiencing a more complex Epilepsy. In this the neurosurgeon places the electrode directly into or onto the brain's surface. The electrodes are called strip or grid or stereo-EEG electrodes. It is done to find out where exactly the seizures are coming up from. Another part of it is cortical mapping that is done to check which part of brain is responsible for memory or speech and this is done to reduce the risk of complications after the surgery.

After detection of Epilepsy using EEG certain lifestyle changes have to be made by an individual depending on the frequency of seizures. Generally people must never skip medications prescribed and the timing of taking medications daily must be consistent in nature. Activities like drinking and smoking must be avoided during this phase. Also one must go for checkups as prescribed by the doctor, for change in the AEDs must be considered very seriously. On the whole these drugs might promote sleep and depression hence exercise, a good diet along with mental strength are very crucial steps in surviving and overcoming this disease.

Considering all the advantageous points mentioned above about EEG it can be considered as highly effective but it is not a sure way of determining whether a person is Epileptic or not. Sometimes people who have Epilepsy are tested as normal while the others not having Epilepsy are tested the other way around. This is simply because the EEG test results show activity of the brain when the EEG test is being done. EEG records the brain waves that are present between seizures. These waves that are present between seizures are called interictal brain waves. To detect abnormal brain activity a neurologist looks for spikes in the EEG report but even if these sharp waves are absent, it does not mean a person cannot be Epileptic. Suppose an unusual activity is picked up in an EEG test report it would require a highly skilled neurologist to identify the type of Epileptic seizure a person may experience. If in the reports a focal spike is recorded a partial seizure is taking place while if in reports if a generalised seizure is taking place the focal points are highly generalised. However, the type of seizure cannot be determined here by a doctor with complete certainness and that may lead to a delay in medication which may lead to complexities with delay in time. Hence this is a major milestone that medical science needs to overcome and deep learning techniques can provide a major level of assistance in this domain.

PREVENTION BETTER THAN CURE

Generally, expectation of a person with Epilepsy coincides with the belief of having no seizures and side effects, but this statement remains partially true even with today's advancements and expert medical care. Although there are many ways to treat Epilepsy but most common of them still remains Medication. Most of the Epileptic and Genetic Syndromes cause seizures and are treated adequately with medication. The good news remains is that if the seizures get identified properly and are prescribed with right kind of medication, most people with Epilepsy will do well. However, the reality is that many doctors fail to recognize specific Epilepsy syndromes and do not use the right medicine to treat them for if the patient is on the improper drug, it is likely that seizures would continue to happen. Hence receiving expert care is very important. Some of the Anti-Epileptic Drugs (AEDs) used in treatment of Epilepsy are (National Health Service, 2020):

- Narrow-spectrum AEDs-carbamazepine, diazepam, divalproex, eslicarbazepine acetate, ethosuximide etc.
- Broad spectrum AEDs- clonazepam, clorazepate, ezogabine, felbamate, lamotrigine etc.

These drugs although effective in controlling seizures may leave the patient experiencing various side-effects like tiredness, dizziness, drowsiness, loss of co-ordination, weight loss. Even mental problems like confusion, slowed thinking, trouble concentrating or paying attention, nervousness, language/speech problems, etc are some other side effects.

In order to avoid the above stated side-effects we must look back to our ancient practices and take precautions to prevent Epilepsy in the first case and even if one does suffer from Epilepsy Yoga has the power to overcome all the above stated side effects .Although Yoga as a practice for preventing, curing and treating Epilepsy has not received a scientific seal but still its power cannot be denied for Yoga(Panebianco et al., 2017) holds the key to almost any and every problem a person suffers from be it mental or physical.

AEDs stated above can although control Epilepsy but about 25%-40% of people treated by them cannot totally prevent Epileptic seizures that occur and this is all because of the fact that the body of the people who get treated with AEDs (Galanopoulou et al., 2012) become resistant to the drugs and their bodies no longer respond to treatments. Hence it is suggested that people who suffer from Epilepsy and even in everyday life of an individual Yoga must be an essential part.

Yoga has always been an integral part of Indian culture that has the power to bestow good health be it physical, mental and spiritual on the practitioner. Exercises(asanas), Breath Control(pranayama) and Meditation (Dharna &Dhyana) all combine to form the true essence of Yoga. As the result of meditation, reduction in stress levels was found as indicated by changes in skin resistance and levels of blood lactate and urinary vanillylmandelic acid. Also, according to a study conducted even practice of Sahaja Yoga (a simple form of Yoga) has the power to reduce the number of seizures an Epileptic person suffers from(Jain, 2019). Also, it is estimated that about 70% of people with Epilepsy can lead a life close that of a normal person on AEDs however 30%have to suffer and cannot live a fulfilled life hence Yoga has been recommended for them as it has long lasting effects on the people. Yoga also proves to be a significant factor in improving the functioning of the nervous system by reducing stress and anxiety which are some of the root causes of Epilepsy. Also triggers of Epilepsy can be reduced or even finished as Hatha Yoga helps in calming down the nervous system and aid in bringing balance between the activity of the neurons. There are many Yoga exercises that aid in preventing, treating and curing Epilepsy but below we shall discus some of them:

- Anulom Vilom (Alternate Nostril Breathing)-It is a breathing exercise without retention. A person has to do breathing in four counts from left nostril and then breathing out immediately eight counts through the right nostril. This completes round one and then the process has to be repeated over and over again. Once a person starts feeling comfortable an eight-count retention after the inhalation may also be done.

- Shashankasana (Balasana or Child's Pose)- While in this pose, we enter into the rest and regenerate state of the nervous system. In this exercise a person rests forehead on the mat and breathes smoothly and comfortably. A very gentle pressure on the forehead is very calming in nature. In this posture however one needs to be sure of the position that the head rests on the bolster while the buttocks rests on heels or on a cushion.

- Salamba Sarvangasana (Supported Shoulder stand against the wall)-Shoulder stand is a very relaxing pose indeed for it increases the blood flow towards the head and pressure in the throat region, triggering a physical reflex referred to as the baroreflex. It is one of the many triggers that we have in our body, that impact our parasympathetic nervous system. Also, this pose is more accessible and safer for people with Epilepsy.

- Paschimottanasana (Seated Forward Bend)-This pose eases up the natural tension present in the lower back and hips for it stretches the entire back side of the body. In this pose maximum flexion with back is allowed till the forehead rests on knees(or on a support).Once in the pose the person must try to relax while breathing into the lower belly and lower back.

- Supta Eka Pada Kapotasana(Sleeping Pigeon Pose)-The Sleeping pigeon is aimed at releasing the tension that is present inside the buttocks(the glutes and piriformis) and the hip flexors(quadriceps femoris and psoas)while giving enough space to breathe into the body and check in with how a person feels. The paoas is considered to be a storehouse for stress and anxiety and gently stretching and releasing long stored stress helps a person emotionally.

- Seal Pose(Yin Yoga)-This exercise or pose has been adapted from the Cobra pose. This pose can be held up for about 3-5 minutes as the posture proves to be extremely beneficial for the spine. It is almost analogue to giving a massage to the spine. The sacral-lumbar arch is not only great for the spine but it also stimulates all the abdominal organs.

- Garland Pose(Malasana)-Garland pose is most commonly known as the Yogic squat where a balance between activation and relaxation needs to be seeked.In this posture the heels of the person are pushing into the ground while elbows are being pushed out and reaching the top of the head. In this posture the Achilles heels are allowed to relax while inner thighs and calves lengthen. In this posture one must make sure that the heels are resting and if necessary, support them with a folded mat or a block.

- Vrkshasana(Tree Pose)-The tree pose strongly aims to develop focus, concentration with a clear and calming mind. In this pose a person has to look up to a certain point and maintain focus while looking at it and gently maintaining the gaze. If one is struggling to focus, directing focus to the breath directly is the most ideal scenario.

Also, these Yogic postures are not only helpful in dealing with Epilepsy but are indeed also very helpful in dealing with the aftermath of a seizure and calming a person. For after experiencing a seizure a person may not remember anything, experience immense tiredness with headaches or be in a completely blank state with a lot of anxiety .Hence practicing these few exercises would not only calm a person but also bring the person back to the original state .Thus from above stated facts we can say that practicing Yoga along with medication would not only reduce seizures in an Epileptic person but can also completely eradicate them and reduce the side effects of AEDs (Tsubouchi et al., 2019)simultaneously.

DEEP LEARNING FOR DETECTION OF EPILEPSY

Detection of Epileptic Seizures in a timely manner is very important or else frequent seizures may pose a risk of mental decline and memory related issues. As discussed above EEG has been the most common method through which the neurologists recognise an Epileptic seizure activity by visual inspection. However, one dimensional convolutional neural network-long short-term memory(1D CNN-LSTM) model for automatic recognition of Epilepsy has been used in this chapter. The approach followed for this detection is that firstly any raw EEG data is pre-processed and normalised. Then a convolutional model is used to extract features from the normalised EEG data sequence. Then for the further extraction of the temporal features LSTM(Kong et al., 2019) layers are used. After that for final seizure recognition the features are fed into fully connected layers for final Epileptic Seizure Recognition. The performance of the proposed 1D CNN LSTM model is tested on UCI Epileptic Seizure Recognition data set. The experiments showcased very high accuracies of 99.39% and 82% on binary and five class epileptic seizure recognition(Jiang et al.,2017b) tasks. Usage of the above methods hold significant superiority over of simple machine learning algorithms like k nearest neighbours, support vector machines and decision trees when compared.

Deep Learning has also developed exponentially over the past few decades and its impact in various fields has been enormous. Convolutional Neural Network(CNN) has been one of the most popular deep learning models. This is because Convolutional Neural Network is a very powerful deep learning model that plays a very important part in extraction by using its filters in fully connected convolutional layers, pooling layers, normalization layers that increase performance of many tasks. However, the drawback that CNN faces is to memorise the various time series patterns and hence it becomes very difficult for convolutional network to directly learn from EEG signals. Also, relationship between CNN and raw EEG signals(San-Segundo et al., 2019) is a difficult one to construct and is not very well suited for Epileptic Seizure Recognition Results.

Recurrent Neural Network(RNN),(Schmidhuber, 2015) are on the other hand a specific type of neural networks that use previous outputs as inputs. These neural networks have a special quality that they can remember information from the past. Also, RNN based models have found their place in even very important applications. LSTM(Long Short-Term Memory) is also one of RNN architectures that has been widely adopted for time series processing(Hanson et al.,2016). The basic model of RNN suffers from a gradient vanishing problem but Long Short-Term Memory helps to learn long term dependencies. These Long-term Dependencies help to acquire temporal feature of sequential data more effectively. Hence combining qualities of CNN and LSTM we can make a better model that will improve performance of CNN-LSTM model that is proposed for feature extraction of EEG signals and automatic recognition and detection.(Cura et al.,2020)

DESCRIPTION OF DATASETS

The data set that is being used is the public UCI epileptic seizure recognition data set . Original data set contained five different folders and each folder had 100 files . Each file represents a recording sample of the brain activity from one subject. In each file, there is a recording of brain activity with 4097 data points, which is sampled for 23.5 s. That is to say, there is a total of 500 subjects in this data set, each has a recording sample with 4097 data points.

The original dataset is first pre-processed by the UCI and then published online. Each sample with 4097 data points is divided into 23 data chunks and each chunk has 178 data points of 1 s. After that, the 23 data chunks are shuffled. Finally, for the 500 subjects, 11,500 time-series EEG signal data samples are obtained.

There are five health conditions in the UCI epileptic seizure recognition data set, they include one epileptic seizure condition and four normal conditions where subjects do not have epileptic seizures. The details of them are as follows(Andrzejak et al.,2001):

- Epileptic seizure condition: the recordings of subjects who have epileptic seizures;
- First normal condition: the recordings of subjects who opened their eyes when they were recording the EEG signals;
- Second normal condition: the recordings of subjects who closed their eyes when they were recording the EEG signals;
- Third normal condition: the recordings of EEG signals collected from the healthy brain area of subjects;
- Fourth normal condition: the recordings of EEG signals collected from the tumour area in the brain of subjects.

The raw EEG signal data of the subjects' five health conditions is shown as stated above. The difference between the raw EEG signal waveform of the Epileptic seizure condition and the normal condition can be easily observed, while the difference between the raw EEG signal waveform of the different normal conditions can hardly be observed. Therefore, binary and five-class epileptic seizure recognition tasks are both considered in order to thoroughly evaluate the performance of the proposed method. (Adeli et al.,2007)

Figure 1. The image in figure 1 presents the five health conditions according to UCI epileptic seizure recognition data set.

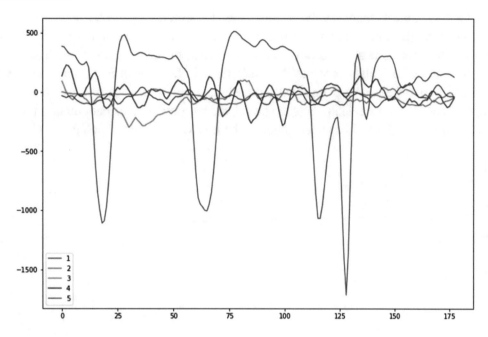

PROPOSED METHOD

Here in this chapter 1D CNN LSTM is used for Epileptic Seizure Recognition. In this process firstly raw EEG signal data is pre-processed then the one-dimensional convolutional neural network model-long short-term memory are introduced finally.

DATA-PREPROCESSING

It had been already mentioned that the original dataset had been restructured and processed by a UCI official when mentioning about the data. Hence in process of data pre-processing EEG signals need to be only normalised before they are fed into the neural network(LeCun et al.,2020).

1D CONVOLUTIONAL NEURAL NETWORK (CNN)

The 1 D CNN can extract the most impactful, effective and representative features of 1D time-series that can sequence data through performing 1D convolutional operations using multiple filters. To match the one-dimensional characteristics of the raw EEG signal data all the filters and feature maps used are completely one dimensional. Also, CNN has the ability to extract number of robust and discriminative features for Epileptic Seizure Recognition tasks if the number of convolutional layers is deepened(Radenovic et al.,2019).

LSTM STRUCTURE

In a particular LSTM block, there are always four gates. These gates are the cell state gate that remembers the information over a period of time, forget gates z^f that controls the extent to which the values are kept in the cell, the input gate z^i that controls value in cell and the output gate z^o which can be used for computing the output. Each and every one of these gates have fully connected layers and an activation function. In addition to these gates there are also three inputs (cell state c^{t-1}, previously hidden state h^{t-1}, current input x^t) as well as three outputs (cell state c^t, hidden state h^{t-1}, current output y^t) in the LSTM block. Below various mathematical formulations of the LSTM units are discussed:

$$z^f = \sigma(W^f[x_t, h_{t-1}])$$

$$z^i = \sigma(W^i[x_t, h_{t-1}])$$

$$z = \tanh(W[x_t, h_{t-1}])$$

$$z^o = \sigma(W^o[x_t, h_{t-1}])$$

$$c^t = z^f * c^{t-1} + z^i * z$$

$$h^t = z^o * \tanh(c^t)$$

$$y^t = \sigma(W^t h_t)$$

1D CNN-LSTM MODEL

- The proposed 1D CNN-LSTM model has the following structure(Sun et al., 2019). It has been composed of four convolutional layers, one pooling layer, an input layer along with four fully connected layers and a SoftMax output layer. 1D EEG Signal Data is firstly passed as the input of the proposed model. The size of input data passed in the first convolutional layer is 178*1. This layer extracts the most abstract features from the raw EEG signal data. Every 1-D layer consists of convolutional kernels. Here the size of layer 1 is 64 while the size of each kernel is 3*1. Also stride of convolutional kernels is 1. This structure is further followed by Rectified Linear Unit (ReLU) as the activation layer which can overcome the problem of overfitting. After the activation and convolutional, about 64 feature maps are extracted. These feature maps have a size of 176*1. After that output is received from convolutional layer1 it is then passed through max pooling layer. Here max pooling is done to extract the most prominent features of the previous feature map. The pooling operation selects maximum element from the region of feature map that is covered by a filter. The size of pooling window is 2 and the stride of windows is also 2. Hence max pooling significantly reduces number of training parameters to accelerate the training process. About 64 feature maps with size 88*1 are outputted. After the process convolutional layers further extract higher level features that further facilitate classification. About three more layers are present named so

Conv Layer2, Conv Layer3 and Conv Layer4 respectively, these convolutional layers have about 128 kernels with shape of 3*1 in Conv Layer2, 512 kernels in the same shape in Conv Layer3, and about 1024 kernels in same shape in the Conv Layer4.These convolutional operations are same as that performed in Conv Layer 1.Also ReLU is applied for non-linear activation.

- On passing the feature maps through all 1D convolutional layers about 1024 feature maps are obtained nearly with the size 82*1 .These features maps will be fed into FC layer with 256 neurons. After that dropout is applied to the output of the FC layer also layer1 has the ability to reduce dimensions of feature maps in order to fit input of LSTM layers. FC layer1 and dropout can also alleviate overfitting concerns to some extent by concatenating the outputs from the previous layers.

- LSTM include four gates cell gate, forget gate, input gate, output gate that work together to store the previous information and further improve ability of model to work in time series forecasting problems. This model has output features fed into the LSTM layers that is very much capable of avoiding long term dependency. This collaborative model has been proven very useful in EEG time series data analysis in which we have 64 neurons fed in both LSTM Layer1 and LSTM Layer2.

- The output obtained above is then passed through LSTM layers, the output features will then be fed into three FC layers. These FC layers are FC layer1, FC layer2, FC layer3 and FC layer4 respectively. Then in a proposed model finally a SoftMax output layer is added for final recognition.

Figure 2. The image in Figure 2 presents the CNN-LSTM model.

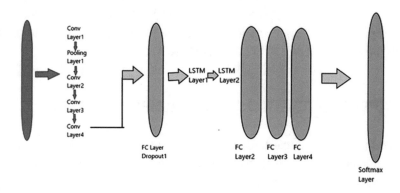

EXPERIMENTAL SETUP

- While doing this experiment the data was divided into two parts training and testing. In this analysis we trained the model using 90% of the data and tested the model based on 10% of the data. Also, in the CNN and, 1D convolutional LSTM models, number of training epochs is set as 100. In order to improve generalisation and overcome problems of overfitting dropout technique had been used in the suggested model.

- Also, it must be noted that data had been randomly shuffled before training and was then fed into the network. After the outputs had been calculated based on proposed 1D CNN-LSTM model training data set and test data set are both calculated to help us evaluate if the model is overfitting and thereby verifying the generalization ability of the current model. Also, in addition to these, checkpoints during training had also been added to further improve the generalisation ability of the proposed model but even if it does not improve after 10 training processes, the learning rate will be changed.

- If the proposed model (CNN -LSTM model) is further compared to DNN (Deep Neural Network) and CNN models(Sainath et al.,2015), we analyse that DNN and CNN models have similar accuracy while the proposed 1D CNN-LSTM model obtains best recognition performance regardless of different recognition task. DNN has fastest convergence speed while training and testing loss of the proposed model needs more training time. While on the other side training and testing loss of proposed model is smaller obviously than the DNN model thus obtaining better training and testing accuracies. All the training performances of the CNN model are very similar to that of the proposed model however the testing performance using a standard CNN degraded seriously after early stages of training process which is significantly inferior to the proposed model. In order to compare the models more deeply their accuracies on binary data had also been compared and even in this binary process the proposed model outperforms the two other models suggested. Also, it is noted that proposed model significantly outperforms the DNN and CNN model in all of the metrics in Five Class Recognition Task .(Jiang et al., 2015)

Although the proposed model achieves a considerable progress in area of Epileptic Seizure Detection but scope of improvement still remains as there are limitations that need to be addressed further(Jiang et al.,2017a). This is because supervised training model requires large amount of EEG signals. However, collecting this information every time is time consuming and laborious work. Hence the future model (Jiang et al.,2020a) can still be modified and optimised further in order to improve its performance on the more complex Epileptic Seizure recognition Tasks that will improve not only the performance of the model but also the classification ability(Yuan et al.,2020).

SUDDEN UNEXPECTED DEATH DUE TO EPILEPSY (SUDEP)

A very accurate detection of Epilepsy can be done by the above-stated model using deep learning techniques that will not only aid in fast but, also a correct diagnosis that results to be lifesaving. This is because if timely treatment is not received sometimes seizures due to Epilepsy can even be deadly that are commonly referred to as SUDEP (Sudden Unexpected Death in Epilepsy).SUDEP is the sudden unexpected death of someone with Epilepsy who was otherwise healthy. In SUDEP people with Epilepsy are often found dead in bed and don't have any convulsive seizure. The cause that a person experiences SUDEP is however quite uncertain and is not even found in the post-mortem report for cause of death in SUDEP may differ. Over one-third of times, there always has been a seizure or is a witnessed seizure and most of the times they are found lying face down. SUDEP death is also estimated to be nearly twenty-four times more likely in Epilepsy than in the general population. However, death rates in children due to SUDEP are much lower. SUDEP has an uncertain cause and so the best way is to lower the risk by controlling seizures. Every year more than one in thousand people with Epilepsy die from SUDEP .People with poorly controlled Epilepsy are at a greater risk of dying from SUDEP.As discussed above people don't know what causes SUDEP and how it happens but some areas are being looked at like breathing, heart rhythm and brain function problems that occur during a seizure, they are discussed as below(Centres for disease Control and Prevention, 2021):

- Breathing

When a person tackles with a seizure a state known as Apnea may be reached. This state causes a person to stop breathing temporarily and this further contributes in reducing the amount of oxygen that reaches to the heart and brain. A lack of oxygen can also be life threatening if not treated immediately as a person's airway may get blocked during convulsive seizure that would ultimately lead to suffocation(inability to breathe).

- Heart Rhythm

A seizure can also rarely cause a dangerous heart rhythm that may lead to a cardiac arrest.

- Brain Function

Seizures can very easily interfere with important areas of brain that may sometimes suppress or aggravate vital aspects in a brain stream. As a result, changes in brain function could cause dangerous breathing and heart rate.

- Genetic

Some of the studies also suggest that genetic factors may play a role but no concrete evidence has yet been found.

SUDEP can prove to be deadly for people having Tonic Clonic Seizures, Night Time Seizures and also for those people who miss prescribed medications(Anti-Epileptic Drugs) and fail to take it regularly at the same time. Although till date no sure way to prevent SUDEP has been discovered but certain methods that have been prescribed to avoid it, have been suggested as below:

- One must take the best seizure control drug possible without any sort of delays. Taking Anti-Epileptic Drugs consistently and around the same time may help prevent seizure even more.
- Keeping a record of when seizures happen may help to show if there is a pattern in seizures to the neurologist. It might also help in showing how the medications work for a particular patient. This is because if triggers of a seizure are recognised, they can be treated timely. This pattern may show triggers of a patient happening when patient is either sleep deprived, taking drugs, in stress and for women during menstrual cycle.
- Also, if an Epileptic person experiences seizures during sleep it may be an indication toward SUDEP. So, a seizure alarm that alerts someone to help the patient might prove to very useful and may also save a life.
- Eating a healthy and well-balanced diet, getting enough rest, regular exercise, not taking any sorts of recreational drugs, avoiding drinking and too much stress are ways to reduce Epilepsy.
- Also, one must remain seizure safe and make sure family and co-workers must know what to do for seizure first aid. Extra precautions however must be taken by the person when swimming or bathing.
- Also understanding how a patient undergoes SUDEP also plays a great role in reducing risk of sudden death. When a patient's body undergoes seizures there are changes seen in brain, lungs and

in heart .It is also very common to see flattening brain waves known as post ictal generalised EEG suppression or PGES and so far, this is one of the patterns that has been identified in EEG recordings of people who have died of SUDEP during EEG monitoring. Since brain is an organ that controls the very functioning of all the other organs the strange rhythmic signals cause abnormal breathing in lungs and can also reduce blood flow towards brain. This increases the carbon dioxide level in the blood with low oxygen, for pumping of fresh blood by heart had also been tapered by the unusual reflexes of the brain. Sometimes if important steps are taken, death due to SUDEP can also be prevented by the nurses and the medical staff for it may shorten the time of seizure and help the patient to return to normal thereby saving a life. The actions include turning patient to the side, suctioning the mouth, giving oxygen and quickly performing a CPR when needed. If suction devices are not available nearby then simple steps like waking a person and adjusting their position after the seizure may help in saving a life. SUDEP is a terrible tragedy and is often made worse by unexplained nature of loss. Although not many things are known about SUDEP but researchers are making a great deal of effort to study it.

MYTHS AND MISCONCEPTIONS

There are many false ideas that still exist in community regarding Epilepsy. Lack of awareness can contribute to the stigma and discrimination faced by Epileptic patients. Also, it can make a person very uncomfortable to talk about their Epilepsy even when they need to or want to. Below certain myths regarding Epilepsy have been discussed (Schachter et al, 2017):

- All people with Epilepsy lose consciousness and have convolutions is by far the most overstated misconception. The most common form of seizure we see and is stereotypically shown on TV is the Tonic Clonic Seizure where a person falls to the ground and starts to shake. In fact, Tonic Clonic Seizures are one of over 40 different seizure types, some of which include quick muscle twitches, brief loss of awareness, confusion or disorientation.
- Epilepsy is a lifelong disease. While currently we see no cure for Epilepsy, some childhood symptoms are outgrown and around 70% of people with Epilepsy become Seizure free with medication. Epilepsy is considered to be resolved in some cases that had not experienced seizure in 10 years and been able to stop medication or treatment for the last five of those years.
- If a person has Epilepsy, then they cannot dive is one of the misconceptions that most people have however people with Epilepsy can obtain a driving license if their seizures are well controlled with medication or they meet the requirement set out by relevant authority.
- Restraining someone during a seizure is not a way to control a seizure. For restraining it, plays a reverse role and is more likely to agitate or harm the person as a seizure will run its course and restraining it will not slow or stop it down.
- Some people even believe that putting something in a person's mouth to stop them from swallowing their tongue is a good idea during a seizure however it is physically impossible to swallow one's tongue. Hence one must not put anything in patients' mouth, as the person first of all is unable to control muscle movements during a seizure and may bite down on the object and break their teeth or injure their own jaw or mouth.

- All seizures do not require hospitalisation and this is a complete myth. Most often the patient who suffered from a seizure will just need some time to rest and recover after a seizure.
- People also think about it as a contagious disease however Epilepsy is not at all contagious in nature.
- People with Epilepsy can't work and are disabled and believing this, is a completely vague scenario for to work one needs to have ability and intelligence .People with seizure disorders are found in all walks of life and at all levels in business, government, arts and other professions. Our society is still not aware about this because even today people suffering from Epilepsy do not talk about it, thinking about the fear of what other people may think about them. This leaves them feeling bounded and stressed in their daily lives.
- Some people believe that if they suffer from a seizure, they have Epilepsy but this is not true because a person can only be called Epileptic if that person has two or more unprovoked seizures that occur 24 hours apart. But when something provokes a seizure, such as drinking, sleep deprivation or a new medication it is not related to Epilepsy at all.
- Detection of a seizure is not possible before the seizures begin to happen. However, Research is being done so that before a seizure a patient can be aware about it.
- One of the myths about Epilepsy is also that Seizures hurt but this is not true for being unconscious does not cause any pain during most seizures. However afterward a patient could feel discomfort if he or she falls down, has muscle aches or if he or she bit their tongue (during grand mal seizure).

CONCLUSION

Coping with Epilepsy is difficult and different for anyone and everyone and this problem is the same, even for those people who suffer from well controlled seizures or those suffering from poorly controlled seizures. Also taking a lot of Anti-Epileptic drugs can affect very well how the people think, feel and their ability to cope with effects of Epilepsy. Living a life with Epilepsy is not a very smooth sailing journey but actually a bumpy road for one does not know when a person is going to experience an Epileptic attack and feels worried continuously. Also, sometime a person with Epilepsy can have a good life but have everything disrupted in the other split second. Hence one needs to be greatly motivated and it may need a new way of looking at life with Epilepsy .It is necessary to fall in love with life in order to overcome any obstacle that these ideas may bring. Epilepsy can also strain families and the patient itself in various ways. Family members also need to support the patient greatly and remain as the source of strength for each other at the same time. Family must align with the patient to overcome all the negative feelings and fears. Epilepsy is not to feel shy about or to be ashamed at any point and this is the main agenda that drives the spirit of this chapter. This chapter raises concerns about how in an unsaid way the patient feels stressed, worried, bounded and fearful. Also, it has been observed that many people shy away from neurological disorders and do not receive timely medical treatment due to certain myths and misconceptions about them. Hence together we even need to create a considerate environment so that people do not consider it as a taboo but just consider it as another ailment that can happen with anyone irrespective of region, sex, or age so that person suffering from it is considered normal and not looked down upon. The present-day society really needs to build itself and support such people rather leaving them to face discrimination in the society and this message drives the ultimate conclusion about improvement in the psychological system of not only those who suffer from Epilepsy but a greater improvement in the so-called pseudo mentality and intelligence of the normal individuals in the present-day community.

REFERENCES

Acharya, U. R., Vinitha Sree, S., Swapna, G., Martis, R. J., & Suri, J. S. (2013). Automated EEG analysis of epilepsy: A review. *Knowledge-Based Systems*, *45*, 147–165. doi:10.1016/j.knosys.2013.02.014

Adeli, H., Ghosh-Dastidar, S., & Dadmehr, N. (2007). A wavelet-chaos methodology for analysis of EEGs and EEG subbands to detect seizure and epilepsy. *IEEE Transactions on Biomedical Engineering*, *54*(2), 205–211. doi:10.1109/TBME.2006.886855 PMID:17278577

Andrzejak, R. G., Lehnertz, K., Rieke, C., Mormann, F., David, P., & Elger, C. E. (2001). Indications of nonlinear deterministic and finite dimensional structures in time series of brain electrical activity: Dependence on recording region and brain state. *Physical Review E: Statistical, Nonlinear, and Soft Matter Physics*, *64*(6), 061907. doi:10.1103/PhysRevE.64.061907 PMID:11736210

Centres for disease Control and Prevention. (2021). Sudden Unexpected Death in Epilepsy (SUDEP). *Epilepsy Features*. https://www.cdc.gov/epilepsy/communications/SUDEP

Choi, E., Schuetz, A., Stewart, W. F., & Sun, J. (2016). Using recurrent neural network models for early detection of heart failure onset. *Journal of the American Medical Informatics Association: JAMIA*, *24*(2), 361–370. doi:10.1093/jamia/ocw112 PMID:27521897

Cura, A., Kucuk, H., Ergen, E., & Oksuzoglu, I. B. (2020). Driver profiling using long short term memory (LSTM) and convolutional neural network (CNN) methods. In *Preceding of the IEEE Transactions on Intelligent Transportation Systems (Early Access)* (pp. 1–11). IEEE. doi:10.1109/TITS.2020.2995722

Galanopoulou, A. S., Buckmaster, P. S., Staley, K. J., Moshé, S. L., Perucca, E., Engel, J. Jr, Löscher, W., Noebels, J. L., Pitkänen, A., Stables, J., White, H. S., O'Brien, T. J., & Simonato for the American Epilepsy, M. (2012). Simonato for the American epilepsy, identification of new epilepsy treatments: Issues in preclinical methodology. *Epilepsia*, *53*(3), 571–582. doi:10.1111/j.1528-1167.2011.03391.x PMID:22292566

Hanson, J., Yang, Y., Paliwal, K., & Zhou, Y. (2016). Improving protein disorder prediction by deep bidirectional long short-term memory recurrent neural networks. *Bioinformatics (Oxford, England)*, *33*, 685–692. doi:10.1093/bioinformatics/btw678 PMID:28011771

Holmes, M. D. (2008). Dense array EEG: Methodology and new hypothesis on epilepsy syndromes. *Epilepsia*, *49*(s3), 3–14. doi:10.1111/j.1528-1167.2008.01505.x PMID:18304251

Jain, R. (2019). Yoga & Epilepsy – What a Yoga Teacher Should Know. *Yoga and physical / mental health*. https://www.arhantayoga.org/blog/yoga-poses-epilepsy/

Jiang, Y., Chung, F.-L., Wang, S., Deng, Z., Wang, J., & Qian, P. (2015). Collaborative fuzzy clustering from multiple weighted views. *IEEE Transactions on Cybernetics*, *45*(4), 688–701. doi:10.1109/TCYB.2014.2334595 PMID:25069132

Jiang, Y., Deng, Z., Chung, F.-L., Wang, G., Qian, P., Choi, K.-S., & Wang, S. (2017a). Recognition of Epileptic EEG signals using a novel multi-view TSK fuzzy system. *IEEE Transactions on Fuzzy Systems*, *25*(1), 3–20. doi:10.1109/TFUZZ.2016.2637405

Jiang, Y., Gu, X., Wu, D., Hang, W., Xue, J., & Qiu, S. (2020a). Novel negative-transfer-resistant fuzzy clustering model with a shared cross-domain transfer latent space and its application to brain CT image segmentation. In *Preceding of the IEEE/ACM Transactions on Computational Biology and Bioinformatics*. IEEE. doi:10.1109/TCBB.2019.2963873

Jiang, Y., Wu, D., Deng, Z., Qian, P., Wang, J., Wang, G., Chung, F.-L., Choi, K.-S., & Wang, S. (2017b). Seizure classification from EEG signals using transfer learning, semi-supervised learning and TSK fuzzy system. *IEEE Transactions on Neural Systems and Rehabilitation Engineering*, *25*(12), 2270–2284. doi:10.1109/TNSRE.2017.2748388 PMID:28880184

Kong, W., Dong, Z. Y., Jia, Y., Hill, D. J., Xu, Y., & Zhang, Y. (2019). Short-term residential load forecasting based on LSTM recurrent neural network. *IEEE Transactions on Smart Grid*, *10*(1), 841–851. doi:10.1109/TSG.2017.2753802

LeCun, Y., Bengio, Y., & Hinton, G. (2015). Deep learning. *Nature*, *521*(7553), 436–444. doi:10.1038/nature14539 PMID:26017442

Mao, W. L., Fathurrahman, H. I. K., Lee, Y., & Chang, T. W. (2020). EEG dataset classification using CNN method. *Journal of Physics: Conference Series*, *1456*(1), 012017. doi:10.1088/1742-6596/1456/1/012017

National Health Service. (2020). Epilepsy Treatment. *Conditions*. https://www.nhs.uk/conditions/epilepsy/treatment/

Panebianco, Sridharan, Ramaratnam, & Cochrane Epilepsy Group. (2017). *Yoga for Epilepsy. In The Cochrane Collaboration*. John Wiley & Sons, Ltd. doi:10.1002/14651858.CD001524.pub3

Radenovic, F., Tolias, G., & Chum, O. (2019). Fine-tuning CNN image retrieval with no human annotation. *IEEE Transactions on Pattern Analysis and Machine Intelligence*, *41*(7), 1655–1668. doi:10.1109/TPAMI.2018.2846566 PMID:29994246

Sainath, T. N., Vinyals, O., Senior, A., & Sak, H. (2015). Convolutional, long short-term memory, fully connected deep neural networks, ICASSP. *Preceding of the IEEE International Conference on Acoustics, Speech and Signal Processing (ICASSP)*, 4580–4584.

San-Segundo, R., Gil-Martín, M., D'Haro-Enríquez, L. F., & Pardo, J. M. (2019). Classification of epileptic EEG recordings using signal transforms and convolutional neural networks. *Computers in Biology and Medicine*, *109*, 148–158. doi:10.1016/j.compbiomed.2019.04.031 PMID:31055181

Schachter & Shafer. (2017). Challenges with Epilepsy. *Social Concerns of Seizures*. https://www.epilepsy.com/learn/challenges-epilepsy/social-concerns

Schmidhuber, J. (2015). Deep Learning in neural networks: An overview. *Neural Networks*, *61*, 5–117. doi:10.1016/j.neunet.2014.09.003 PMID:25462637

Sirven & Shafer. (2014). What is Epilepsy. *Epilepsy. Foundation*.https://www.epilepsy.com/learn/about-epilepsy-basics/what-epilepsy

Smith, S. J. M. (2005). EEG in the diagnosis, classification, and management of patients with epilepsy. *Journal of Neurology, Neurosurgery, and Psychiatry*, *76*(suppl_2), ii2–ii7. doi:10.1136/jnnp.2005.069245 PMID:15961864

Sun, Y., Lo, F. P.-W., & Lo, B. (2019). EEG-based user identification system using 1D-convolutional long short-term memory neural networks. *Expert Systems with Applications*, *125*, 259–267. doi:10.1016/j.eswa.2019.01.080

Tsubouchi, Y., Tanabe, A., Saito, Y., Noma, H., & Maegaki, Y. (2019). Long−term prognosis of epilepsy in patients with cerebral palsy. *Developmental Medicine and Child Neurology*, *61*(9), 1067–1073. doi:10.1111/dmcn.14188 PMID:30854645

Yuan, X., Li, L., & Wang, Y. (2020). Nonlinear dynamic soft sensor modeling with supervised long short-term memory network. In *Preceding of the IEEE Transactions on Industrial Informatics* (pp. 3168–3176). IEEE. doi:10.1109/TII.2019.2902129

Chapter 5
Computational Statistics on Stress Patients With Happiness and Radiation Indices by Vedic Homa Therapy:
A Knowledge–Based Approach to Get Insights in a Global Pandemic

Rohit Rastogi

https://orcid.org/0000-0002-6402-7638

Dayalbagh Educational Institute, India & ABES Engineering College, India

Sheelu Sagar

Amity University, Noida, India

Neeti Tandon

Vikram University, Ujjain, India

Bhavna Singh

G.S. Ayurved Medical College and Hospital, Pilkhuwa, India

T. Rajeshwari

Gayatri Chetna Kendra, Kolkata, India

ABSTRACT

The happiness programs and seeking their various means are popular across the globe. Many cultures and races are using them in different ways through carnivals, festivals, and occasions. In India, the Yajna, Mantra, Pranayama, and Yoga-like alternate therapies are now drawing attention of researchers, socio behavioral scientists, and philosophers by their scientific divinity. The chapter is an honest effort to identify the logical progress on happiness indices and reduction in radiation of electronic gadgets. The visualizations propound evidence that the ancient Vedic rituals and activities were effective in maintaining the mental balance. The data set was collected after a specified protocol followed and analyzed through various scientific data analysis tools.

DOI: 10.4018/978-1-7998-8929-8.ch005

INTRODUCTION

Pregnancy and Issues With Global and Indian Females Related to Health

Many scientific studies have now shown that if a mother is stressed, anxious or depressed while pregnant, her child is at increased risk for having a range of diseases like ADHD, conduct disorder and impaired cognitive development, including emotional problems. Thus it is important to keep a healthy body with a healthy and peaceful mind during natal and prenatal stage (Cameron, A.J. et al., 2003).

Women's health during the reproductive or fertile years (between the ages of 15 and 49 years) is relevant not only to women themselves but it also impacts on the health and development of the next generation. Pregnancy and childbearing are especially risky for women who have high blood pressure, high cholesterol levels, tobacco use, obesity, which are the very common resultant of modern lifestyle. These factors contribute to poor reproductive outcomes for both mother and infant and are direct causes of other health problems for women. Another main cause is malnutrition and especially anemia which make various complications during pregnancy. More than half a million maternal deaths occur every year and, of these, 99% happen in developing countries (Chaturvedi, D.K. et al., 2013).

However, there is nothing inevitable about these deaths. In industrialized countries, there are on average nine maternal deaths per 100,000 live births, whereas this figure can be as high as 1000 or more per 100 000 live births in the most disadvantaged countries. In settings where high fertility is the norm, women face such risks with each pregnancy. With the appropriate care, maternal mortality is in fact a very rare event (Chaturvedi, D.K. et al., 2013a); (Chaturvedi, D.K. et al., 2013b); (Saeed, S. et al., 2018).

On account of modernization and urbanization, different kinds of changes in our lifestyle are the main cause of most of the gynecological disorders and infertility is also one of them. Infertility has become a very challenging problem for working class ladies as well as common housewives. Many lifestyle factors such as the age at which to start a family, nutrition, weight, exercise, psychological stress, environmental and occupational exposures, can have substantial effects on fertility. Other lifestyle factors such as cigarette smoking, illicit drug use, and alcohol and caffeine consumption can negatively influence fertility (Gunavathi, C., et al., 2014).

All these factors are associated with a range of poor pregnancy outcomes, including reduced fertility, an increased risk of pregnancy complications and impaired infant and child development. It has been estimated that the number of infertile people in the world may be as high as 15%, particularly in industrialized nations (Jain, G. et al., 2017); (Saeed, S. et al., 2021).

Figure 1. Garbhasth Gayatri Mantra, a Rhythmic group of Syllabels for pregnant ladies to protect the womb

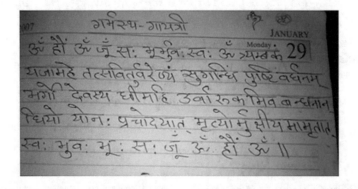

Pain and Its Own World

Studies have shown that the mantra chanting, meditation, Pranayama, Yoga and other practices are much useful for all the humans of different age groups, especially to females and aged persons. For females, pregnant ladies are specially getting immense benefit for themselves as well as for their baby in their womb (Kim., K. J. et al., 2019).

Scientific experiments are being conducted with help of different sensors and latest electronic gadgets to record the benefits of Yajna, mantra and meditation over these issues (Pl. refer Fig. 2 and Fig. 3).

Figure 2. (A World of Pain", National Geographic Magazine, vol. 1, issue-1, pp. 32-57, (January 2020))
Source:https://www.nationalgeographic.com/magazine/2020/01/scientists-are-unraveling-the-mysteries-of-pain-feature/

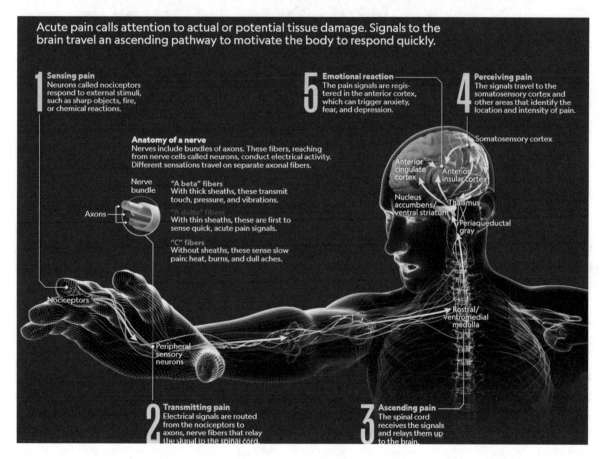

Figure 3. (A World of Pain", National Geographic Magazine, vol. 1, issue-1, pp. 32-57, (January 2020))

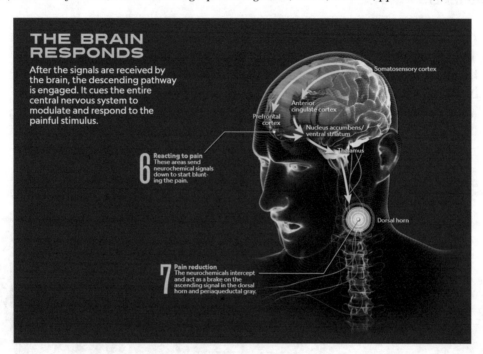

Chemical Property of Ghee (Clove Butter)

Chemically, Ghee is essentially composed of a mixture of triglycerides extracted from acidic acids such as polymitic, oleic, meristic and stearic. The composition of fatty acid of ghee varies according to the diet of the animal producing it. The Reichert-Missal or Reichert-Wolney number is important in calculating the amount of these acids in the whole balanced ghee (Lahoty, P. et al., 2013).

Chemical Organization of Ghee

Approximately 98% triglyceridase in ghee, 1-2% diglyceridus, 0.1–0.2% monoglycera-eidus, 1–10 mg / 100 gm Ghee free fatty acid (FFA), 0–80 mg / 100 gm phospholipidase, 0.25–0.40% cholesterol And in small amounts, fat soluble vitamins, carbonyl, glyceryl ether and alcohol are found. About 500 fatty acids are found in hGhee, most of which are found to have even-numbered carbon chains (C4–18). Poly-unsaturated Fatty Acids are found in 3-4% in Ghee (Mahajan, P. et al., 2016); (Marjani, M. et al., 2017).

Butyric, palmitic, stearic, tetranoic and pantanoic acids are found in buffalo ghee more than cow ghee. The acid of the series from caproic to myrrheic is found in cow's ghee more than buffalo ghee (Pl. refer Fig. 4).

Figure 4. Chemical compositions of atoms extracted in Yajna

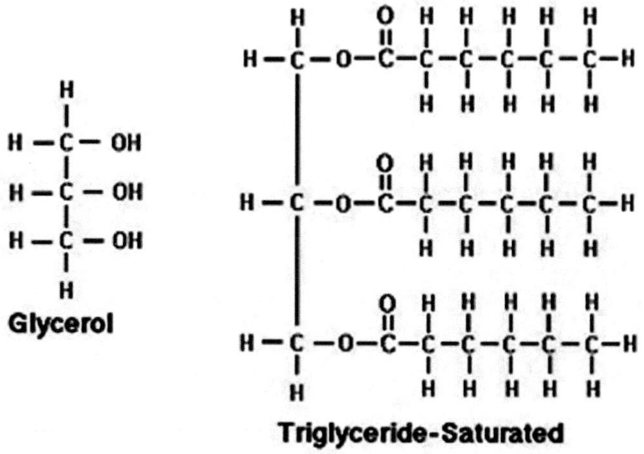

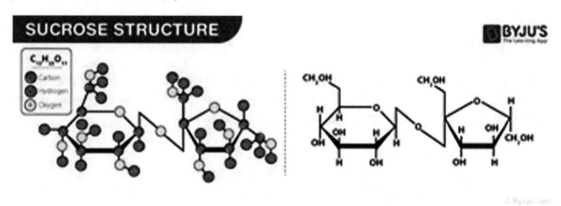

Composition of Fats

Simple triglycerides are those in which each molecule of glycerol is combined with three molecules of one acid—e.g., tripalmitin, $C_3H_5(OCOC_{15}H_{31})_3$, the glyceryl ester of palmitic acid, $C_{15}H_{31}COOH$.

Figure 5. Molecular structure of sucrose

Sugar is sucrose, a molecule composed of 12 atoms of carbon, 22 atoms of hydrogen, and 11 atoms of oxygen ($C_{12}H_{22}O_{11}$). Like all compounds made from these three elements, sugar is a carbohydrate(Pl. refer Fig. 5).

In this way, by sacrificing Yajna, oxygen is not spent but is emitted / produced. At the same time, the environment is purified by Gaseous products made from other chemical reactions and we also get health benefits (Rastogi, R. et al., 2018); (Rastogi, R. et al., 2018a). The remaining ash of Agnihotra increases the fertility of our soil and also works to remove some skin diseases. So there is no harm but benefit from the sacrifice. Yagya in the house everyday and organize big yagyas on festivals, then the world can be free from diseases (Pl. refer Fig. 6).

Figure 6. Analysis of different elements present in emission of Yajna Gaseous vapors

Ultimate Analysis (wt %) and HHV for Selected Solid Biofuels (Dry Basis)							
Biomass	C	H	O	N	S	Ash	HHV (MJ/kg)
Kelp, giant brown, Monterey	26.6	3.7	20.2	2.6	1.1	45.8	10.3
Mango wood	46.2	6.1	44.4	0.3	0.0	3.0	19.2
Maple	50.6	6	41.7	0.3	0.0	1.4	19.9
Oak	49.9	5.9	41.8	0.3	0.0	2.1	19.4
Pine	51.4	6.2	42.1	0.1	0.1	0.1	20.3
Pine, bark	52.3	5.8	38.8	0.2	0.0	2.9	20.4
Poplar, hybrid	50.2	6.1	40.4	0.6	0.0	2.7	19.0
Rice hulls	38.5	5.7	39.8	0.5	0.0	15.5	15.3
Rice straw	39.2	5.1	35.8	0.6	0.1	19.2	15.2
Sudan grass	45.0	5.5	39.6	1.2	0.0	8.7	17.4
Switchgrass, Dakota Leaf, MN	47.4	5.8	42.4	0.7	0.1	3.6	18.6

Source: Bain, R. L., Amos, W. P., Downing, M., and Perlack, R. L., *Biopower Technical Assessment: State of the Industry and the Technology,* NREL Report No. TP-510-33123, National Renewable Energy Laboratory, Department of Energy Laboratory, Golden, CO, 2003.

Yajna With Cow Clove Produces Oxygen

One misconception that is prevailing about Yajna that Yajna with Desi Cow's ghee produces x tons of oxygen. Solution-This is not correct. If at all some oxygen is produced it is produced by photochemical reactions as an interim product which is again consumed in the process.

- The end products are largely CO2 and water vapors.
- This CO2 when escapes in atmosphere is absorbed by plants and trees which in turn give out Oxygen. But this is their usual activity (Rastogi, R. et al., 2018b); (Rastogi, R. et al., 2018c).

- We have observed in our logical and scientific experiments that the level of oxygen is maintained if Havan is done with Gomay Samidha as they have a large amount of oxygen trapped inside (Pl. refer Fig. 7).

Figure 7. Yajna ceremony performed by volunteers at their home or public places like temples

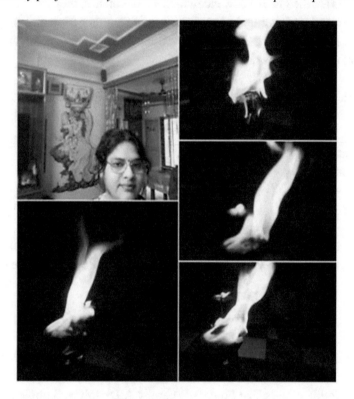

Many countries of the world have done research on Gayatri Mantra and the results they got were surprising. Hence, Gayatri Mantra is the reason the world's most powerful mantra. https://youtu.be/ CrwTLrN2q60

LITERATURE SURVEY

Scientific Aspects of Yajna and related Doubts are presented here. Usually there is a myth and doubt that there is smoke from Yagya, which increases air pollution and oxygen is also spent because something burns only when it gets oxygen. Clarification and solution to this is that there is no pollution by sacrificial fire. It increases more than the amount of oxygen spent. Pollution is cured.

- Yagya is a completely scientific process.
- It is the best act.
- There is no better work than Yagya
- Yajna is also called Agnihotra or Havan.

- Agnihotra means the sacrifices made for the purification of water, earth, air, etc.
- Yajna is not only ritual, but also a medical practice. The various chants that we perform while performing the Yajna have a special effect on our mind, brain, and soul. It also purifies the atmosphere.
- Yajna is also called Havi which means one who defeats poison. According to the theory of science, no substance is destroyed, but yes its form can be changed.
- Havan Ingredients are the ghee of cow etc. which we put on fire, they are like medicines for Havan, they are not destroyed by burning, but are converted to another form and we get it in subtle form. When there was no allopath, there was Aayurved in ancient times. In Aayurved, it was only from these plants that treatment was done.

Among the medicines which are in the incense material, they have qualities like:

1. Disinfectant
2. Aromatic Enhancer
3. Medicinal Action Property
4. Nutritious.
5. Oxygen Booster

When these medicines are burnt in the Havan Kund, they reach not one, but many living animals through the breath in atomic form, which also helps them. The following are the chemical activities in the Yajna.

1. Combustion
2. Sublimation
3. Fumigation Is A Method Of Pest Control That Completely Fills An Area With Smoke, Vapor, Or Gas To Deliver For The Purpose Of Disinfecting Or Of Destroying Pests.
4. Volatilization Volatilization Is The Process Whereby A Dissolved Sample Is Vaporised.

All these chemical activities are beneficial for us. In these, cow's ghee (containing about 8% saturated Fatty Acids and Triglycerides, Diglycerides, Monoglyceride) during combustion reaction intensifies the combustion leading to Complete Combustion.

CO_2 and H_2O are released during the combustion of Fatty Acid. Complete Combustion also reduces CO_2. Pyruvic Acid and Glyoxal ($C_2H_2O_2$) are formed in the combustion of glycerol. Pyruvic Acid increases our metabolism and kills Glyoxal bacteria (Mistry, R. et al., 2020); (Mrunal, R. et al., 2017).

Apart from these, the hydrocarbons that are formed during combustion again go through slow combustion reaction and form methyle, ethyle alcohol, formic acid and formaldehyde etc., which smells like air and is disinfectant. It also has the ability to eliminate H1N1 virus. Now you must be thinking that oxygen is spent when ignition and in a way we harm the environment. But you are wrong. Yajna is the process in which oxygen is spent but oxygen is also produced, as it also produces vapor (H_2O) along with CO_2.

$$CO_2 + H_2O \text{ (G)} + 112000 \text{ Cal} = HCHO \text{ (Farmaldehyde)} + O_2 \text{ (Oxygen)}$$

It is certain that whenever anything burnt, Oxygen will be absorbed and carbon will be emitted. But there are vast difference in carbon emitted by garbage burning and carbon emission from burning fragrant.

Commonly accepted philosophical factors that antidote to a poison is, also a poison derived from another resource. Similarly smoke and poisonous gases emitted by burning garbage, can be reversed back by the fumes produced by aromatic herbs that are offered in the Yagya as oblations (Aahutis).

The carbon that emits during Yagya, through aromatic herbs are in very little amount that are considered necessary to activate certain neurons in the system. Apart from the herbs that are offered in the fire which produces qualities environmental friendly gases, creosote, phenols, acetylene, aldehyde and ozone too assimilate in this. Even if any poisonous substance emitted on a little quantity is immediately evaporated with the oblations given by clarified butter (Ghee) and makes it non poisonous.

EXPERIMENTAL SETUP AND METHODOLOGY

The Experiments to support the science of Yajna and Mantra were conducted through a well defined protocol of 45 minutes where the Mantra Chanting, Pranayama, Yoga and Fitness activities were carried out. The laughing therapy and some alternative therapies like acupressure, Pranik Healing were also used in different time intervals.

Protocol Followed

The readings were being recorded by research team members quantitatively under different parameters and analyzed through various data analytics tool like Python, Tableau, SPSS, and excel. The subjects were asked to fill a small consent form to give their will to participate in the aforesaid experiments and were assured that their identity and data will not be made commercial and misused (Rastogi, R. et al., 2020a); (Rastogi, R. et al., 2020b); (Rastogi, R. et al., 2020c).

The whole experiment was conducted through Online platforms like Google meet, Zoom sessions, MS Team etc. as per convenience of the subjects during the lockdown period and their scores were recorded. The activities were conducted in India of duration of pandemic Sars-Cov'19 peak of 1st April 2020 to 31st Aug. 2020 in the period of 150 days around where a strict lockdown was imposed in India to save the mass from third stage infection of spread of Sars Cov'19.

The Subjects were asked to follow a strict protocol of 45 min. around which included some Asans (sitting, standing, lying front and back postures), some set of Mantra Chanting, Breathing Exercises(Pranayam), Alternate Therapies like Laughing Technique and Shantipath with certain breathing Exercises were followed. Subjects' data was recorded pre and post of the experiment and accordingly comparative study was conducted to check the efficacy of the methodology adopted (Rastogi, R. et al., 2019a); (Rastogi, R. et al., 2019b); (Rastogi, R. et al., 2019c).

Scientific Experiments on the Ash of Yajna and Chemical Analysis

Pl. see Annex for Permission Letter and Scientific Analysis of Different components in the Ash of Yajna
Pinch of consumption of Yagya bhasm as Prasad, was questioned by a person, that created an inquisitiveness which lead to do an experiment on Yagya to understand the components contained in Yagya bhasm, and its composition. With proper letter issued from Sunderpur, Jabalpur, MP. GAYATRI SHAKTIPEETH was sent to Geological survey of India, through Mr. Jayant Gupta of Gayatri Pariwar of Jaipur (Youth wing), an executive at GSI. He approached their director and research on Yagya bhasm

was executed with approval. We extend our heartfelt gratitude to all, who put their efforts to conduct this research and released the appropriate report.

Some scientists from BARC have also agreed to do research on the Yagyaagni. They are interested to study the flames of Yajna beginning temperature, gases released, temperature in the middle and its intensity with gases released, and temperatures at the end when the flames are off with the gases released (Saxena, M. et al. 2008); (Saxena, M. et al. 2018); (Saxena, M. et al. 2020).

RESULTS AND DISCUSSIONS

Happiness Index of Human and Radiation Analysis of Gadgets Analysis

Figure 8. Radiation analysis of electronic gadgest before and after Yajna

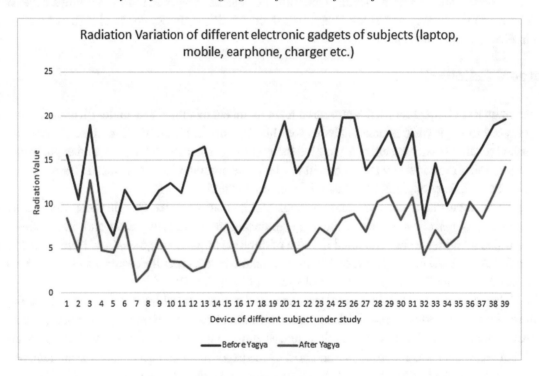

The electronic gadget like mobile, laptop, charger etc. radiations were recorded significantly low after the Yajna Process than before Yajna Rituals (Pl. refer Fig. 8).

Figure 9. Happiness index analysis of human subjects (left hand) before and after Yajna

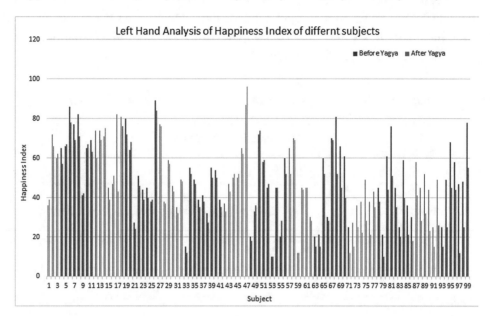

If see and analyze the graphs critically that we can easily see that red graph(After Yajna) is continuous below to blue(Before) graphs through left hand readings which shows the reduction in stress level and increase in happiness Index measured by Happiness Meter of the subjects participated in Yajna Ceremony and chanting of mantra (Pl. refer Fig. 9).

Figure 10. Happiness index analysis of human subjects (right hand) before and after Yajna

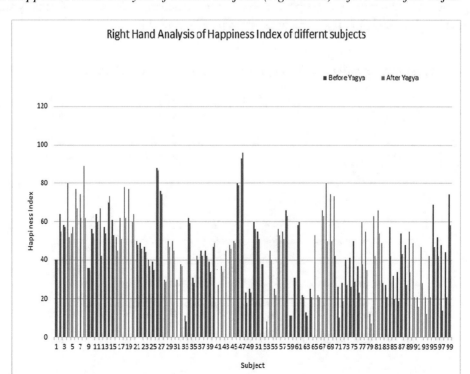

If see and analyze the graphs critically that we can easily see that red graph(After Yajna) is continuous below to blue(Before) graph through right hand readings which shows the reduction in stress level and increase in happiness Index measured by Happiness Meter of the subjects participated in Yajna Ceremony and chanting of mantra (Pl. refer Fig. 10).

Figure 11. Age vs. happiness index analysis of human subjects(right hand) in Yajna

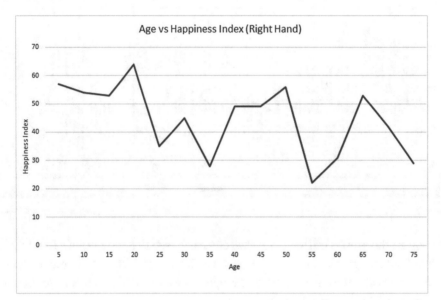

The participants Happiness counted through right hand w.r.t age is reflected above and shows that there is significant fluctuation in happiness index as per increasing rate of age. It totally depends on mental fitness, cool and calf life style and inner strength (Pl. refer Fig. 11).

Figure 12. Age vs. happiness index analysis of human subjects (left hand) in Yajna

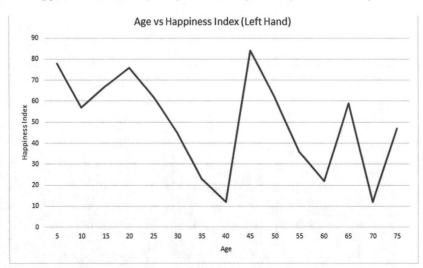

The participants Happiness counted through left hand w.r.t age is refected above and shows that there is significant fluctuation in happiness index as per increasing rate of age. It totally depends on mental fitness, cool and calf life style and inner strength (Pl. refer Fig. 12).

RECOMMENDATIONS

The main recommendations from Indian culture is Yagya Pita- Gayatri Mata(Yajna Father, Gayatri Mother)

According to science, heat, sound and light have been the fundamental units of power. Mantra is only the sound. The word is expected to travel at the speed of heat and light. To make the mantra wider, heat and light have to be combined with it as Yagya, only then it becomes more powerful and universal (Knowledge of Yagya, science, Yugrishi Shriram Sharma Acharya) (Rastogi, R. et al., 2018) and (Rastogi, R. et al., 2018).

One of the main reasons is said to be the delay in enforcing restrictions in Italy. After China, Now it is fully blown up epidemic in Italy and Spain and it is moving to other European countries as declared by WHO. This is third stage in Italy and Europe and second stage in USA.

In India, we are passing through 1st stage and 2nd stage is very near. China has shown the way to the world (Sharma, S., 2013; 2015a, 2015b; 2015c; 2015d).

NOVELTY

Yagyopathy was an integral part of the Vedik Period and it was vanished during the medieval period. Now the Yagyopathy has been developing as a Yagya Therapy for solving various issues. Evoking of the Inner power, Establishment of Spiritual Environmental place, development of wholesome culture, cleansing of micro environment, benefit on humanity are various new domains which are ipening for human race. The need is to get the benefit and explot this knowledge to address the current threats for this planet (Shrivastava, V. et al., 2019); (Srikant et al., 2019).

FUTURE RESEARCH DIRECTIONS

Many more research is needed in the domain of Meditation with Pranayama. Diseases are caused by the weakness of life force. Power comes in the body due to the strength in life. It is impossible to happen that power comes in the soul due to strength in the body. That is why it is said that Pranayama (the action - which exercises the souls and which makes the soul strong) increases age and sage muni by this will. They used to live long (Yajna: a holistic healing process, Yugrishi Shriram Sharma Acharya).

Divine powers strengthened to destroy demonic powers, to force the constructive powers (Yajna is a means: a holistic healing process, Yugrishi Shriram Sharma Acharya) (Sri Vedmata Gayatri Trust, 2011); (Strate School of Design; 2016); (Verma, S. et al., 2018).

CONCLUSION

Aim of Yajna science is for many dimensions in which the main aspects are fortification and balance of environment, rain of water with energy(Pranik Urja), improvement of health, treatment of illness, reviving through Yagyopathy.

Param Pujya Pt. SriRam Sharma Acharya ji, founder of All world Gayatri Parivar, revived the Yajna and Yagyopathy. Brahmvarchas research Center and Shantikunj Haridwar are conducting researches from past 40 years. Dev Sanskriti University Haridwar was added as a feather in its cap in year 2002. Several PhDs and research works are being enlightened in the field of human consciousness upliftment through ancient Vedik Sciences for Human Health and Environment is being conducted here.

The present Manuscripts also present the happiness measurement through Yagyopathy. Much more research is possible through this in coming future.

ACKNOWLEDGMENT

The Team of authors would love to pay our deep sense of gratitude to the ABES Engineering College, Ghaziabad & Amity International Business School, Amity University, and Noida for arranging us all the facilities, the direct-indirect supporters for their timely help and valuable suggestions and the almighty for blessing us throughout. We would also like to extend the vote of thanks to IIT Delhi, IIT Roorkee, Dev Sanskriti Vishwavidyalaya, Haridwar, Patanjali Foundation and Ayurveda Institute, Dehradun for their support and guidance in accomplishing our research paper.

REFERENCES

Cameron, Zimmet, Dunstan, Dalton, Shaw, Welborn, Owen, Salmon, & Jolly. (2003). *Overweight and obesity in Australia: the 1999–2000 Australian Diabetes, Obesity and Lifestyle Study (AusDiab)*. doi:10.5694/j.1326-5377.2003.tb05283.x

Chaturvedi, D. K., & Arya, M. (2013a). A Study of Correlation between Consciousness Level and Performance of Worker, *Industrial. Engineering Journal (New York)*, 6(8), 40–43.

Chaturvedi, D. K., & Arya, M. (2013b). Correlation between Human Performance and Consciousness. *IEEE-International Conference on Human Computer Interaction*.

Chaturvedi, D. K., & Satsangi, R. (2013). The Correlation between Student Performance and Consciousness Level. *International Conference on Advanced Computing and Communication Technologies (ICACCT™-2013)*, 200-203.

Gunavathi, C., & Premalatha, K. (2014). A Comparative Analysis of Swarm Intelligence Techniques for Feature Selection in Cancer Classification. *TheScientificWorldJournal*, *14*, 12. doi:10.1155/2014/693831 PMID:25157377

Jain, G. (2017). *Hawan for Cleansing the Environment*. medium.com/@giftofforest192/hawan-for-cleansing-the-environment-a9e1746e38e0

Kim, K.J., &Tagkopoulos, L. (2019). Application of Machine Learning Rheumatic Disease Research. *Korean J. Intern Med.,34,* 2.

Lahoty, P., & Rana, M. (2013). Agnihotra organic farming. *Popular Kheti, 1*(4), 49-54.

Mahajan, P. (2016). Application of Pattern Recognition Algorithm in Health and Medicine: a review. *International Journal of Engineering and Computer Science, 5*(5), 16580-83.

Marjani, M., Nasaruddin, F., Gani, A., Karim, A., Hashem, I. A. T., Siddiqa, A., & Yakoob, I. (2017, March). Big IoT Data Analytics: Architecture, Opportunities, and Open Research Challenges. *IEEE Access: Practical Innovations, Open Solutions, 5,* 5247–5261. doi:10.1109/ACCESS.2017.2689040

Mistry, R., Tanwar, S., Tyagi, S., & Kumar, N. (2020). Blockchain for 5G-Enabled IoT for Industrial Automation: A Systematic Review, Solutions, and Challenges. *Mechanical Systems and Signal Processing, 135,* 1–19. doi:10.1016/j.ymssp.2019.106382

Rastogi, R. (2012). Current Approaches for Researches in Naturopathy: How far is its Evidence Base? *J of Homeopathy & Ayurvedic Medicine, 1*(2), 1–107. doi:10.4172/2167-1206.1000107

Rastogi, R., Chaturvedi, D. K., Satya, S., Arora, N., Sirohi, H., Singh, M., Verma, P., & Singh, V. (2018b). Which One is Best: Electromyography Biofeedback Efficacy Analysis on Audio, Visual and Audio-Visual Modes for Chronic TTH on Different Characteristics. *Proceedings of International Conference on Computational Intelligence &IoT (ICCIIoT) 2018.*

Rastogi, R., Chaturvedi, D. K., Satya, S., Arora, N., Gupta, M., Verma, H., & Saini, H. (2020c). An Optimized Biofeedback EMG and GSR Biofeedback Therapy for Chronic TTH on SF-36 Scores of Different MMBD Modes on Various Medical Symptoms. Studies Comp. Intelligence, 841. doi:10.1007/978-981-13-8930-6_8

Rastogi, R., Chaturvedi, D. K., Satya, S., Arora, N., Saini, H., & Verma, H. (2018c). Comparative Efficacy Analysis of Electromyography and Galvanic Skin Resistance Biofeedback on Audio Mode for Chronic TTH on Various Indicators. *Proceedings of International Conference on Computational Intelligence &IoT (ICCIIoT) 2018.*

Rastogi, R., Chaturvedi, D. K., Sharma, S., Bansal, A., & Agrawal, A. (2018a). Audio Visual EMG & GSR Biofeedback Analysis for Effect of Spiritual Techniques on Human Behaviour and Psychic Challenges. *Proceedings of the 12th INDIACom,* 252-258.

Rastogi, R., Chaturvedi, D. K., Verma, H., Mishra, Y., & Gupta, M. (2020a). Identifying Better? Analytical Trends to Check Subjects' Medications Using Biofeedback Therapies. *International Journal of Applied Research on Public Health Management, 5*(1). https://www.igi-global.com/article/identifying-better/240753 doi:10.4018/IJARPHM.2020010102

Rastogi, R., Gupta, M., & Chaturvedi, D.K. (2020b). Efficacy of Study for Correlation of TTH vs Age and Gender Factors using EMG Biofeedback Technique. *International Journal of Applied Research on Public Health Management, 5*(1), 49-66. doi:10.4018/IJARPHM.2020010104

Rastogi, R., Saxena, M., Gupta, U. S., Sharma, S., Chaturvedi, D. K., Singhal, P., Gupta, M., Garg, P., Gupta, M., & Maheshwari, M. (2019b). Yajna and Mantra Therapy Applications on Diabetic Subjects: Computational Intelligence Based Experimental Approach. *Proceedings of The 2nd edition of International Conference on Industry Interactive Innovations in Science, Engineering and Technology (I3SET2K19)*. https://papers.ssrn.com/sol3/papers.cfm?abstract_id=3515800

Rastogi, R., Saxena, M., Sharma, S. K., Muralidharan, S., Beriwal, V. K., Singhal, P., Rastogi, M., & Shrivastava, R. (2019a). Evaluation of efficacy of Yagya therapy on t2- diabetes mellitus patients. *Proceedings of the 2nd edition of International Conference on Industry Interactive Innovations in Science, Engineering and Technology (I3SET2K19)*. https://papers.ssrn.com/sol3/papers.cfm?abstract_id=3514326

Rastogi, R., Saxena, M., Sharma, S. K., Murlidharan, S., Berival, V. K., Jaiswal, D., Sharma, A., & Mishra, A. (2019c). Statistical Analysis on Efficacy of Yagya Therapy for Type-2 Diabetic Mellitus Patients through Various Parameters. In On Computational Intelligence in Pattern Recognition (CIPR). doi:10.1007/978-981-15-2449-3_15

Saeed, S., & Abdullah, A. (20121). Statistical Analysis the Pre and Post-Surgery of health care sector using High Dimension Segmentation. *Machine Learning Healthcare: Handling and Managing Data, 1*(1), 1-25.

Saeed, S., & Naqvi, S. M. (2018). Impact of Data Mining Techniques to Analyze Health Care Data. *Journal of Medical Sciences and Health.*

Saxena, M., Kumar, B., & Matharu, S. (2018). Impact of Yagya on Particulate Matters. *Interdisciplinary Journal of Yagya Research, 1*(1), 1-8.

Saxena, M., Sengupta, B., & Pandya, P. (2008, September). Controlling the Microflora in Outdoor Environment: Effect of Yagya. *Indian Journal of Air Pollution Control, 8*(2), 30–36.

Saxena, M., Sharma, S. K., Muralidharan, S., Beriwal, V., Rastogi, R., Singhal, P., Sharma, V., & Sangam, U. (2020). Statistical Analysis Of Efficacy Of Yagya Therapy On Type-2 Diabetic Mellitus Patients on Various Parameters. *Proceedings Of 2ⁿᵈ International Conference on Computational Intelligence In Pattern Recognition (CIPR – 2020).*

Sharma, S.R. (2013). Shabd Brahma—Naad Brahm. *BrahmVarchas, Shantikunj,* 55.

Sharma, S.R. (2015a). Shabd Brahma—Naad Brahm. *BrahmVarchas, Shantikunj,* 98.

Sharma, S.R. (2015b). Gayatri MahaVigyan. *BrahmVarchas, Shantikunj,* 235.

Sharma, S.R. (2015c). Shabd Brahma—Naad Brahm. *BrahmVarchas, Shantikunj,* 34

Sharma, S.R. (2015d). Shabd Brahma—Naad Brahm. *BrahmVarchas, Shantikunj,* 61

Shenwai & Tare. (2017). Integrated Approach towards Holistic Health: Current Trends and Future Scope. *Int. J. of Cur. Rec. Rev., 9*(7), 11-14.

Shrivastava, V., Batham, L., Mishra, A. (2019). Yagyopathy (Yagya Therapy) for Various Diseases - An Overview. *Ayurveda Evam Samagra Swasthya Shodhamala, 1*(1), 1-11.

Srikanth. (2019). *15 Benefits of Machine Learning in Health Care*. https://techiexpert.com/benefits-of-machine-learning-in-health-care/

Srivedmata Gayatri Trust. Gayatri Parivar, UK. (2011). *Yagya's Effect On The Environment*. https://home.awgpuk.org/index.php/yagya/42-yagya-s-effect-on-the-environment

Strate School of Design. Paris and Singapore. (2016). *IoT applications in healthcare, Supporting Robust Health and Medical Practices*. https://www.strate.education/gallery/news/healthcare-iot

Verma, S., Mishra, A., & Shrivastava, V. (2018). Yagya Therapy in Vedic and Ayurvedic Literature: A Preliminary exploration. *Interdisciplinary Journal of Yagya Research, 1*(1), 15-20. http://ijyr.dsvv.ac.in/index.php/ijyr/article/view/7/13

APPENDIX

Questionnaire From Sheelu Sagar, Ph. D Scholar Amity University, Noida, Uttar Pradesh
Objective: To investigate the effects of Gayatri Mantra on Wellness and in lowering of Stress level in Working and Non Working Women during Pregnancy Period of First Trimester.

1. Your education level is:
    a. Undergraduate
    b. Graduate
    c. Post Graduate
2. How stressed do you feel on a daily basis during this time ? (1-10 are stress level)
    1 2 3 4 5 6 7 8 9 10
3. What are the usual causes of stress in your life? (Select all that apply)
    a. Financial issues
    b. Studies issues
    c. Family issues
    d. Friend's issues
    e. Work (job-related) issues
    f. Health Related Issues
    g. Any other
4. What are the usual Behavioral effects of stress you've noticed in yourself? (Select all that apply)
    a. Change in activity levels
    b. Decreased efficiency and effectiveness
    c. Difficulty communicating
    d. Irritability, outbursts of anger, frequent arguments
    e. Inability to rest, relax or let down
    f. Change in eating habits
    g. Avoidance of activities or places that trigger memories
5. What are the usual Psychological or Emotional effects of stress you've noticed in yourself? (Select all that apply)
    a. Feeling heroic, euphoric or invulnerable
    b. Anxiety or fear
    c. Worry about safety of self or others
    d. Feeling overwhelmed, helpless or hopeless
    e. Sadness, moodiness, grief or depression
    f. Restlessness
    g. Feeling isolated, lost, lonely or abandoned
    h. Feeling misunderstood or unappreciated
    i. Other
6. What are the usual social effects of stress you've noticed in yourself? (Select all that apply)
    a. Withdrawing or isolating from people
    b. Difficulty listening
    c. Difficulty in giving or accepting support or help

      d.   Impatient with or disrespectful to others

      e.   None of the Above

      f.   Other

7.   What are your personal methods to relieve stress? (Select all that apply)

      a.   Reading Books

      b.   Listening to Music

      c.   Chanting Mantra

      d.   Eating

      e.   Sleeping

      f.   Drugs

      g.   Sports / Exercise

      h.   Talking with someone

      i.   Shopping

      j.   Social Media

      k.   Other

8.   What are the most pressing stress factors in your current phase of life ? Select all that apply.

      a.   Workload

      b.   Lot of domestic responsibilities

      c.   Financial pressure

      d.   Life balance between office and home

      e.   Relationship with office colleagues

      f.   Relationship with family members

9.   Do you Practice Yoga?

      a.   Yes

      b.   No

10.   Do you see yourself involved in spirituality?

      a.   Involved as minimal or casual

      b.   Involved with ideas and practices

      c.   Deeply involved with ideas and practices

      d.   I provide spiritual guidance, coaching / therapies .

11.   Do you practice meditation or some other form of spiritual technique?

      a.   Often

      b.   Regularly

      c.   Sometimes

      d.   Rarely

      e.   Never

12.   I prefer chanting of Gayatri Mantra in morning before I eat my breakfast

      a.   Strongly Agree

      b.   Strongly Disagree

      c.   Natural

13.   Almost all the religions and faiths globally may achieve healthy body, mind and soul, through the practice of some technique of meditation.

      a.   Yes I very much agree

b.   Yes I agree

c.   Neutral Cannot say

d.   No I disagree

e.   No I totally disagree

14. How much do you practice Gayatri Mantra in terms of number and time .

a.   108 times 5 Minutes

b.   648 times 30 Minutes

c.   1296 times 01 hour

d.   Nil

15. Since How long have you have being practicing Gayatri Mantra ?

a.   Over 2 Years

b.   Less than 1 years

c.   I have recently started this practice

d.   I have never done this practice

16. How do you feel after Chanting or listening to Mantra ?

a.   Very Happy and very satisfied

b.   Happy somewhat satisfied

c.   Neutral

d.   Unhappy and unsatisfied

e.   Very unhappy and unsatisfied

17. Do you think that for maximum result of Meditation time should be early Morning

a.   Agree

b.   Somewhat agree

c.   Disagree

d.   Neutral

18. How happy are you at your workplace?

a.   Very Happy at workplace

b.   Somewhat Happy

c.   Neutral

d.   Very Unhappy

e.   Unhappy

19. Are you satisfied with the career growth in your organization?

a.   Very Satisfied.

b.   Satisfied.

c.   Neutral.

d.   Dissatisfied.

e.   Very Dissatisfied.

Consent to Take Part in Research

TOPIC: "Holistic Health Management through Vedic Processes."

I…………………………………………………………………………Age……………Years voluntarily agree to participate in this research Study for my Wellness through Recitation & Meditation of Vedic Mantra (Gayatri Mantra) during my Maternity Period

I agree to participate in the research study. I understand the purpose and nature of this study and I am participating voluntarily. I understand that I can withdraw from the study at any time, without any penalty or consequences.

a) Yes b) NO.

I grant permission for the data generated from this interview to be used in the researcher's publications on this topic. a) Yes b) No

Signature of research participant --

DATE:

Signature of researcher -------------------------------------

I believe the participant is giving informed consent to participate in this study

DATE:

Agreement Letter

I_____Son/Daughter_____age _____, of_____ _____want to do my own clinical examination/ Examinations, and request for necessary medicines from the Yagyopathy Research Center, essential medical / treatment etc.

I declare that I am over 18 years of age.

I will follow all the instructions given by the physicians of Yagyopathy Research Center during the course of treatment.

I give my consent to receive therapy / treatment from the Yagyopathy Research Center. The nature and purpose of therapy / treatment is explained to me. I have been given due information for all the inherent risks involved in clinical investigation, medicines and medical / treatment. I have been duly informed, and with a proper understanding of all these risks, I will do my investigation, medicines and give my consent to the necessary medical / treatment. I will be fully responsible for all results of Medical / Treatment.

I have voluntarily given this consent without any pressure.

Date: Signature of the patient

Consent for Research Purposes

At the beginning of therapy / treatment for medical, scientific, educational and research purposes, and finally, I have no objection to photography and videography of my condition. Along with publishing this information, its scientific observations in scientific journals presenting the data and using it in conferences / seminars / workshops without using my name, I give my consent for submission.

Patient's signature:
(Agree) / (Disagree)

The Readings Collected for Different Experiments

Table 1 (a). Happiness index

Happiness Index				Index			
S.No.	Name	Gender	Age	20 Minutes Prior to Yagya		20 Minutes After Yagya	
				Left Hand	Right Hand	Left Hand	Right Hand
1	Anuj Yadav	Male	19	36	40	39	40
2	Yatharth Katyaya	Male	19	72	64	66	55
3	Lalit Mohan	Male	21	60	58	62	57
4	Chetan Garg	Male	20	65	80	57	52
5	Mayank	Male	20	66	54	67	57
6	Aarsh Verma	Male	19	86	77	78	67
7	Akash Patel	Male	20	77	74	69	62
8	Nishit Kumar	Male	20	82	89	71	62
9	Mohit Chauhan	Male	20	41	36	42	36
10	Yash Thakur	Male	20	65	56	67	54
11	Vibhor Kaushal	Male	20	69	64	63	60
12	Akhand	Male	20	74	67	60	42
13	Pankaj Kumar	Male	20	74	57	69	54
14	Ritik	Male	20	71	70	75	73
15	Deepanshu Srivastava	Male	21	45	61	39	53
16	Sanjeev Sagar	Male	21	47	52	51	45
17	Deepesh Yadav	Male	21	82	62	43	51
18	Mridul	Male	20	81	78	76	62
19	Divik Yadav	Male	20	80	77	72	72
20	Utkarsh Saini	Male	20	64	60	68	64

Table 1 (b). Happiness index

09-03-2020 at Gayatri Shaktipeeth HariharGanj Fatehpur							
1	Aasha Tripathi	F	57	27	50	24	48
2	Chaaya	F	55	51	49	46	46
3	Suneeta Gupta	F	57	44	47	39	44
4	Nirmala	F	76	45	40	40	37
5	Rupa	F	60	38	39	39	35
6	Shikha	F	32	89	88	84	87
7	Sandhya	F	45	77	76	76	74
8	Laxmi	F	52	38	30	37	29
9	Vandana	F	48	59	50	57	47
10	Ajay	M	55	46	50	43	45
11	Ishwar	M	53	35	30	32	27
12	Nema	F	45	49	38	48	37
13	Shivam	M	22	15	11	12	8
14	Anurag	M	48	55	62	52	59
15	Asaha	F	55	49	31	47	28
16	RamSwaroop Gupta	M	68	39	42	35	40
17	Gomti	F	64	41	45	38	42
18	Padma	F	58	32	45	27	42
19	SP Shukla	M	76	55	39	50	34
20	Meera	F	72	54	47	50	49
21	Vijay Laxmi	F	62	39	24	35	27
22	GL Gupta	M	75	37	37	33	34
23	Rajdesh	M	58	47	45	43	42
24	Ranjana Rastogi	F	60	50	48	52	46
25	Anamika Dubey	F	37	50	50	52	49
26	Rohit Rastogi	M	39	65	80	62	79
27	Mukund Rastogi	M	19	87	93	96	96
28	Suneel Kumar Rastogi	M	51	20	23	18	18
29	Anoop Mishra	M	44	33	25	36	23
30	Ashu Dwivedi	M	32	72	60	74	56
31	Rishi Mishra	M	48	58	55	59	51
32	Tarashankar Mishra	M	42	45	38	47	38

Continued on following page

Table 1 (b). Continued

33	Dr. Sharda Mishra	F	75		10	8	10	8
34	Susheela Dubey	F	58		45	45	45	40
35	Avartika Dubey	F	37		20	25	28	22
36	Radhika	F	27		60	56	52	53
37	Meetu Rastogi	F	44		65	55	52	51
38	Sejal	F	20		70	66	69	63
39	Motilal Rastogi	M	75		12	11	12	11
40	Rishabh Rastogi	M	25		45	31	44	31
41	Sanjay Rastogi	M	55		45	58	45	60
42	Anupam Rastogi	F	60		30	22	28	21
43	Shyam Babu Rastogi	M	56		20	13	15	11
44	Rekha	F	45		21	25	15	21
45	Ajay Rastogi	M	58		60	56	52	53
46	Kumkum Rastogi	F	55		30	22	28	21
47	Archit Rastogi	M	26		70	66	69	63

Table 1 (c). Happiness index

13-03-2020 BY MUKUND							
48	Sahil Verma	M	19	81	80	52	50
49	Kamal Kant Mishra	M	20	66	74	45	50
50	Yash Rastogi	M	19	61	73	40	42
51	Archana Mishra	F	52	25	26	12	10
52	Dev Narayana Mishra	M	54	27	28	15	19
53	Aishwarya Mishra	F	18	36	40	25	27
54	Jay Prakash Verma	M	45	38	41	22	26
55	Sunita Verma	F	40	49	50	28	29
56	RadheShyam	M	43	38	37	21	23
57	Geeta Devi	F	39	43	60	35	38
58	Vinod Verma	M	50	45	55	38	35
59	Neetu	F	45	21	12	10	7
60	Muskan Verma	F	21	61	63	44	42
61	Vishwas Verma	M	16	76	66	51	54
62	Bharat Rastogi	M	58	45	49	35	28
63	Shubhra Rastogi	F	45	25	27	20	21
64	Raghav Rastogi	M	22	59	57	40	42
65	Anju Rastogi	F	58	36	32	21	20
66	Goverdhan Rastogi	M	63	30	34	18	19
67	Satyam Rastogi	M	27	58	54	41	43
68	Anshita Rastogi	F	32	45	48	28	27
69	Smriti Rastogi	F	19	52	55	32	34
70	Stuti Rastogi	F	23	44	49	23	21
71	Babita Rastogi	F	49	25	21	15	16
72	Abhishek Gupta	M	22	49	47	26	28
73	Shikhar Rastogi	M	23	25	21	15	12
74	Shishir Mishra	M	24	49	42	25	21
75	Pradyumn	M	21	68	69	45	47
76	Ankit Kumar Mishra	M	26	58	52	44	42
77	Punit Kumar	M	25	47	48	12	14
78	Prateek Kumar	M	21	48	44	25	21
79	Pushp Raj	M	24	78	74	55	58

Table 2. Radiation analysis

S.No.	Radiation Value	(-By Pradeep Kumar, phone no:7388083531, email ID: pradeep.18bcs1099@abes.ac.in)				
	Device Used	Date	Time	Location	Before Yagya	After Yagya
1	Mobile Phone	3/1/2020	6:00 AM	ABES EC Hostel	15.62	8.42
2	Headphone	3/2/2020	6:00 AM	ABES EC Hostel	10.58	4.67
3	Laptop of Pradeep	3/3/2020	6:00 AM	ABES EC Hostel	18.95	12.73
4	Watch	3/4/2020	6:00 AM	ABES EC Hostel	9.23	4.79
5	Charger	3/5/2020	6:00 AM	ABES EC Hostel	6.55	4.61
6	Speaker	3/6/2020	6:00 AM	ABES EC Hostel	11.65	7.83
09-03-2020 at Gayatri Shaktipeeth HariharGanj Fatehpur						
Mobiles						
	Aasha Tripathi				9.45	1.31
	Chaaya				9.59	2.64
	Suneeta Gupta				11.54	6.08
	Nirmala				12.45	3.54
	Rupa				11.34	3.45
	Shikha				15.89	2.47
	Sandhya				16.56	2.95
	Laxmi				11.4	6.32
	Vandana				8.9	7.7
	Ajay				6.7	3.1
	Ishwar				8.9	3.57
	Nema				11.5	6.27
	Shivam				15.56	7.5
	Anurag				19.38	8.86
	Asaha				13.56	4.57
	RamSwaroop Gupta					2.18
10-03-2020 at Chowk Fatehpur By Rr						
All Mobiles	RR Motorola				15.56	5.4
	Anamika MI				19.67	7.32
	Rr Jio				12.64	6.43

Continued on following page

Table 2. Continued

S.No.	Radiation Value	(-By Pradeep Kumar, phone no:7388083531, email ID: pradeep.18bcs1099@abes.ac.in)				
	Device Used	Date	Time	Location	Before Yagya	After Yagya
	Tarashankar Mishra Jio				19.85	8.44
	Annop Mishra Samsung				19.83	8.95
	Aashu Dwivedi Samsung				13.89	6.89
	Rishabh Rastogi Samsung				15.88	10.32
	Sejal Rastogi Micromax				18.31	11.1
13-03-2020 by Mukund						
	Yash Rastogi motorola				14.54	8.25
	Kamal Kant Mishra Realme3				18.26	10.85
	Sahil Verma Redmi 5A				8.47	4.29
	Raghav Rastogi Redmi note 5 pro				14.68	7.14
	Mukund Rastogi Samsung j3 pro				9.87	5.21
	Prateek Kumar Samsung j7				12.58	6.46
	Abhishek Gupta Nokia 6.1				14.29	10.28
	Shishir Mishra Lenovo k3 note				16.54	8.49
	Pushpraj yadav vivo				18.98	11.25
	Anurag Nagar Oppo f1				19.68	14.27

Table 3.

09-03-2020 at Gayatri Shaktipeeth HariharGanj Fatehpur			
Before	**After Yagya**	**Before**	**After Yagya**
Mukund Laptop		RR Laptop	
11.98	5.6	14.01	5.5

Chapter 6
Deep Learning

Khalid A. Al Afandy

ⓘ https://orcid.org/0000-0003-1465-4446

National School for Applied Science (ENSA), Abdelmalek Essaadi University, Tetouan, Morocco

Hicham Omara

Faculty of Science (FS), Abdelmalek Essaadi University, Tetouan, Morocco

Mohamed Lazaar

ENSIAS, Mohammed V University, Rabat, Morocco

Mohammed Al Achhab

National School for Applied Science (ENSA), Abdelmalek Essaadi University, Tetouan, Morocco

ABSTRACT

This chapter provides a comprehensive explanation of deep learning including an introduction to ANNs, improving the deep NNs, CNNs, classic networks, and some technical tricks for image classification using deep learning. ANNs, mathematical models for one node ANN, and multi-layers/multi-nodes ANNs are explained followed by the ANNs training algorithm followed by the loss function, the cost function, the activation function with its derivatives, and the back-propagation algorithm. This chapter also outlines the most common training problems with the most common solutions and ANNs improvements. CNNs are explained in this chapter with the convolution filters, pooling filters, stride, padding, and the CNNs mathematical models. This chapter explains the four most commonly used classic networks and ends with some technical tricks that can be used in CNNs model training.

INTRODUCTION

Deep learning enabled people to create brand new products and businesses and ways of helping from better healthcare, by getting really good at reading images, to delivering personalized education, to precision agriculture, to even self-driving cars and many others. One of the most common applications of deep learning is image classification which has made tremendous progress in this field. Deep learning is a branch of machine learning which is completely based on NNs (Gaur et al., 2021a; Du et al., 2016).

DOI: 10.4018/978-1-7998-8929-8.ch006

Human brain approximately contains 100 billion neurons each neuron is connected through thousands of their neighbors. Thus, NNs are going to mimic the human brain and can also be called ANNs so deep learning is also a kind of mimic of the human brain. There's been a lot of hype about NNs given how well they're working. But it turns out that so far, almost all the economic value created by NNs has been through one type of machine learning which is supervised learning. The necessity of rising ANNs' right predictions in upgrading the ANNs structures, it causes the appearance of specific NNs such as CNNs (Du et al., 2016; Bengio et al., 2017). CNNs are derived from NNs but its layers are not fully connected like ANNs layers; it has an exciting rapid advance in computer vision. It is based on some blocks that can be applied on an image as filters and then extract convolution object features from this image that can be used in solving many of computer vision problems, one of these problems is classification. The need of processing the huge data, which appeared with the advent of the high resolution color images and its rapid development, produced the need of CNNs deep architectures that can produce a high accuracy in classification. It caused the appearance of the classic networks (Du et al., 2016; Bengio et al., 2017). There are many classic networks that are mentioned in research papers which can be used in image classification.

THE ANNS

The ANNs approach is an algorithm that tries to mimic the human brain in which the use of the ANNs as a supervised classifier is based on the structure of the biological NNs (Shanmuganathan, 2016; Gaur et al., 2021b). The structure of ANNs depends on the data that flow through this network. The accuracy and the performance of the ANNs are highly dependent on the network structure. The ANNs computational rate is high but the network takes a huge time for training and there is some difficulty to choose the network structure because the network design is based on intuition (Du et al., 2016; AlAfandy et al., 2019).

NNs are deemed as nonlinear statistical data modeling tools where the complex relationships between inputs and outputs are modeled. NNs are formed of a sequence of layers; each layer contains a set of neurons. The input and the output layers are the first and the last layers, where the internal layers are treated as the hidden layers. Neurons in the preceding and the succeeding layers are connected by weighted connections called the weights (Du et al., 2016). In the ANNs models, the given dataset inputs and outputs must have a mathematical relation in which the outputs are predicted within discrete function for classification models or continuous function for regression models; this mathematical model is based on the ANNs structure and design. This mathematical model is the calculation of the prediction $\hat{y}$ which is a function of weights W, bias b, and input features X (Bengio et al., 2017).

Figure 1. One node ANN structure

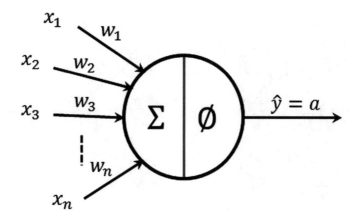

As shown in figure 1, this example is an ANN structure which is consists of one node with input features $X = \{x_1, x_2, x_3, \ldots, x_n\}$, the output in this model is calculated as (Bengio et al., 2017):

$$\hat{y} = a \qquad (1)$$

$$a = \varnothing\left(z\right) \qquad (2)$$

$$z = w^T X + b \qquad (3)$$

where $\hat{y}$ is the ANN output, X is the dataset input, $\varnothing\left(z\right)$ is the activation function, b is the bias, and w is the weight matrix.

$$X = \begin{bmatrix} x_1 \\ x_2 \\ x_3 \\ \vdots \\ x_n \end{bmatrix}, \text{ and } w = \begin{bmatrix} w_1 \\ w_2 \\ w_3 \\ \vdots \\ w_n \end{bmatrix} \qquad (4)$$

In the previous ANN, output calculations are based on one node and one layer only, then in the case of multilayers and multi nodes in each layer the previous calculation can be used with some modification where each layer depends on the output of its preceding layer. Figure 2 shows the ANNs structure with multilayers in which each layer contains multiple nodes (Du et al., 2016).

Figure 2. The ANNs structure with multilayers which each layer contains multiple nodes

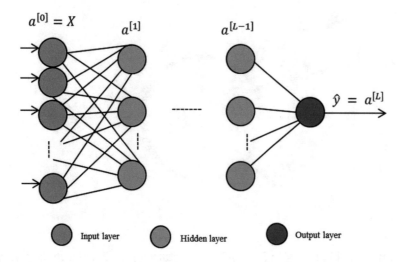

The ANNs structure with multilayers which each layer contains multiple nodes has input layer $X = A^{[0]}$, hidden layers from $A^{[1]}$ to $A^{[L-1]}$, and output layer $\hat{y} = A^{[L]}$

$$X = A^{[0]} = \begin{bmatrix} x_1 \\ x_2 \\ x_3 \\ \vdots \\ x_n \end{bmatrix}, \ A^{[l]} = \begin{bmatrix} a_1^{[l]} \\ a_2^{[l]} \\ a_3^{[l]} \\ \vdots \\ a_{k^{[l]}}^{[l]} \end{bmatrix}, \text{ and } l = \{1,2,...,L\} \tag{5}$$

where L is the ANNs layers, n is the input features, and $k^{[l]}$ is the l th layer nodes.
Then, from (1) to (5), the l th layer output can be calculated as:

$$A^{[l]} = \varnothing^{[l]}\left(Z^{[l]}\right) \tag{6}$$

$$Z^{[l]} = W^{[l]}A^{[l-1]} + b^{[l]} \tag{7}$$

$$Z^{[l]} = \begin{bmatrix} z_1^{[l]} \\ z_2^{[l]} \\ z_3^{[l]} \\ \vdots \\ z_{k^{[l]}}^{[l]} \end{bmatrix}, \ b^{[l]} = \begin{bmatrix} b_1^{[l]} \\ b_2^{[l]} \\ b_3^{[l]} \\ \vdots \\ b_{k^{[l]}}^{[l]} \end{bmatrix}, \text{ and } W^{[l]} = \begin{bmatrix} w_{11}^{[l]} & \cdots & w_{1k^{[l-1]}}^{[l]} \\ \vdots & \ddots & \vdots \\ w_{k^{[l]}1}^{[l]} & \cdots & w_{k^{[l]}k^{[l-1]}}^{[l]} \end{bmatrix} \tag{8}$$

So, the right vectors dimensions are $W^{[l]} = \left(k^{[l]}, k^{[l-1]}\right)$, $b^{[l]} = \left(k^{[l]}, 1\right)$, $Z^{[l]} = \left(k^{[l]}, 1\right)$, and $A^{[l]} = \left(k^{[l]}, 1\right)$.

The $\varnothing^{[l]}$ is the activation function of the l th layer.

Then, the output of the ANN structure is calculated as:

$$\hat{y} = A^{[L]} \tag{9}$$

The network weights W and bias b must be well selected and updated according to the dataset input features X and ANNs structure to achieving the lowest losses that calculated using the loss function $\mathcal{L}(y, \hat{y})$ and the cost function $J(W, b)$ (Bengio et al., 2017).

For training the ANNs model even if this model is regression or classification, there are many steps to finalize the training process.

1. Design the ANNs structure by taking into account that the input layer nodes must equal the dataset input features.
2. Divide the dataset into training dataset, which is 60% from dataset records, validation dataset, which is 20% from dataset records, and the test dataset, which is 20% from dataset records.
3. Initialize the weights W values with random values and the bias b values with zeros. Then, initialize optimization parameters to zeros.
4. Calculate the ANNs output $\hat{y}$ using mathematical models from (5) to (9) for each layer.
5. Calculate the loss functions $\mathcal{L}\left(y_{train}, \hat{y}_{train}\right)$ and $\mathcal{L}\left(y_v, \hat{y}_v\right)$ and the cost function $J(W, b)$ where y_{train} is the training dataset outputs and y_v is the validation dataset outputs, even if using regularization or not.
6. Calculate the ANNs model gradients using the back-propagation calculations.
7. Update the model parameters W and b values using the gradient descent if not using optimization or using the used optimization in the ANNs model.
8. Repeat steps from 4 to 7 with the suggested number of iterations.
9. Determine the iteration number that gives the lowest validation loss value of $\mathcal{L}\left(y_v, \hat{y}_v\right)$.
10. Consider the validation dataset and training dataset as the new training dataset (80% from the dataset records).

11. Repeat steps from 4 to 7 with the number of iterations that gave the lowest loss value of $\mathcal{L}\left(y_v, \hat{y}_v\right)$ using the new training dataset (80% from the dataset records).
12. Calculate the ANNs output $\hat{y}_{test}$ using the final model parameters W and b values and the test dataset input features.
13. Compare the output $\hat{y}_{test}$ with the test dataset known correct outputs y_{test} to assess the learning model performance.

From the previous algorithm steps and calculations, it is necessary to clarify the mentioned used functions and calculations; the activation function, the loss function, the back-propagation calculations, and the gradient descent.

The Activation Functions

There are many activation functions that can be used with the NNs models which can use a different activation function for each layer in the same NNs model. This section illustrates the most used activation functions with its derivatives.

The ReLU Function

The ReLU function is the very popular activation function in deep learning which is the most commonly used for hidden layers. Figure 3 shows the ReLU function output graph. The ReLU function can be calculated as (Rasamoelina et al., 2020):

$$a^{[l]} = \varnothing^{[l]}\left(Z^{[l]}\right) = \max\left(0, Z^{[l]}\right) \tag{10}$$

The derivative of the ReLU function $\dfrac{\partial a}{\partial Z}$ can be calculated by (Rasamoelina et al., 2020):

$$\frac{\partial a^{[l]}}{\partial Z^{[l]}} = \begin{cases} 0, Z^{[l]} < 0 \\ 1, Z^{[l]} \geq 0 \end{cases} \tag{11}$$

Figure 3. The ReLU function output graph

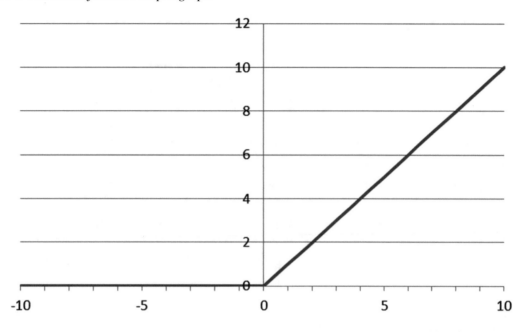

The Sigmoid Function

The Sigmoid function is a popular function in machine learning which is used for output layers. This function output is any real number to the (0, 1) interval as shown in figure 4. If the output is less than 0.5 then the classification output is 0, and if the output is greater than or equal 0.5 then the classification output is 1 (Shanthamallu et al., 2017; Rasamoelina et al., 2020; Mishra et al., 2017). The sigmoid function can be calculated as (Shanthamallu et al., 2017; Rasamoelina et al., 2020):

$$a^{[l]} = \varnothing^{[l]}\left(Z^{[l]}\right) = \frac{1}{1 + e^{-Z^{[l]}}} \qquad (12)$$

The derivative of the sigmoid function $\dfrac{\partial a}{\partial Z}$ can be calculated by (Rasamoelina et al., 2020; Mishra et al., 2017):

$$\frac{\partial a^{[l]}}{\partial Z^{[l]}} = a^{[l]}\left(1 - a^{[l]}\right) \qquad (13)$$

Figure 4. The Sigmoid function output graph

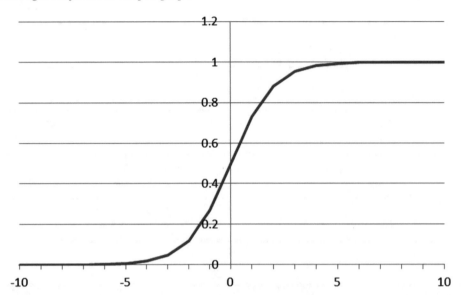

The Tanh Function

The tanh function is one of the popular functions in deep learning which is used for output layers. This function output is any real number to the (-1, 1) interval as shown in figure 5 which leads to works better than the sigmoid function. It is mathematically a shifted version from the sigmoid function. The tanh function can be calculated as (Rasamoelina et al., 2020; Mishra et al., 2017):

$$a^{[l]} = \varnothing^{[l]}\left(Z^{[l]}\right) = \tanh\left(Z^{[l]}\right) \tag{14}$$

$$a^{[l]} = \varnothing^{[l]}\left(Z^{[l]}\right) = \frac{e^{Z^{[l]}} - e^{-Z^{[l]}}}{e^{Z^{[l]}} + e^{-Z^{[l]}}} \tag{15}$$

The derivative of the tanh function $\dfrac{\partial a}{\partial Z}$ can be calculated by (Rasamoelina et al., 2020; Mishra et al., 2017):

$$\frac{\partial a^{[l]}}{\partial Z^{[l]}} = 1 - a^{[l]2} \tag{16}$$

Figure 5. The Tanh function output graph

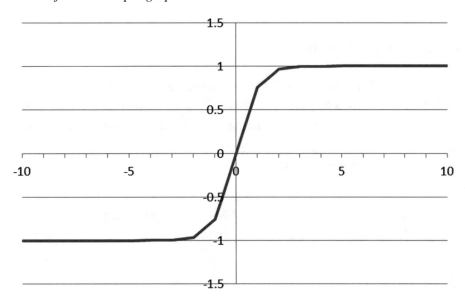

The Softmax Function

The softmax function is the very popular activation function in deep learning which is the most commonly used for output layers for the NNs classification models. It is a vector-to-vector transformation whose output is always in the (0, 1) interval. The softmax output can be considered as a probability distribution over a finite set of outcomes which used for the multi-class logistic regression. Then, for the $q^{[l]}$ th class in the $k^{[l]}$ th classes in the l th layers' ANNs classification model, the softmax function can be calculated as (Kanai et al., 2018):

$$\hat{y} = a_q^{[l]} = \varnothing^{[l]}\left(Z_q^{[l]}\right) = \frac{e^{z_q^{[l]}}}{\sum_{j=1}^{k^{[l]}} e^{z_j^{[l]}}} \tag{17}$$

The derivative of the softmax function $\dfrac{\partial a}{\partial Z}$ can be calculated by (Kanai et al., 2018):

$$\frac{\partial a_q^{[l]}}{\partial Z_q^{[l]}} = \frac{e^{z_q^{[l]}} \left(\sum_{j=1}^{k^{[l]}} e^{z_j^{[l]}} - e^{z_q^{[l]}} \right)}{\left(\sum_{j=1}^{k^{[l]}} e^{z_j^{[l]}} \right)^2} \qquad (18)$$

The Loss and the Cost Functions

Through the training stage for ANNs models, two outputs can be used to test the learning model performance; the dataset known correct output y and the prediction ANNs output $\hat{y}$ where the loss function is based on these two outputs. Thus, the loss function $\mathcal{L}(y, \hat{y})$ can be calculated as (Singh et al., 2014):

$$\mathcal{L}(y, \hat{y}) = -\left((y \log \hat{y}) + (1 - y) \log(1 - \hat{y}) \right) \qquad (19)$$

where y is the correct dataset output and $\hat{y}$ is the ANNs model prediction output.

The cost function $J(W, b)$ is given by (Singh et al., 2014):

$$J(W, b) = \frac{1}{m} \sum_{i=1}^{m} \mathcal{L}\left(y^{(i)}, \hat{y}^{(i)} \right) \qquad (20)$$

The Back-Propagation Calculations

The back-propagation is a widely used algorithm for training the ANNs learning models. The back-propagation computes the gradients of the loss function with respect to the ANNs weights W and bias b. The back-propagation process is the reverse direction calculation for the ANNs prediction results; the start is the last layer derivative $dA^{[L]}$ ending with the first hidden layer derivative $dA^{[1]}$ by using the derivative calculations. The end is the first hidden layer derivative $dA^{[1]}$ because there is no need to calculate the input layer derivative $dA^{[0]}$ (Li et al., 2012; Ooyen & Nienhuis, 1992; Paola & Schowengerdt, 1995). Figure 6 shows the forward-propagation and back-propagation process in the ANNs models.

Figure 6. The forward-propagation and back-propagation process in the ANNs models

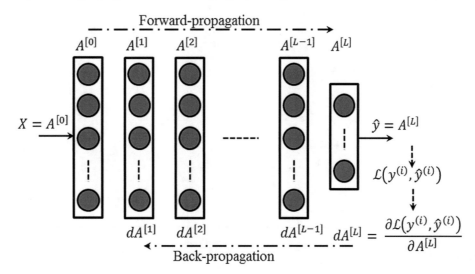

In the forward-propagation, the mathematical models from (5) to (9) illustrate that the inputs are $A^{[l-1]}$, $W^{[l]}$, and $b^{[l]}$ and the output is $A^{[l]}$. Thus, the reverse mathematical models illustrate that the back-propagation input is $dA^{[l]}$ and the outputs are $dA^{[l-1]}$, $dW^{[l]}$, and $db^{[l]}$. So, the goal from the back-propagation calculations is to obtain dW and db values for all ANNs layers. The back-propagation for the lth layer in ANNs model that have L layers can be represented as (Li et al., 2012; Ooyen & Nienhuis, 1992; Paola & Schowengerdt, 1995):

$$dA^{[L]} = \frac{\partial \mathcal{L}(y, \hat{y})}{\partial A^{[L]}} \tag{21}$$

$$dA^{[L]} = -\frac{y}{\hat{y}} + \frac{1-y}{1-\hat{y}} \tag{22}$$

$$dZ^{[l]} = dA^{[l]} \varnothing^{[l]'}\left(Z^{[l]}\right) \tag{23}$$

$$\varnothing^{[l]'}\left(Z^{[l]}\right) = \frac{\partial \varnothing^{[l]}\left(Z^{[l]}\right)}{\partial Z^{[l]}} \tag{24}$$

$$dW^{[l]} = \frac{\partial J}{\partial W^{[l]}} \tag{25}$$

$$dW^{[l]} = \frac{1}{m} dZ^{[l]} A^{[l-1]T} \tag{26}$$

$$db^{[l]} = \frac{\partial J}{\partial b^{[l]}} \tag{27}$$

$$db^{[l]} = \frac{1}{m} \sum dZ^{[l]} \tag{28}$$

$$dA^{[l-1]} = W^{[l]T} dZ^{[l]} \tag{29}$$

The Gradient Descent

The target of the training stage in any learning NNs model is the high correct predictions for the input data. The loss function and the cost function minimization is the guarantee to achieve that. So, the goal of iterate the previous calculations is to achieve the optimum model parameters (weights W and bias b). As mentioned before, the start with initializing these parameters; weights with random values and bias with zeros. Then, the forward-propagation, loss function, and back-propagation are used to update these model parameters through the gradient descent to achieve the targeted minimum loss value (Bottou, 1991; Dubey et al., 2019). The gradient descent can be considered as an optimization method for improving the learning models (including NNs) which is also called batch gradient descent optimization. The gradient descent can be represented by (Bottou, 1991; Dubey et al., 2019):

$$W^{[l]} = W^{[l]} - \alpha \frac{\partial J}{\partial W^{[l]}} \tag{30}$$

$$W^{[l]} = W^{[l]} - \alpha dW^{[l]} \tag{31}$$

$$b^{[l]} = b^{[l]} - \alpha \frac{\partial J}{\partial b^{[l]}} \tag{32}$$

$$b^{[l]} = b^{[l]} - \alpha db^{[l]} \qquad\qquad (33)$$

where α is the learning rate, it must be notice that the selection of α value is based on self-intuition where it is preferred to select a small value that must be less than 1 (Ruder, 2016; Bottou, 1991; Dubey et al., 2019).

The Learning Models Problems

Through running a learning algorithm, it may doesn't do as well as hoped, almost all the time, it will be because it has either a high bias problem or a high variance problem, in other words, either an under-fitting problem or an over-fitting problem. These two problems are considered as the main problems that can occur in supervised machine learning algorithms. To deal with these problems in the learning model, it is must divide the used dataset into training dataset which is 60% from dataset records, validation dataset which is 20% from dataset records, and test dataset which is 20% from dataset records. After solving the problem, the training dataset and the validation dataset, which are 80% from the dataset records, are together the training dataset, and then retrain the model with the suggested problem solution (Hawkins, 2004; Jabbar & Khan, 2015).

The Over-Fitting Problem

The over-fitting problem is that the learning model can fit 100% of training data well through prediction after the training process but can't predict the test data well. In this problem, the training set loss values will be low and the validation set loss values will be much greater than the training set loss values, it can be shown in the learning curves. There are three main solutions for these problems; the first solution is done by reducing the training features, the first layer neurons, thus it must fine select the features to be removed that can't affect the required data to train. This selection can be done manually or by model selection algorithm. The second solution is done by reducing the number of network layers and/or reducing neurons in one or more hidden layers. The Third solution is the regularization where it will be mentioned later in the ANNs improvements. There is another solution which is the increase of training data by using data augmentation; data augmentation will be mentioned later in the ANNs improvements (Hawkins, 2004; H. Zhang et al., 2019).

The Under-Fitting Problem

The under-fitting problem is that the learning model fails to predict the training data well after the training process. In this problem, the training set and validation set loss values will be high. There are three main solutions for these problems; the first solution is done by increasing the training features, the first layer neurons. It can be done by selecting some features and adding these features as new features after mathematical modification such as square or any other mathematical function. The second solution is done by increasing the training set data. It can be done by getting more training data. The third solution is done by increasing the number of network layers and/or increasing neurons in one or more hidden layers. There is another solution which is the decrease of the regularization hyper-parameters values if these values are high (Jabbar & Khan, 2015; H. Zhang et al., 2019).

IMPROVING DEEP NNS

Improving the NNs building models is very important to build high performance models. Whereas, it is essential to avoid problems of learning models to build well functioned models of NNs, this is done with these improvements. There are many stages that can be used to improve the NNs models; these stages can be used all or some of them according to the model problems and results. These stages are the regularizations and the optimization algorithms. This section illustrates these stages and the most commonly used hyper-parameters, regularizations, and optimizations in building the NNs learning models.

The Hyper-Parameters

There are many hyper-parameters which are used in learning models such as the learning rate α which is used in gradient descent, the suggested numbers of iterations, and regularization and optimization hyper-parameters. These hyper-parameters' values are determined by self-intuition. As mentioned before, it is preferred to select a small value for the learning rate α that must be less than 1. The other hyper-parameters will be mentioned later in the regularizations and optimizations sections where every hyper-parameter will be mentioned in the section that has been used in it with its preferred values.

The Regularization

The regularization is always used to prevent the over-fitting problem or high variance in learning models. There are many regularization methods that can be used through training NNs models; the widely used regularization methods are L1 and L2 regularization, the dropout regularization, data augmentation, and data normalization.

The L1 and L2 Regularization

The L1 and L2 regularizations are added terms to the cost function that depends on the network weights values. From (20) the cost function with L1 regularization can be represented as (Dialameh et al., 2020; Ng, 2004):

$$J\left(W,b\right) = \frac{1}{m}\sum_{i=1}^{m}\mathcal{L}\left(y^{(i)},\hat{y}^{(i)}\right) + \frac{\lambda}{2m}\sum_{l=1}^{L}W^{[l]} \tag{34}$$

$$W^{[l]} = \sum_{i=1}^{n^{[l]}}\sum_{j=1}^{n^{[l-1]}}\left(W_{ij}^{[l]}\right) \tag{35}$$

As well, the cost function with L2 regularization can be represented as (Dialameh et al., 2020; Ng, 2004):

$$J(W,b) = \frac{1}{m}\sum_{i=1}^{m}\mathcal{L}\left(y^{(i)},\hat{y}^{(i)}\right) + \frac{\lambda}{2m}\sum_{l=1}^{L}W^{[l]2} \tag{36}$$

$$W^{[l]2} = \sum_{i=1}^{n^{[l]}}\sum_{j=1}^{n^{[l-1]}}\left(W_{ij}^{[l]}\right)^2 \tag{37}$$

where L is the NNs layers, $n^{[l]}$ is the layer neurons, m is the training dataset records, λ is the regularization parameter and $W^{[l]}$ is the l th layer weights with dimension $\left(n^{[l]},n^{[l-1]}\right)$. The regularization parameter λ is considered as one of the used hyper-parameters for learning NNs models; it is determined by intuition as mentioned before. Increasing this parameter lead to increasing the cost function value then with using back-propagation and gradient descent the W and b will be small, on the other hand through training iterations the cost function $J(W,b)$ decreases monotonically after every elevation of gradient descent. It must be noticed that the L2 regularization is actually the more widely used regularization technique than the L1 regularization in training deep learning modules (Dialameh et al., 2020; Ng, 2004).

The Dropout Regularization

Dropout is a regularization method that approximates training a large number of NNs with different architectures in parallel which prevents the over-fitting problem and speeds up the training process at the same time. It looks like a crazy technique because the idea of dropout regularization is the random ignoring of some number of layer nodes "drop out" during the training of the NNs model. This has the effect of making the layer look-like and be treated-like a layer with a different number of nodes and connectivity to the prior layer. In effect, each update to a layer during training is performed with a different structure of the configured layer. That means it is a temporary removal for nodes through the training phase which is not used after training when making a prediction with the fit network (Srivastava et al., 2014). Dropout has the effect of making the training process noisy, forcing nodes within a layer to probabilistically take on more or less responsibility for the inputs. This conceptualization suggests that perhaps dropout breaks-up situations where network layers co-adapt to correct mistakes from prior layers, in turn making the model more robust (Srivastava et al., 2014). Like the L1 and L2 regularizations which implemented with a regularization parameter λ for each layer in the NNs, Dropout is implemented per-layer in NNs and the dropout rate also can vary from layer to layer in the same network. The dropout rate is considered as a one of the used hyper-parameters for learning NNs models; it is determined by intuition as mentioned before which indicates the ignored rate of layer neurons (Srivastava et al., 2014).

Data Augmentation

One way of preventing the over-fitting problems and the under-fitting problems is increasing the training data, but sometimes there is no data available for use in training or providing additional data has high cost. Thus, the data augmentation is the solution in this situation. So, data augmentation are techniques used to increase the amount of data by adding slightly modified copies of already existing data or newly created synthetic data from existing data which is widely used in computer vision (Shorten & Khoshgoftaar, 2019). Image data augmentation is perhaps the most well-known type of data augmentation and involves creating transformed versions of images in the training dataset that belong to the same class as the original image. Transforms include a range of operations from the field of image manipulation, such as shifts, flips, zooms, color modification, random cropping, rotation, noise injection, and much more. Image data augmentation is typically only applied to the training dataset, and not to the validation or test dataset. This is different from data preparation such as image resizing and pixel scaling; they must be performed consistently across all datasets that interact with the model (Shorten & Khoshgoftaar, 2019).

Data Normalization

Normalization is a technique often applied as part of data preparation for deep learning. The goal of normalization is to change the features values in the dataset to use a common scale, without distorting differences in the ranges of values or losing information. It is considered as one of the techniques that will speed up the training process. It is necessary to use the same scale for training records and test records in the dataset for the same NNs model. The input normalization can be represented as (Patro & Sahu, 2015):

$$X_{normalized} = \frac{X - \mu}{\sigma} \tag{38}$$

$$\mu = \frac{1}{m}\sum_{i=1}^{m}X^{(i)} \tag{39}$$

$$\sigma^2 = \frac{1}{m}\sum_{i=1}^{m}X^{(i)2} \tag{40}$$

where μ is the mean value and σ is the standard deviation.

The Optimization Algorithms

Optimization algorithm is a procedure which is executed iteratively by comparing various solutions till an optimum or a satisfactory solution is found. For deep learning, Optimization is the problem of finding a set of inputs to an objective function that is results in a maximum or minimum function evaluation (Maggiori et al., 2017; Qian, 1999; Kingma & Ba, 2015). The purpose of optimization is to achieve a high performance learning model that is has high ratio correct predictions. There are many optimization algorithms in deep learning; this section illustrates the widely used optimization algorithms in NNs models.

Mini-Batch Gradient Descent and SGD

The gradient descent, which is illustrated in section 2.4, is used to achieve the optimum values for the weights W and bias b. The model parameters updates are based on scanning all the training dataset records one time per iteration which is called batch gradient descent. So, in batch gradient descent, all the training data is taken into consideration to take a single step (iteration). The SGD is the same gradient descent calculations with a difference that just one record from the training dataset is considered as a single step, and then one scanning for all training dataset records is considered as one epoch (Maggiori et al., 2017). The mini-batch gradient descent is based on splitting the training dataset records into smaller training dataset records batches which is less than the actual dataset and called mini batches. The training algorithm that using mini-batch gradient descent is the same training algorithm that mentioned in section 2 but with some modifications as follows (Maggiori et al., 2017; Qian, 1999; Kingma & Ba, 2015):

1. Before step 4, the training dataset records are split into mini batches which each mini batch size is less than the actual training dataset records.
2. The steps from step 4 to step 7 are done for each mini batch.
3. The cost function calculation is done as mentioned before for each mini batch, and then the average cost function is calculated using (41).
4. The model parameters are updated for each mini bath using gradient descent.
5. The steps from step 8 to step 13 are done with the replacement of iterations by epochs.

In the mini-batch gradient descent the average cost function is calculated as (Maggiori et al., 2017):

$$J_{average}\left(W,b\right) = \frac{1}{T}\sum_{t=1}^{T} J_t\left(W,b\right) \qquad (41)$$

where T is the total number of mini batches and $J_t\left(W,b\right)$ is the cost function for mini batch t. It must be noticed that, if the mini batch size is one then the gradient descent is called SGD

SGD With Momentum

SGD with momentum is a method which helps accelerate gradient vectors in the right directions, thus leading to faster convergence. The SGD always works faster than the standard gradient descent algorithm (Maggiori et al., 2017; Qian, 1999). The main idea of SGD with momentum is to calculate the exponentially weighted average of model gradients and then use it to update the model parameters. It functions faster than the regular algorithm for the gradient descent. The exponentially weighted average is a type of moving average that places a greater weight and significance on the most recent data points (Maggiori et al., 2017; Qian, 1999). The exponentially weighted average deals with sequences of noisy data numbers S that required some kind of moving average to de-noise the data and bring it closer to the original function. So, the exponentially weighted averages define a new sequence V after removing noise as (Maggiori et al., 2017; Qian, 1999):

$$V_t = \beta V_{t-1} + \left(1 - \beta\right) S_t \tag{42}$$

where V_t is the tth number of new sequence data, S_t is the original sequence, β is random number where $\beta \in \left[0,1\right]$.

The SGD with momentum can be calculated by applying the exponentially weighted averages for NNs. As the new sequence calculations in the exponentially weighted averages, the velocity V is defined calculated as (Maggiori et al., 2017; Qian, 1999):

$$V_{dW}^{[l]} = \beta V_{dW}^{[l]} + \left(1 - \beta\right) dW^{[l]} \tag{43}$$

$$V_{db}^{[l]} = \beta V_{db}^{[l]} + \left(1 - \beta\right) db^{[l]} \tag{44}$$

where V_{dW} is the weight gradient velocity and V_{db} is the bias gradient velocity which are initialized by zero in the first epoch, β is considered as momentum hyper-parameter which is determined by intuition as mentioned before where $\beta \in \left[0,1\right]$, and l is the NNs layer number. Then, the model parameters are updated using the SGD with momentum as (Maggiori et al., 2017; Qian, 1999):

$$W^{[l]} = W^{[l]} - \alpha V_{dW}^{[l]} \tag{45}$$

$$b^{[l]} = b^{[l]} - \alpha V_{db}^{[l]} \tag{46}$$

where α is the leaning rate.

Adam Optimizer

In 2015, Kingma and Ba (2015) proposed the Adam optimizer, which can be used instead of the SGD to update network weights iteratively based on training data, in their ICLR 2015 conference paper (poster presented). The algorithm is called Adam which this name is derived from adaptive moment estimation. The Adam optimization algorithm is an extension to the SGD that has recently seen broader adoption for deep learning applications in computer vision and natural language processing. Adam is described as a combination of the advantages of two other extensions of SGD which realizes the benefits of both; AdaGrad and RMSprop (Maggiori et al., 2017; Kingma & Ba, 2015). The AdaGrad maintains a per-parameter learning rate that improves performance on problems with sparse gradients (e.g. natural language and computer vision problems) and the RMSProp maintains per-parameter learning rates that are adapted based on the average of recent magnitudes of the gradients for the weight (e.g. how quickly it is changing) (Maggiori et al., 2017; Kingma & Ba, 2015). Instead of the SGD with momentum, Adam algorithm defines the average of the first moments (the mean) and the average of the second moments (the un-centered variance) of the gradients. The Adam algorithm calculates an exponential moving average of the gradient V and an exponential moving average of the squared gradient S, which the parameters β_1 and β_2 control the decay rates of these moving averages. These calculations are represented as (Maggiori et al., 2017; Kingma & Ba, 2015):

$$V_{dW}^{[l]} = \beta_1 V_{dW}^{[l]} + \left(1 - \beta_1\right) dW^{[l]} \tag{47}$$

$$V_{db}^{[l]} = \beta_1 V_{db}^{[l]} + \left(1 - \beta_1\right) db^{[l]} \tag{48}$$

$$S_{dW}^{[l]} = \beta_2 S_{dW}^{[l]} + \left(1 - \beta_2\right) dW^{[l]2} \tag{49}$$

$$S_{db}^{[l]} = \beta_2 S_{db}^{[l]} + \left(1 - \beta_2\right) db^{[l]2} \tag{50}$$

where V_{dW} is the weight gradient moving average, V_{db} is the bias gradient moving average, S_{dW} is the weight squared gradient moving average, and S_{db} is the bias squared gradient moving average which are initialized by zero in the first epoch, β_1 and β_2 are considered as momentum hyper-parameter which are determined by intuition as mentioned before where $\beta_1, \beta_2 \in \left[0,1\right]$, and l is the NNs layer number.

Then, it must implement the gradients correction. So, the corrected average of the gradient $V^{corrected}$ and moving average of the squared gradient $S^{corrected}$ are calculated by (Maggiori et al., 2017; Kingma & Ba, 2015):

$$V_{dW}^{[l]\ corrected} = \frac{V_{dW}^{[l]}}{\left(1 - \beta_1^{\ t}\right)} \tag{51}$$

$$V_{db}^{[l]corrected} = \frac{V_{db}^{[l]}}{\left(1 - \beta_1^{\ t}\right)} \tag{52}$$

$$S_{dW}^{[l]\ corrected} = \frac{S_{dW}^{[l]}}{\left(1 - \beta_2^{\ t}\right)} \tag{53}$$

$$S_{db}^{[l]corrected} = \frac{S_{db}^{[l]}}{\left(1 - \beta_2^{~t}\right)} \tag{54}$$

where t is the iteration (epoch) number if t iterations (epochs) are done. Then the model parameters are updated using the Adam optimizer as (Maggiori et al., 2017; Kingma & Ba, 2015):

$$W^{[l]} = W^{[l]} - \alpha \frac{V_{dW}^{[l]~corrected}}{\sqrt{S_{dW}^{[l]~corrected}} - \varepsilon} \tag{55}$$

$$b^{[l]} = b^{[l]} - \alpha \frac{V_{db}^{[l]corrected}}{\sqrt{S_{db}^{[l]corrected}} - \varepsilon} \tag{56}$$

where α is the leaning rate and ε is one of Adam's optimizer hyper-parameters. Finally, it must be notified that the authors that proposed the Adam optimizer paper recommended some hyper-parameters values; these values are $\beta_1 = 0.9$, $\beta_2 = 0.999$, and $\varepsilon = 10^{-8}$, but these recommendations are not binding, that means the model designer can change any of these values according to the model design (Kingma & Ba, 2015).

THE CNNS

The CNNs are possessed from the ANNs with the exclusion that there are not fully connected layers (Yamashita et al., 2018). CNNs are considered as the magic solution for many computer vision problems. The CNNs depend on some filters that reduce the image height and width and increase the number of channels, then producing the output with FC layers which reduce the input layer neurons, reduce training time, and increase the training model performance (Yamashita et al., 2018). These filter values are initialized with many random functions which can be optimized. The filters design is based on the use of self-intuition as with the ANNs structure design and learning hyper-parameters coefficient choice, which increases the difficulty to reach the best solution for the learning problems (Yamashita et al., 2018; AlAfandy et al., 2020a).

Like the ANNs, the CNNs are deemed as nonlinear statistical data modeling tools where the complex relationships between inputs and outputs are modeled. The CNNs network consists of some blocks each block contains a set of filters which are in different types, ending with one or more FC layers. Filters' types are the convolution filters, the activation filters, and the pooling filters where each block can consist of one or more filters from one or more types (Yamashita et al., 2018; Albawi et al., 2017). Thus, the first convolution filter in the first block is considered CNNs input and the last FC layer is considered CNNs output. Like the ANNs, the given dataset inputs and outputs must have a mathematical relation which the outputs are predicted within discrete function for classification models or continuous function for regression models where this mathematical model is also based on the CNNs structure, design, filters types and values, stride, and padding (Yamashita et al., 2018; Albawi et al., 2017; AlAfandy et al., 2020b).

- **Stride** is the number of pixels shifts over the input matrix, then filters are moved to s pixels at a time where s is the stride number. In CNNs stride denotes how many moving pixels in each step in convolution (Albawi et al., 2017). Figure 7 shows convolution stride with $s = 2$.

Figure 7. Convolution stride with $s = 2$

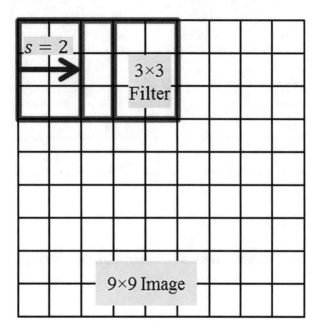

- **Padding** is a term relevant to CNNs as it refers to the amount of pixels added to an image when it is being processed by the kernel of a CNN. For example, if the padding in a CNN is set to zero, then every pixel value that is added will be of value zero. With "SAME" padding; if using a stride of 1, the layer's outputs will have the same spatial dimensions as its inputs where with "VALID" padding; there are no "made-up" padding inputs. The layer only uses valid input data (Albawi et al., 2017). Figure 8 shows one layer zero padding.

Figure 8. One more layer "SAME" padding example

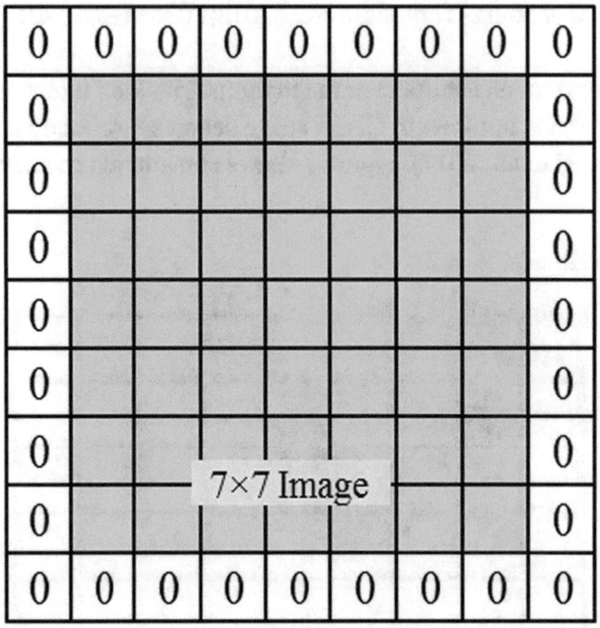

0	0	0	0	0	0	0	0	0
0								0
0								0
0								0
0								0
0								0
0			7×7 Image					0
0								0
0	0	0	0	0	0	0	0	0

The Layers Types in CNNs

Before elucidating the CNNs and its structure and mathematics, the layers types that used in CNNs must be demonstrated.

Activation Layer

The activation layers are a non-linear transformation building block of CNNs structure, which can use any of the activation functions that are mentioned in section 2.1. In CNNs, it is usually applied on convolution layers outputs. ReLU is the most commonly used activation in CNNs.

Convolution Layer

The convolution layers are the main building block of CNNs structure, which are small matrices that are slid over the image. For applying convolution filter with shape (f, f), which convolution filter shape f must be an odd number, on a (n, n) matrix with padding p and stride s the output shape is (z, z) where (Gad, 2018)

$$z = \text{floor}(z) \tag{57}$$

$$z = \frac{n + 2p - f}{s} + 1 \qquad\qquad (58)$$

Figure 9. How the convolution filters work

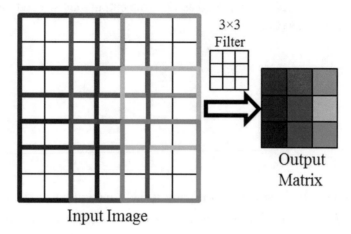

The idea of convolution filters is taken from the edge detection with the difference that the used convolution filters values in the CNNs are initialized by random values then are updated by back-propagation and optimization algorithms not as edge detection which uses one of some known filters with known values. Each cell in the output matrix after applying a convolution filter is calculated as shown in figure 9 (Gad, 2018). Figure 10 presents a numerical example of applying convolution on a $(6,6)$ matrix with a $(3,3)$ convolution filter and $s = 1$.

Figure 10. A numerical example of applying convolution

3	0	2	1	7	4
1	5	8	2	6	9
2	7	2	8	5	10
0	1	3	9	14	9
4	2	1	7	5	13
2	4	5	13	8	6

×

1	0	-1
1	0	-1
1	0	1

=

-6	1	-6	-12
-10	-6	-12	-9
0	-14	-18	-8
-3	-22	-18	1

In the case of applying convolution on an RGB image with shape $(n, n, 3)$, the used convolution filter's shape must be $(f, f, 3)$. So, the convolution filter must have the same image channels. It can be used more than one convolution filter on the same image but it must have the same shape, in the case of using n_C convolution filters, the output shape is $\left(z, z, n_C\right)$ (Yamashita et al., 2018; Gad, 2018). Figure 11 shows an example of using convolution filters on an RGB image.

The convolution layer in the CNNs mathematical model is similar to the ANNs mathematical model with the difference that the convolution layers are not fully connected. So, for input matrix $A^{[l-1]}$, convolution filters are applied which considered as $W^{[l]}$, the output must added to bias $b^{[l]}$, and then the activation layer must applied as (Gad, 2018):

$$A^{[l]} = \varnothing\left(W^{[l]} * A^{[l-1]} + b^{[l]}\right) \tag{59}$$

$$A^{[l]} = \varnothing\left(Z^{[l]}\right) \tag{60}$$

where $\varnothing$ is the activation function which is usually ReLU function but it can be another activation function according to design and $Z^{[l]}$ is the convolution output without activation.

Figure 11. An example of using convolution filters on an RGB image

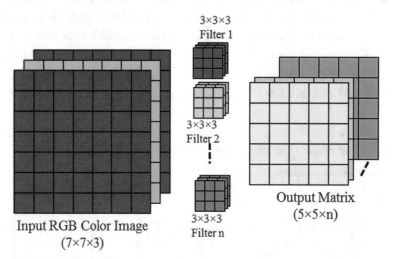

Then the convolution channel output by using one convolution filter CF with shape $\left(f, f\right)$ can be represented as (Yamashita et al., 2018; Gad, 2018):

$$A^{[l]}_{ij} = \varnothing\left(\sum_{fi=0}^{f^{[l]}-1}\sum_{fj=0}^{f^{[l]}-1}\sum_{c=1}^{n_C^{[l-1]}}\left(CF_{fi,fj,c} * A^{[l-1]}_{i+fi,j+fj,c}\right) + b^{[l]}\right) \tag{61}$$

It results that the convolution output channels are equal to the number of the used filters. So, for convolution layer l where $f^{[l]}$ is filter size, $p^{[l]}$ is padding, $s^{[l]}$ is stride, $n_C^{[l]}$ is number of filters, m is the input dataset records, $\left(f^{[l]}, f^{[l]}, n_C^{[l-1]}\right)$ is the shape of each filter for $n_C^{[l]}$ filters, and input $A^{[l-1]}$ shape is $\left(m, n_H^{[l-1]}, n_W^{[l-1]}, n_C^{[l-1]}\right)$, and the results shapes are $\left(f^{[l]}, f^{[l]}, n_C^{[l-1]}, n_C^{[l]}\right)$ for weights $W^{[l]}$, $\left(1,1,1,n_C^{[l]}\right)$ for bias $b^{[l]}$, and $\left(m, n_H^{[l]}, n_W^{[l]}, n_C^{[l]}\right)$ for convolution output or activations $A^{[l]}$ (Albawi et al., 2017; Gad, 2018). $n_H^{[l]}$ and $n_W^{[l]}$ are calculated as (Lecun et al., 1998):

$$n_H^{[l]} = \frac{n_H^{[l-1]} + 2p^{[l]} - f^{[l]}}{s^{[l]}} + 1 \tag{62}$$

$$n_W^{[l]} = \frac{n_W^{[l-1]} + 2p^{[l]} - f^{[l]}}{s^{[l]}} + 1 \tag{63}$$

The learning parameters here are $W^{[l]}$ and $b^{[l]}$. Thus, it must be well selected to achieve a high performance learning model (Yamashita et al., 2018; Albawi et al., 2017; Gad, 2018).

Pooling Layer

The pooling layers are another building block of CNNs structure. Pooling is a function that progressively reduces the spatial size of the representation to reduce the amount of parameters and speed the computation in the network. Pooling layer is added after the convolutional layer and the activation layer, it has been applied to the convolutional output and operates on each feature map independently (Yamashita et al., 2018; Gad, 2018). The pooling filter can act as maximum pooling or average pooling. For applying pooling $\left(f, f\right)$ filter, which pooling filters shape f can be an odd or even number, on a $\left(n, n\right)$ matrix with padding p and stride s the output shape is $\left(z, z\right)$ where can be calculated as (57) and (58). Each cell in the output matrix after applying maximum or average pooling filter is calculated as shown in figure 12 (Gad, 2018).

Figure 12. How the pooling filters work

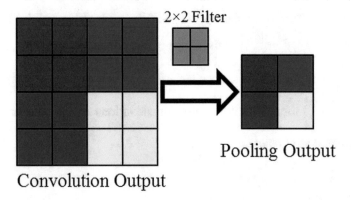

2×2 Filter

Pooling Output

Convolution Output

Figures 13 and 14 present a numerical example of applying maximum pooling and a numerical example of applying average pooling respectively, with $(2,2)$ pooling filter and $s=2$, on the convolution output matrix that is in figure 10.

Figure 13. An example of applying maximum pooling

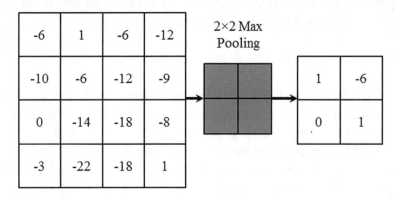

Figure 14. An example of applying average pooling

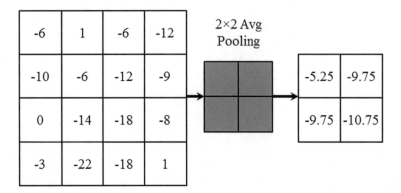

In the case of applying maximum or average pooling on a multi-channels matrix with shape $\left(n, n, n_C\right)$, the used pooling filter's shape must $\left(f, f, n_C\right)$. So, the pooling filter must have the same matrix channels number, the output shape is $\left(z, z, n_C\right)$ (Gad, 2018). Figure 15 shows an example of using pooling filters on a multi-channels matrix.

For pooling layer l where $f^{[l]}$ is filter size, $p^{[l]}$ is padding, $s^{[l]}$ is stride, $n_C^{[l]}$ is number of filters, m is the input dataset records, $\left(f^{[l]}, f^{[l]}, n_C^{[l]}\right)$ is the pooling filter shape, and input $A^{[l-1]}$ shape is $\left(m, n_H^{[l-1]}, n_W^{[l-1]}, n_C^{[l]}\right)$, the result shape is $\left(m, n_H^{[l]}, n_W^{[l]}, n_C^{[l]}\right)$ for pooling output $A^{[l]}$ where $n_H^{[l]}$ and $n_W^{[l]}$ are calculated as (62) and (63) (Yamashita et al., 2018; Albawi et al., 2017; Gad, 2018; Lecun et al., 1998). The padding in pooling layers is very rarely used which is usually equal to zero. In pooling layers, there are no parameters to learn. On the other hand there are two other pooling types that can be applied on multi-channels matrices; global maximum pooling and global average pooling whose results are one dimensional array, each cell is equal to the average or the maximum of each channel according to the used pooling type. So, in case of applying global maximum pooling or global average pooling on a multi-channels matrix with shape $\left(n, n, n_C\right)$ the output shape is $\left(1, n_C\right)$ which is one dimension array (Yamashita et al., 2018; Gad, 2018).

Figure 15. An example of using pooling filters on a convoluted RGB image

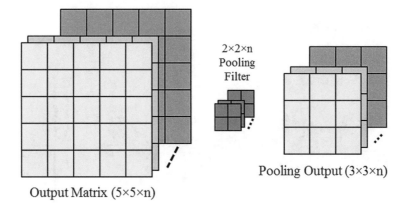

Output Matrix (5×5×n)

2×2×n Pooling Filter

Pooling Output (3×3×n)

Simple CNNs Model Example

This section offers a simple example of CNNs network; this network is quite similar to one of classic networks called LeNet (Lecun et al., 1998). The input image shape is $\left(32, 32, 3\right)$. The first layer consists of 6 convolution filters (Conv1), with ReLU activation, with shape $\left(5, 5\right)$ and stride $= 1$ which results a matrix with shape $\left(28, 28, 6\right)$, and then max pooling filter (Pool1) with shape $\left(2, 2\right)$ and stride $= 2$ which results a matrix with shape $\left(14, 14, 6\right)$. The second layer consists of 16 convolution filters (Conv2), with ReLU activation, with shape $\left(5, 5\right)$ and stride $= 1$ which results a matrix with shape $\left(10, 10, 16\right)$, and then max pooling filter (Pool2) with shape $(2,2)$ and stride $= 2$ which results a matrix with shape $(5,5,16)$. The second layer output is flattened which results 400 neurons, then the third layer is a FC layer (FC3) with 120 neurons and ReLU activation, then the fourth layer is a FC layer (FC4) with 84 neurons and ReLU activation, and then the output layer is a FC layer ($\hat{y}$) with 10 neurons (classes) and softmax activation. Table 1 and figure 16 show this simple example.

Table 1. A CNNs simple example

Layers	The CNNs	Activation	Output Shape	Output Size
Input	RGB image (32,32)		(32,32,3)	3072
Conv1	5×5 conv 6, stride 1	ReLU	(28,28,6)	4704
Pool1	2×2 max pool, stride 2		(14,14,6)	1176
Conv2	5×5 conv 16, stride 1	ReLU	(10,10,16)	1600
Pool2	2×2 max pool, stride 2		(5,5,16)	400
FC3	FC with 120 neurons	ReLU	(1,120)	120
FC4	FC with 84 neurons	ReLU	(1,84)	84
Output	FC with 10 neurons	Softmax	(1,10)	10

Figure 16. A CNNs simple example

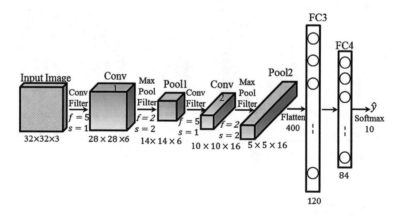

CNNs Back-Propagation

The learning parameters for CNNs $W^{[l]}$ and $b^{[l]}$, that mentioned in section 4.1.2, must be optimized to achieve high performance learning models. Thus, back-propagation algorithms can also be used for the CNNs as in the ANNs case. Back-propagation is rarely used for CNNs where it is used for sophisticated models. In the CNNs, the back-propagation algorithm is the same in the ANNs that mentioned in section 2.3 with the difference that the convolution layers and the pooling layers derivative calculations where the CNNs contain convolution layers and pooling layers in addition with FC layers and activation layers such as the ANNs (Wei et al., 2017; Z. Zhang, 2016).

For the convolution layer, by using (60) and (61) the convolution derivative can be represented as (Wei et al., 2017; Z. Zhang, 2016):

$$dW^{[l]}_{f,f} = \frac{\partial J}{\partial W^{[l]}_{f,f}} = \sum_{i=0}^{n_H^{[l-1]}}\sum_{j=0}^{n_W^{[l-1]}} \frac{\partial J}{\partial A^{[l]}_{i,j}} \frac{\partial A^{[l]}_{i,j}}{\partial W^{[l]}_{f,f}} \tag{64}$$

$$dW^{[l]}_{f,f} = \sum_{i=0}^{n_H^{[l-1]}}\sum_{j=0}^{n_W^{[l-1]}} \Delta^{[l]}_{i,j} \frac{\partial A^{[l]}_{i,j}}{\partial W^{[l]}_{f,f}} \tag{65}$$

$$db^{[l]} = \frac{\partial J}{\partial b^{[l]}} = \sum_{i=0}^{n_H^{[l-1]}}\sum_{j=0}^{n_W^{[l-1]}} \frac{\partial J}{\partial A^{[l]}_{i,j}} \frac{\partial A^{[l]}_{i,j}}{\partial b^{[l]}} \tag{66}$$

where $\Delta^{[l]}_{i,j} = \frac{\partial J}{\partial A^{[l]}_{i,j}}$ and refer to the change in the input single pixel (in image) or single cell (in matrix) which affected by the loss function and $\frac{\partial A^{[l]}_{i,j}}{\partial b^{[l]}} = 1$ (Wei et al., 2017; Z. Zhang, 2016).

$$\frac{\partial A^{[l]}_{ij}}{\partial W^{[l]}_{f,f}} = \frac{\partial}{\partial W^{[l]}_{f,f}}\left(\sum_{fi=0}^{f^{[l]}-1}\sum_{fj=0}^{f^{[l]}-1}\sum_{c=1}^{n_C^{[l-1]}}\left(CF_{fi,fj,c} * A^{[l-1]}_{i+fi,j+fj,c}\right) + b^{[l]}\right) \tag{67}$$

$$\frac{\partial A^{[l]}_{ij}}{\partial W^{[l]}_{f,f}} = A^{[l-1]}_{i+f,j+f} \tag{68}$$

$$dW^{[l]}_{f,f} = \frac{\partial J}{\partial W^{[l]}_{f,f}} = \sum_{i=0}^{n_H^{[l-1]}}\sum_{j=0}^{n_W^{[l-1]}} \Delta^{[l]}_{i,j} * A^{[l-1]}_{i+f,j+f} \tag{69}$$

$$db^{[l]} = \sum_{i=0}^{n_H^{[l-1]}} \sum_{j=0}^{n_W^{[l-1]}} \Delta^{[l]}_{i,j} \tag{70}$$

From (64) and (65) we found that (Wei et al., 2017; Z. Zhang, 2016):

$$\Delta^{[l]}_{i,j} = \sum_{fi=0}^{f-1} \sum_{fj=0}^{f-1} \Delta^{[l+1]}_{i-fi,j-fj} W^{[l+1]}_{fi,fj} A^{[l]}_{ij} \tag{71}$$

As mentioned before, there are no parameters to be learned in pooling layers. Finally, the learning parameters updates can be done as in ANNs.

CLASSIC NETWORKS

Classic networks have seemed as CNNs deep networks with particular construction, which can give rise to rising precisions in the classification issues, this chapter will utilize four well-known classic networks; these networks are the VGG model, the ResNet model, the DenseNet model, and the NASNet model.

The VGG Models

Simonyan and Zisserman (2015) proposed the VGG network in the ICLR conference. The first step was to look at how the depth of the convolution network affected its accuracy in the context of large-scale image interpretation. Authors tested the deeper network architecture with extremely small (3,3) convolution filters, and found that expanding the depth to 16-19 weight layers yields in expressive increase over prior-art setups.

VGG models are deep convolutional networks that have been trained using the ImageNet dataset. The network's input images are shaped (224,224,3). This network is made up of five convolution blocks, each of which has convolution layers and a pooling layer, followed by two FC hidden layers with ReLU activation (each layer has 4096 neurons) and a softmax output layer (1000 classes). Table 2 shows the VGG models architecture with the ImageNet pre-trained weights, every convolution layer is followed by ReLU activation layer.

Table 2. The VGG models structures

A	A-LRN	B	C	D	E
11 weights layers	11 weights layers	13 weights layers	16 weights layers	16 weights layers	19 weights layers
133 parameters	133 parameters	133 parameters	134 parameters	138 parameters	144 parameters
Input Image (224×224×3)					
Conv3-64 stride = 1	Conv3-64 LRN stride = 1	Conv3-64 Conv3-64 stride = 1	Conv3-64 Conv3-64 stride = 1	Conv3-64 Conv3-64 stride = 1	Conv3-64 Conv3-64 stride = 1
Conv3-128 stride = 1	Conv3-128 stride = 1	Conv3-128 Conv3-128 stride = 1	Conv3-128 Conv3-128 stride = 1	Conv3-128 Conv3-128 stride = 1	Conv3-128 Conv3-128 stride = 1
Max pool, 2×2, stride = 2					
Conv3-256 Conv3-256 stride = 1	Conv3-256 Conv3-256 stride = 1	Conv3-256 Conv3-256 stride = 1	Conv3-256 Conv3-256 Conv1-256 stride = 1	Conv3-256 Conv3-256 Conv3-256 stride = 1	Conv3-256 Conv3-256 Conv3-256 Conv3-256 stride = 1
Max pool, 2×2, stride = 2					
Conv3-512 Conv3-512 stride = 1	Conv3-512 Conv3-512 stride = 1	Conv3-512 Conv3-512 stride = 1	Conv3-512 Conv3-512 Conv1-512 stride = 1	Conv3-512 Conv3-512 Conv3-512 stride = 1	Conv3-512 Conv3-512 Conv3-512 Conv3-512 stride = 1
Max pool, 2×2, stride = 2					
Conv3-512 Conv3-512 stride = 1	Conv3-512 Conv3-512 stride = 1	Conv3-512 Conv3-512 stride = 1	Conv3-512 Conv3-512 Conv1-512 stride = 1	Conv3-512 Conv3-512 Conv3-512 stride = 1	Conv3-512 Conv3-512 Conv3-512 Conv3-512 stride = 1
Max pool, 2×2, stride = 2					
FC-4096					
FC-4096					
FC-1000 (Softmax)					

The ResNet Models

He et al. (2016) proposed the ResNet models in the CPVR conference. A deep residual learning framework is exhibited by authors. From authors' suggestion, authors hope to make it easier to train networks in a more in-depth manner than before. This proposed learning paradigm can help with the problem of degradation. Authors permitted these layers to deliberately appropriate a residual mapping rather than assuming that every small number of stacked layers clearly appropriated the ideal underlying mapping.

Figure 17. One building block in the ResNet model

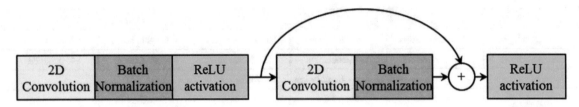

ResNet is based on the concept of creating bypass connections, which connect the deep layers while bypassing non-linear transformation layers. The block output $H(X)$ is the sum of these connections' outputs and the outputs of the network stack layers.

$$H(X) = F(X) + X \qquad (72)$$

where X is the connections' outputs and $F(X)$ is the network stack layer's outputs.

The one building block in the ResNet models is shown in figure 17 and the ResNet models structure with the ImageNet pre-trained weights are presented in tables 3 where all convolution filters are with stride of 2.

Table 3. The ResNet models structures

Layer Name	18-layer	34-layer	50-layer	101-layer	152-layer
Input layer	Input Image (224×224×3)				
Conv_1_x	Conv7-64, stride = 2				
	Max pool, 3×3, stride = 2				
Conv_2_x	$\begin{bmatrix} \text{Conv3}-64 \\ \text{Conv3}-64 \end{bmatrix} \times 2$	$\begin{bmatrix} \text{Conv3}-64 \\ \text{Conv3}-64 \end{bmatrix} \times 3$	$\begin{bmatrix} \text{Conv1}-64 \\ \text{Conv3}-64 \\ \text{Conv1}-256 \end{bmatrix} \times 3$	$\begin{bmatrix} \text{Conv1}-64 \\ \text{Conv3}-64 \\ \text{Conv1}-256 \end{bmatrix} \times 3$	$\begin{bmatrix} \text{Conv1}-64 \\ \text{Conv3}-64 \\ \text{Conv1}-256 \end{bmatrix} \times 3$
Conv_3_x	$\begin{bmatrix} \text{Conv3}-128 \\ \text{Conv3}-128 \end{bmatrix} \times 2$	$\begin{bmatrix} \text{Conv3}-128 \\ \text{Conv3}-128 \end{bmatrix} \times 4$	$\begin{bmatrix} \text{Conv1}-128 \\ \text{Conv3}-128 \\ \text{Conv1}-512 \end{bmatrix} \times 4$	$\begin{bmatrix} \text{Conv1}-128 \\ \text{Conv3}-128 \\ \text{Conv1}-512 \end{bmatrix} \times 4$	$\begin{bmatrix} \text{Conv1}-128 \\ \text{Conv3}-128 \\ \text{Conv1}-512 \end{bmatrix} \times 8$
Conv_4_x	$\begin{bmatrix} \text{Conv3}-256 \\ \text{Conv3}-256 \end{bmatrix} \times 2$	$\begin{bmatrix} \text{Conv3}-256 \\ \text{Conv3}-256 \end{bmatrix} \times 6$	$\begin{bmatrix} \text{Conv1}-128 \\ \text{Conv3}-128 \\ \text{Conv1}-1024 \end{bmatrix} \times 6$	$\begin{bmatrix} \text{Conv1}-256 \\ \text{Conv3}-256 \\ \text{Conv1}-1024 \end{bmatrix} \times 23$	$\begin{bmatrix} \text{Conv1}-256 \\ \text{Conv3}-256 \\ \text{Conv1}-1024 \end{bmatrix} \times 36$
Conv_5_x	$\begin{bmatrix} \text{Conv3}-512 \\ \text{Conv3}-512 \end{bmatrix} \times 2$	$\begin{bmatrix} \text{Conv3}-512 \\ \text{Conv3}-512 \end{bmatrix} \times 3$	$\begin{bmatrix} \text{Conv1}-512 \\ \text{Conv3}-512 \\ \text{Conv1}-2048 \end{bmatrix} \times 3$	$\begin{bmatrix} \text{Conv1}-512 \\ \text{Conv3}-512 \\ \text{Conv1}-2048 \end{bmatrix} \times 3$	$\begin{bmatrix} \text{Conv1}-512 \\ \text{Conv3}-512 \\ \text{Conv1}-2048 \end{bmatrix} \times 3$
Classification layer	Global average pool, 7×7				
	FC-1000 (Softmax)				

The DenseNet Models

Huang et al. (2017) proposed the DenseNet models in the CPVR conference. The first step was to conduct a study on the impact of any linkages between CNN layers, which was prepared by the authors. The authors then attempted to build deep CNNs with shorter links between layers near the input and output. Deep CNNs models, which have shorter links between layers, are more effective and precise to train, according to the results (the closest example is The ResNets). The ResNets have skip-connections among deep layers which bypass nonlinear transformation layers. Other than the ResNets, the DenseNets have full layers connections. Any layer in DenseNets has direct connections to the other subsequent layers. So the lth layer obtains the function charts of all previous layers X_0 to X_{l-1} as:

$$X_l = H_l\big([X_0, X_1, \ldots, X_{l-1}]\big) \tag{73}$$

where $[X_0, X_1, \ldots, X_{l-1}]$ refers to the feature-map spectrum produced in the layers $0, 1, \ldots, l-1$.

Figure 18. One building block in the DenseNet model

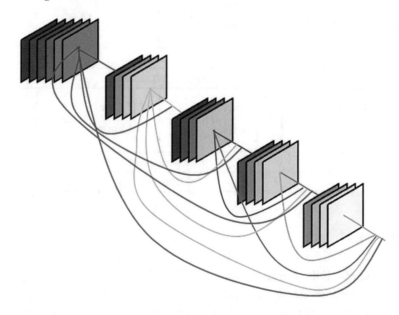

Table 4 shows the DenseNet models structure with the ImageNet pre-trained weights which The growth rate for all the networks was $k = 32$. Figure 18 shows the 5-layers dense block structure.

Table 4. The DenseNet models structures

Layer Name	DenseNet-121	DenseNet-169	DenseNet-201	DenseNet-264
Input layer	\multicolumn{4}{Input Image (224×224×3)}
Convolution	Conv7, stride = 2			
Pooling	Max pool, 3×3, stride = 2			
Denseblock (1)	$\begin{bmatrix} \text{Conv1} \\ \text{Conv3} \end{bmatrix} \times 6$	$\begin{bmatrix} \text{Conv1} \\ \text{Conv3} \end{bmatrix} \times 6$	$\begin{bmatrix} \text{Conv1} \\ \text{Conv3} \end{bmatrix} \times 6$	$\begin{bmatrix} \text{Conv1} \\ \text{Conv3} \end{bmatrix} \times 6$
Transition layer (1)	Conv1			
	Avg pool, 2×2, stride = 2			
Denseblock (2)	$\begin{bmatrix} \text{Conv1} \\ \text{Conv3} \end{bmatrix} \times 12$	$\begin{bmatrix} \text{Conv1} \\ \text{Conv3} \end{bmatrix} \times 12$	$\begin{bmatrix} \text{Conv1} \\ \text{Conv3} \end{bmatrix} \times 12$	$\begin{bmatrix} \text{Conv1} \\ \text{Conv3} \end{bmatrix} \times 12$
Transition layer (2)	Conv1			
	Avg pool, 2×2, stride = 2			
Denseblock (3)	$\begin{bmatrix} \text{Conv1} \\ \text{Conv3} \end{bmatrix} \times 24$	$\begin{bmatrix} \text{Conv1} \\ \text{Conv3} \end{bmatrix} \times 32$	$\begin{bmatrix} \text{Conv1} \\ \text{Conv3} \end{bmatrix} \times 48$	$\begin{bmatrix} \text{Conv1} \\ \text{Conv3} \end{bmatrix} \times 64$
Transition layer (3)	Conv1			
	Avg pool, 2×2, stride = 2			
Denseblock (4)	$\begin{bmatrix} \text{Conv1} \\ \text{Conv3} \end{bmatrix} \times 16$	$\begin{bmatrix} \text{Conv1} \\ \text{Conv3} \end{bmatrix} \times 32$	$\begin{bmatrix} \text{Conv1} \\ \text{Conv3} \end{bmatrix} \times 32$	$\begin{bmatrix} \text{Conv1} \\ \text{Conv3} \end{bmatrix} \times 48$
Classification layer	Global average pool, 7×7			
	FC-1000 (Softmax)			

The NASNet Models

Zoph and Le (2017) proposed the NASNet models in the ICLR conference. Authors studied a method to learn the model architectures directly on the dataset of interest. Therefore, authors proposed to search an architectural building block on a small dataset then transfer the block to a large dataset. They utilized the reinforcement learning search method to search for the best convolutional layer or cell on CIFAR-10 first, and then apply this cell to the ImageNet by stacking together more copies of this cell. The used cells in these achieved architectures are called normal cell and reduction cell. Normal cells are convolutional cells that return a feature map of the same dimension where reduction cells are convolutional cells that return a feature map where the feature map height and width is reduced by a factor of two. The controller RNNs is utilized to search the architectures of normal and reduction cells only. Figure 19 shows the controller model architecture for recursively constructing one block of a convolutional cell. For the ImageNet dataset achieved architecture.

Figure 19. The controller model architecture for recursively constructing one block of a convolutional cell

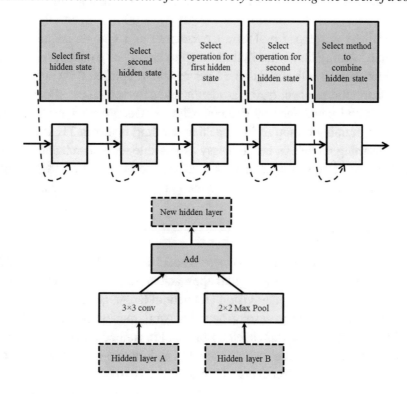

TECHNICAL TRICKS

In deep learning, it turns out that a lot of NNs are finicky to replicate because more things such as a lot of details about tuning of the hyper-parameters like the learning decay, optimization algorithms, activation functions, the required huge amount of data for training, the sophisticated hardware required for training, and other things that make some difference to the performance. It is not recommended to train a learning model from scratch; it may take many days, weeks, or months with the condition that the required hardware and huge training data are available. So, this section outlines some technical tricks which can be used to facilitate and to accelerate the learning process.

Open Source Implementations

Open source is an expression referred to open source software. Open source software is a code that is designed to be publicly accessible for free. So, anyone can see, modify, and distribute this code. In machine learning and deep learning, a lot of researchers routinely open source their work on the Internet, such as on GitHub. On the other hand there are open source libraries for machine learning and deep learning such as TF, Scikit-learn, and Keras. These libraries are available and easy to deal with the widely used programming languages such as MATLAB and Python.

TF is an open-source end-to-end platform for creating machine learning and deep learning applications which is created by the Google Brain team. It is a symbolic math library that uses dataflow and differentiable programming to perform various tasks focused on training and inference of the DNNs (Gad, 2018).

Scikit-learn is initially developed by David Cournapeau as a Google summer of code project in 2007. It a free machine learning library for Python and provides a range of supervised and unsupervised machine learning algorithms. It is licensed under a permissive simplified BSD license and is distributed under many Linux distributions, encouraging academic and commercial use (Pedregosa et al., 2011).

Keras is developed and maintained by François Chollet (Google Engineer). It is a deep learning API written in Python, running on top of the machine learning platform TF. It is developed to make implementing deep learning models as fast and easy as possible for research and development. It runs on Python 3.3 to 3.8, operating system Windows 7 or later or Mac 10.12.6 (Sierra) or later, and can seamlessly execute on GPUs and CPUs given the underlying frameworks (Ketkar, 2017).

Transfer Learning

Transfer learning is a machine learning method where a model developed for a task is reused as the starting point for a model on a second task. It is a popular approach in deep learning where pre-trained models are used as the starting point on computer vision and natural language processing tasks given the vast compute and time resources required to develop neural network models on these problems and from the huge jumps in skill that they provide on related problems. Pre-trained models are learning models that were trained with a large dataset where saving the model and the pre-trained weights for use in future; the widely used dataset is the ImageNet dataset (Pan & Yang, 2010).

The idea of transfer learning is based on removing the output layer with softmax activation function, alone or with some preceding layers, from the pre-trained model and freezing the other layers with its weights, then adding a softmax output layer or more and then training the additional layers only with the required dataset. It is possible to remove one or more layers from the last hidden layers according to the required task and the pre-trained model original task (Pan & Yang, 2010).

Figure 20 shows the applying of transfer learning in the CNNs example that mentioned in section 4.2 which remove the softmax output layer $\hat{y}$, that contains 10 neurons (output classes) and the last hidden layer, that contains 84 neurons, freeze other previous layers, and adding a softmax output layer $\widehat{y_T}$, with 5 output classes, directly to the FC3 layer that contains 120 neurons. For computer vision tasks, it is common to use pre-trained deep learning models for a large and challenging image classification task such as the ImageNet dataset which contains 1.2 million images with 1000 classes.

Figure 20. The applying of transfer learning

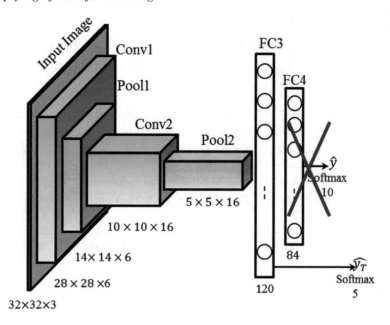

REFERENCES

AlAfandy, K. A., Omara, H., Lazaar, M., & Al Achhab, M. (Eds.). (2019). Artificial Neural Networks Optimization and Convolution Neural Networks to Classifying Images in Remote Sensing: A Review. *Proceeding of The 4th International Conference on Big Data and Internet of Things (BDIoT'19)*. 10.1145/3372938.3372945

AlAfandy, K. A., Omara, H., Lazaar, M., & Al Achhab, M. (2020a). Investment of Classic Deep CNNs and SVM for Classifying Remote Sensing Images. *Advances in Science, Technology and Engineering Systems Journal, 5*(5), 652-659. doi:10.25046/aj050580

AlAfandy, K. A., Omara, H., Lazaar, M., & Al Achhab, M. (2020b). Using Classic Networks for Classifying Remote Sensing Images: Comparative Study. *Advances in Science, Technology and Engineering Systems Journal, 5*(5), 770-780. doi:10.25046/aj050594

Bengio, Y., Goodfellow, I., & Courville, A. (2017). *Deep Learning*. MIT Press.

Bottou, L. (Ed.). (1991). Stochastic Gradient Learning in Neural Networks. In *Proceedings of the Neuro-Nîmes* (pp. 12-23). Academic Press.

(2016). Deep Residual Learning for Image Recognition. In K. He, X. Zhang, S. Ren, & J. Sun (Eds.), Proceeding of the 2016 IEEE Conference on Computer Vision and Pattern Recognition (CVPR 2016) (pp. 770–778). IEEE. https://doi.org/10.1109/CVPR.2016.90.

Densely Connected Convolutional Networks. (2017). In G. Huang, Z. Liu, L. V. D. Maaten, & K. Q. Weinberger (Eds.), Proceeding of the 2017 IEEE Conference on Computer Vision and Pattern Recognition (CVPR 2017) (pp. 2261–2269). IEEE. https://doi.org/10.1109/CVPR.2017.243.

Dialameh, M., Hamzeh, A., & Rahmani, H. (2020). *DL-Reg: A Deep Learning Regularization Technique using Linear Regression.* https://arxiv.org/abs/2011.00368

X. Du, Y. Cai, S. Wang, & L. Zhang (Eds.). (2016). Overview of Deep Learning. In *Proceeding of the 31st Youth Academic Annual Conference of Chinese Association of Automation (YAC).* IEEE. 10.1109/ YAC.2016.7804882

Dubey, S. R., Chakraborty, S., Roy, S. K., Mukherjee, S., Singh, S. K., & Chaudhuri, B. B. (2019). diffGrad: An Optimization Method for Convolutional Neural Networks. *IEEE Transactions on Neural Networks and Learning Systems, 31*(11), 4500–4511. https://doi.org/10.1109/TNNLS.2019.2955777

Feature Selection, L1 Vs. L2 Regularization, and Rotational Invariance. (2004). In A. Ng (Ed.), Proceedings of the 21st International Conference on Machine Learning (ICML '04) (pp. 78–85). ACM. https:// doi.org/10.1145/1015330.1015435.

Gad, A. F. (2018). *Practical Computer Vision Applications Using Deep Learning with CNNs.* Apress. doi:10.1007/978-1-4842-4167-7

Gaur, L., Singh, G., & Agarwal, V. (2021a). Leveraging Artificial Intelligence Tools to Combat the CO-VID-19 Crisis. In P. K. Singh, G. Veselov, V. Vyatkin, A. Pljonkin, J. M. Dodero, & Y. Kumar (Eds.), *Futuristic Trends in Network and Communication Technologies. FTNCT 2020. Communications in Computer and Information Science* (Vol. 1395). Springer. doi:10.1007/978-981-16-1480-4_28

Gaur, L., Solanki, A., Wamba, S. F., & Jhanjhi, N. Z. (2021b). *Advanced AI Techniques and Applications in Bioinformatics.* CRC Press. doi:10.1201/9781003126164

Hawkins, D. M. (2004). The Problem of Overfitting. *Journal of Chemical Information and Computer Sciences, ACM, 44*(1), 1–12. https://doi.org/10.1021/ci0342472

Jabbar, H. K., & Khan, R. Z. (2015). Methods to Avoid Over-fitting and Under-fitting in Supervised Machine Learning (Comparative Study). *Computer Science, Communication and Instrumentation Devices*, 163-172. doi:10.3850/978-981-09-5247-1_017

Kanai, S., Fujiwara, Y., Yamanaka, Y., & Adachi, S. (2018). *Sigsoftmax: Reanalysis of the softmax bottleneck.* arXiv preprint arXiv:1805.10829.

Ketkar, N. (2017). Introduction to Keras. In *Deep Learning with Python* (pp. 97-111). Apress. doi:10.1007/978-1-4842-2766-4_7

Kingma, D. P., & Ba, J. L. (Eds.). (2015). Adam: A Method for Stochastic Optimization. *Proceeding of the 3rd International Conference on Learning Representations (ICLR 2015).* https://arxiv.org/abs/1406.3269

Lecun, Y., Bottou, L., Bengio, Y., & Haffner, P. (1998). Gradient-based Learning Applied to Document Recognition. *Proceedings of the IEEE, 86*(11), 2278–2324. https://doi.org/10.1109/5.726791

Li, J., Cheng, J., Shi, J., & Huang, F. (2012). Brief Introduction of Back Propagation (BP) Neural Network Algorithm and Its Improvement. In D. Jin & S. Lin (Eds.), Advances in Computer Science and Information Engineering (pp. 553–558). Springer. https://doi.org/10.1007/978-3-642-30223-7_87.

Maggiori, E., Tarabalka, Y., Charpiat, G., & Alliez, P. (2017). Convolutional Neural Networks for Large-Scale Remote-Sensing Image Classification. *IEEE Transactions on Geoscience and Remote Sensing, 55*(2), 645–657. https://doi.org/10.1109/TGRS.2016.2612821

Mishra, A., Chandra, P., Ghose, U., & Sodhi, S. S. (2017). Bi-modal Derivative Adaptive Activation Function Sigmoidal Feedforward Artificial Neural Networks. *Applied Soft Computing, Elsevier, 61*, 983–994. doi:10.1016/j.asoc.2017.09.002

Ooyen, A. V., & Nienhuis, B. (1992). Improving the Convergence of the Back-propagation Algorithm. *Neural Networks, 5*(3), 465-471. doi:10.1016/0893-6080(92)90008-7

(2019). Overfitting and Underfitting Analysis for Deep Learning Based End-to-end Communication Systems. In H. Zhang, L. Zhang, & Y. Jiang (Eds.), Proceeding of the 11th International Conference on Wireless Communications and Signal Processing (WCSP) (pp. 1–6). IEEE. https://doi.org/10.1109/WCSP.2019.8927876.

Pan, S. J., & Yang, Q. (2010). A Survey on Transfer Learning. *IEEE Transactions on Knowledge and Data Engineering, 22*(10), 1345–1359. https://doi.org/10.1109/TKDE.2009.191

Paola, J. D., & Schowengerdt, R. A. (1995). A Review and Analysis of Backpropagation Neural Networks for Classification of Remotely-sensed Multi-spectral Imagery. *International Journal of Remote Sensing, 16*(16), 3033-3058. doi:10.1080/01431169508954607

Patro, S. G. K., & Sahu, K. K. (2015). *Normalization: A Preprocessing Stage.* arXiv e-prints arXiv:1503.06462.

Pedregosa, F., Varoquaux, G., Gramfort, A., Michel, V., Thirion, B., Grisel, O., Blondel, M., Prettenhofer, P., Weiss, R., Dubourg, V., Vanderplas, J., Passos, A., Cournapeau, D., Brucher, M., Perrot, M., & Duchesnay, É. (2011). Scikit-learn: Machine Learning in Python. *Journal of Machine Learning Research, 12*, 2825–2830.

Qian, N. (1999). On the Momentum Term in Gradient Descent Learning Algorithms. *Neural Networks, 12*(1), 145-151. doi:10.1016/S0893-6080(98)00116-6

A. D. Rasamoelina, F. Adjailia, & P. Sinčák (Eds.). (2020). A Review of Activation Function for Artificial Neural Network. In *Proceeding of the 2020 IEEE 18th World Symposium on Applied Machine Intelligence and Informatics (SAMI).* IEEE. 10.1109/SAMI48414.2020.9108717

Ruder, S. (2016). *An Overview of Gradient Descent Optimization Algorithms.* arXiv preprint arXiv:1609.04747.

Shanmuganathan, S. (2016). Artificial Neural Network Modelling: An Introduction. In S. Shanmuganathan & S. Samarasinghe (Eds.), *Artificial Neural Network Modelling* (pp. 1–14). Springer. doi:10.1007/978-3-319-28495-8_1

U. S. Shanthamallu, A. Spanias, C. Tepedelenlioglu, & M. Stanley (Eds.). (2017). A Brief Survey of Machine Learning Methods and Their Sensor and IoT Applications. In *Proceeding of the 8th International Conference on Information, Intelligence, Systems & Applications (IISA).* IEEE. 10.1109/IISA.2017.8316459

Shorten, C., & Khoshgoftaar, T. M. (2019). A Survey on Image Data Augmentation for Deep Learning. *Journal of Big Data, 6*(1), 1–48. https://doi.org/10.1186/s40537-019-0197-0

Simonyan, K., & Zisserman, A. (Eds.). (2015). Very deep convolutional networks for large-scale image recognition. *Proceeding of the 3rd International Conference on Learning Representations (ICLR 2015).* https://arxiv.org/abs/1409.1556

Singh, A., Pokharel, R., & Principe, J. (2014). The C-loss Function for Pattern Classification. *Pattern Recognition, 47*(1), 441-453. doi:10.1016/j.patcog.2013.07.017

Srivastava, N., Hinton, G., Krizhevsky, A., Sutskever, I., & Salakhutdinov, R. (2014). Dropout: A Simple Way to Prevent Neural Networks from Overfitting. *Journal of Machine Learning Research, 15*, 1929–1958.

(2017). Understanding of a Convolutional Neural Network. In S. Albawi, T. A. Mohammed, & S. Al-Zawi (Eds.), Proceeding of the 2017 International Conference on Engineering and Technology (ICET) (pp. 1–6). IEEE. https://doi.org/10.1109/ICEngTechnol.2017.8308186.

Wei, B., Sun, X., Ren, X., & Xu, J. (2017). *Minimal Effort Back Propagation for Convolutional Neural Networks.* arXiv preprint arXiv:1709.05804.

Yamashita, R., Nishio, M., Do, R. K. G., & Togashi, K. (2018). Convolutional Neural Networks: An Overview and Application in Radiology. *Insights into Imaging, 9*, 611-629. doi:10.1007/s13244-018-0639-9

Zhang, Z. (2016). *Derivation of Backpropagation in Convolutional Neural Network (CNN).* University of Tennessee.

Zoph, B., & Le, Q. V. (Eds.). (2017). Neural Architecture Search with Reinforcement Learning. *Proceeding of the 5th International Conference on Learning Representations (ICLR 2017).* https://openreview.net/forum?id=r1Ue8Hcxg

APPENDIX: ABBREVIATIONS

AdaGrad: Adaptive Gradient Algorithm
Adam: Adaptive Moment Estimation
ANNs: Artificial Neural Networks
API: Application Programming Interface
BSD: Berkeley Software Distribution
CNNs: Convolution Neural Networks
CVPR: Conference on Computer Vision and Pattern Recognition
DenseNet: Dense Convolutional Network
DNNs: Deep Neural Networks
FC: Fully Connected
ICLR: International Conference on Learning Representations
LRN: Local Response Normalization
NASNet: Neural Architecture Search Network
NNs: Neural Networks
ReLU: Rectified Linear Unit
ResNet: Residual Network
RMSProp: Root Mean Square Propagation
SGD: Stochastic gradient descent
TF: Tensorflow
VGG: Visual Geometry Group

Chapter 7

A Systematic Mapping Study of Low-Grade Tumor of Brain Cancer and CSF Fluid Detecting in MRI Images Through Multi-Algorithm Techniques

Soobia Saeed
Universiti Teknologi Malaysia, Malaysia

Habibullah Bin Haroon
University Technology Malaysia, Malaysia

Noor Zaman Jhanjhi
(iD) https://orcid.org/0000-0001-8116-4733

Taylor's University, Malaysia

Mehmood Naqvi
Mohawk College, Canada

Muneer Ahmad
National University of Science and Technology, Pakistan

ABSTRACT

Low-grade tumor or CSF fluid, the symptoms of brain tumour and CSF liquid, usually requires image segmentation to evaluate tumour detection in brain images. This research uses systematic literature review (SLR) process for analysis of the different segmentation approach for detecting the low-grade tumor and CSF fluid presence in the brain. This research work investigated how to evaluate and detect the tumor and CSF fluid, supervised machine learning algorithm and segmentation method (3D and 4D segmentation process, supervised segmentation process, Fourier transformation, and Laplace transformation), and mentioned the details of publication selection with the publishing digital libraries bodies. Furthermore, this research discusses selected segmentation techniques to detect the low-grade tumor and CSF fluid in systematic mapping through systematic literature review (SLR) process.

DOI: 10.4018/978-1-7998-8929-8.ch007

INTRODUCTION

The motive of this chapter is to evaluate and use a proper scientific method to spot the research problems in a systematic and organized body of knowledge. This chapter examines various related researches to explain the background of brain cancer, CSF and multiple approach algorithm details to use in segmentation method of MRI and research questions that are mentioned in details.

R1: What is the common symptom of CSF Fluid leak in the brain and Brain Tumor?

The ventricles that surround the brain and the spinal cord are filled with a clear, colourless, and ultra-filtrate of plasma that is known as cerebrospinal fluid. The brain and spinal cord form the central nervous system, which controls, and coordinates the working of all the body parts such as complex thinking and planning, muscle movement, and all organs functions. It acts as a shield and pillow to protect the brain and spinal cord from unexpected injuries. It also helps in waste removal from the brain so that the nervous system will function normally. It performs main functions as if it protects and nourishes the brain and removes the wastage as well (Spector, R. *et al.*, 2015). It gives hydro-mechanical protection of the neuraxis through two mechanisms. In the first mechanism, it acts as a shock absorber that shields the brain against the skull (Telano, L. N., and Baker, S., 2020). CSF is ultra-filtrate of plasma that lies within the brain ventricles and the subarachnoid spaces of the cranium and spine (Sakka, L. *et al.*, 2011). The second mechanism reduces the effective brain weight that makes the brain and the spinal cord buoyant. The volume of CSF in adults is 150 ml; around 25 ml is distributed within the ventricles and 125 ml within the subarachnoid spaces. Choroid plexus secretes CSF, in adults this secretin ranges from 400 ml to 600 ml daily. In an average young person, this constant secretion helps in the detailed renewal of CSF four to five times daily. Aging and various neurodegenerative diseases result due to the addition of metabolites because of a decrease in CSF turnover. Strict management of the CSF composition is essential and any difference can support in diagnosis (Sakka, L. *et al.*, 2011).

Cerebrospinal Fluid Circulation and Leak

Brinker, T. *et al.*, (2014) studied CSF physiology and revealed that CSF is secreted by epithelial cells of the choroid plexus and it flows via the ventricles, then flows in the middle of the subarachnoid space. This literature reviews major developments that lead to the previous theories. Observations using cellular and molecular biology as well as neuroimaging show that CSF physiology is more complicated than it is traditionally assumed. Its circulation does not constitute a directed flow only, but it is a flow with periodic variations that is filled all over the brain and exchanges the local fluid among blood, intestinal fluid, and CSF. Speedy carrier of brain water and CSF homeostasis occurs through astrocytes, aquaporin, and other membranes. The steady exchange of bidirectional fluid yields a flow rate that boosts the choroidal CSF production rate. The CSF circulation enters from the subarachnoid space into the Virchow Robin space. It delivers a site for the interaction between the brain and the immune system and a drainage way so that the water molecules from the brain are cleared. Various physiological functions depend on CSF transportation like regeneration of the brain during sleep, etc. (Brinker, T. *et al.*, 2014).

Among various neurological difficulties, CSF leak is a challenging one because it occurs without any reason also. CSF moves through the ventricles of the brain and the surface of the spine. The condition, when this fluid leaks through a nose or ear due to a tear or a hole in the skull or dura, is called CSF leakage. This tear or hole affects the system of the brain and the sinus badly. CSF openings are generated after the lower back section, also known as a spinal block or spinal anesthesia (S. Saeed *et al.*,2021).

Due to the spinal surgery complications, usually, tear in the dura (brain covering) takes place that causes CSF to leak (Fang, Z. *et al.*, 2017). To stop this leakage, there are various studies for repairing the dural tear but the following new treatments have given promising results:

1. Substitute material may be used to create watertight dural closure.
2. Changing pressure difference along with increasing the epidural space pressure and decreasing the subarachnoid liquid pressure and may slow down the CSF leak.

Sometimes a combination of both methods is used to stop the CSF leakage. (Fang, Z. *et al.*, 2017).

Brain Tumour

All the living things are created of basic units, called cells. In grownups, usually, new cells are not produced unless there is a necessity to replace the damaged or the old cells. In children, new cells are produced so that they can grow well or if there is a need to repair the damaged cells. When any kind of the cells propagate rapidly and unnecessarily, the tumor develops. Central nervous system cancer is developed in the brain and the spinal cord. Tumors can be formed at any stage and in anyone. The brain tumor is of two types, malignant or benign, among these two only malignant is considered as cancerous. Primary cancer originates in the brain tissues, whereas secondary cancer originates in any other organ and spreads to the brain tissues (metastasized). Secondary brain cancer is entitled according to that tissue or organ in which it is originated for example lung cancer with metastatic brain cancer (Soobia Saeed *et al*,2021).

If cells grow and propagate without any check and control by the mechanisms that are entitled to control the normal cells, it forms an abnormal mass of tissues and this kind of brain tumor will be called an intracranial tumor. There are more than 150 kinds of brain tumors, among them primary and metastatic brain tumors are considered as the main groups. Primary brain tumors are formed on and within the brain structures that contain blood vessels, nerves, and glands. These tumors are considered as malignant or benign and glial, that is they are composed of glial cells, or non-glial. Conversely, metastatic brain tumors are developed in other organs like lungs or breasts and spread to the brain through the blood vessels. These tumors are categorized as malignant that are cancerous (Blumenfeld, H., 2010).

R2: How can be investigation of Brian Tumor and CSF fluid leak through segmentation method?

Image Segmentation

Roy, S. *et al.*, (2013) developed the images technique in discrete domains like MRI and in continuous domains like X-ray films. The position of each measurement in 2D is named as a pixel and in 3D is named as a voxel. Sometimes the word pixel is used in both 2D and 3D images. Let 'I' represent the image domain, then the segmentation problem is to find out Sk I sets, which forms the complete image I with its union. Therefore, the sets, which form segmentation, must satisfy the following eq. (Roy, S. *et al.*, 2013).

$$I = \bigcup_{k=1}^{k} sk$$

Here Sk Sj = Ø for k≠j and each Sk is connected. The segmentation method determines the sets, which correlates to clear anatomical structures or sub-regions of the anatomical structures in the image. Finding the sets after the removal of the constraint, with which the regions are connected, is known as pixel classification and the determined sets are named as classes. One of the preferable goals in medical images is pixel classification especially when the identification of the disconnected regions relating to a similar tissue class is required. There are various types of segmentation, with different advantages and disadvantages, for segmenting a brain tumor in MRI. No particular algorithm exists that always gives very good results for all types of brain MRI. So, a quick summation for various types of segmentation is described here. For image segmentation of the brain, the prime difficulties are the perfect selection of features, tissues, and brain and non-brain elements (S. Saeed *et al.*,2021).

Image Segmentation With MRI

Calabrese, C. *et al.*, (2007) presented the analysis of brain tumours is considered as the evolution of abnormal cells of the brain. Primarily, brain tumors are categorized as primary brain tumors as they are developed in the brain and do not spread to other organs (Calabrese, C. *et al.*, 2007). However, sometimes tumors develop and expand into adjacent tissues and regions. They may be categorized as malignant that is cancerous or benign that is non-cancerous. It is not easy to say benign is not harmful because it can cause some serious problems that is why both are considered risky. MRI is an advanced imaging technique, which gives complete and abundant information regarding the anatomy of soft human tissues. The reason why MRI is considered more effective than other imaging techniques is that it is capable to provide 3D data with high contrast between soft tissues (Calabrese, C. *et al.*, 2007). Its tremendous advantage is that helps to examine and diagnose diseases of internal brain lesions. The neurosurgeons need medical images to analyse the growth of a tumor therefore it is essential to know the accurate changes in the images. For this purpose, MR image, segmentation is used to bring out meaningful information from an image. Cerebrospinal fluid (CSF), grey matter (GM), and White matter (WM), all are tissue classes of MRI segmentation (Pradhan, S., 2010).

Image segmentation is a technique in which an image is divided into regions with boundaries along with the same assigned pixels (Pascal, N.E. *et al.*, 2014). To attain a valuable estimation and understanding, the regions must be related to the illustrated structures and details in interest. When random fields and other models are used to shape the gray level and label images, then the segmentation of the image involves extracting hidden data, the labels, from clouded and noisy data and the grey levels (Pascal, N.E. *et al.*, 2014). For measuring the parameters of the appropriate probabilistic models, the expectation-maximization (EM) algorithm is applied extensively. Hidden Markov random field (HMRF) models are widely used to diagnose brain tumors (Pascal, N.E. *et al.*, 2014). These models result in efficient outcomes while segmenting homogeneously noisy areas. Another frequently employed technique is Threshold, which distinguishes the foreground from the background. When an exact threshold value T is assigned, the grey level image is transformed into a binary image (Mustaqeem, A. *et al.*, 2012). The binary image must possess all the necessary details regarding the shape along with the location of the concerned objects. A widely used and easy procedure to convert a grey level image into a binary image is to choose a single threshold value T (Taheri, S. *et al.*, 2010). Now that all the grey level values above this T are labelled as white (1) and the below values as black (0). Thresholding is the simplest image segmentation method, which develops binary images from grayscale images (Al-Amri, S.S. and Kalyankar, N. V., 2010). A few assumptions regarding the shape and size of the tumor are made, which become the basis for morphological operations. Then these operations are employed on the image that is achieved after threshold-based segmentation (Natarajan, P. *et al.*, 2012). Finally, the image subtraction technique is employed so that the accurate tumor region will be acquired. A new method namely, the hybrid method that is a blend of threshold and HMRF methods is presented for brain tumor diagnosis.

R3: How can we utilize the Supervised Segmentation Methods for detecting the brain tumor in MRI images?

Supervised Segmentation Methods

Supervised segmentation methods are also called classification methods as they partition an image feature space by using data with known labels. These image features may be intensity values, texture, or other properties. These methods require manually segmented training images and then proceed these images for automatic segmentation of new images as references. Some of the frequently using supervised segmentation methods are:

K-NN Algorithm

Wang. L (2019), describe that the KNN stands for k nearest neighbour classifications, which uses a mixture of K's most recent history data to identify historical records. KNN is a well-known statistical algorithm for pattern recognition that has been extensively explored over the last 40 years. KNN has been used to categorise text in early research tactics and is one of the benchmark Reuters body's highly operational methodologies. LLSF, decision trees, and neural networks are examples of other techniques. The KNN concept is as follows: Calculate the distance between the new sample and the training sample, then locate the nearest K neighbours; finally, decide the category of the new sample based on the category to which the neighbour belongs, if they all belong to the same category, then the new sample is then placed in this category as well; alternatively, each post-selection category is scored, and the new sample category is selected using specified rules.

Take the unknown sample X's K neighbours and determine which group the K neighbours belong to, then classify X accordingly. That is, K X neighbours are found among the K samples of X. The KNN expands the area around the test sample X until it contains K training samples, at which point it classifies the test sample X as the most frequently occurring category among the most recent K training samples. In the case of K=6, the test sample X is classified as black using the decision rule shown in Fig. 2.6(Wang, L, 2019).

Figure 1. K nearest neighbour

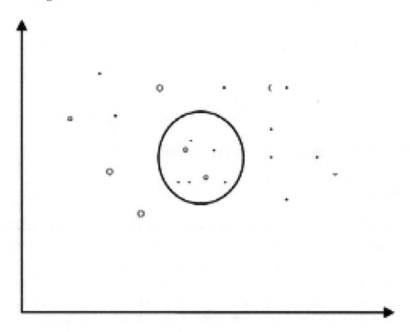

The neighbourhood classification is a lazy learning method based on the eyeball; it maintains all of the training data and recognises that new samples must be classified in order to construct the classification. Decision numbers and backpropagation algorithms, on the other hand, need the construction of a general model before admitting additional samples for classification. Lazy learning is faster than eager learning in terms of training, but it is slower in terms of classification because all calculations are postponed till then (Wang, L, 2019).

R4: How can we investigate the Detection of tumor or CSF fluid through Hidden Markov model and Grab Cut algorithm in 4D Light field segmentation?

Hidden Markov Model

The 3D spatial segmentation method is reiterated for every single time point independently to track the brain tissue segmentation over time (Prastawa, M. *et al.*, 2003). To decide the tissue classes for the current scan it is assumed that improvements can be achieved by using results from earlier and following 3D segmentations. In this research, a unique temporal method is implemented for 4D segmentation of brain MRIs by combining probabilistic reasoning over space and probabilistic reasoning over time. The temporal model is a Dynamic Bayesian Network, especially the hidden Markov model, along with sensor models and image-based transition. We assumed in our 4D image data that each voxel has a lesion status, along with all possible lesion and non-lesion values. The segmenting and tracking lesions over time problems can be designed as an HMM. Xt represents the state of the lesion or non-lesion system and is not observable. Et represents the MR signal intensity at each voxel and is observable. Here 1st order Markov assumption was developed that is to determine the current state from the previous one. This state-to-state transition model is given by Eq. (1) and (2) (Prastawa, M. *et al.*, 2003).

$$P\left(Xt \mid Xt-1\right) = P\left(Xt \mid X0:t-1\right) transition\ model \tag{1}$$

Et being the evidence variable depends on the present state only. This dependency is called the sensor model.

$$P\left(Et \mid Xt\right) = P\left(Et \mid X0:t-1\right) sensor\ model \tag{2}$$

MRF models HMM. Spatial coherence among neighbourhood voxels.

Grab Cut Algorithm in 4D

Segmentation is a significant task and a core subject to study in the computer vision field. The graph-cut algorithm is the most famous and supervised foreground/background segmentation method used for 2D images (Rother, C., *et al.,* 2004). It is a widely used method in various software applications for image editing. It is based upon graph algorithms (Boykov, Y. and Kolmogorov, V., 2004). It applies to data of any dimension like video footage, imagery, and 3D structures (Boykov, Y.Y., and Jolly, M.P., 2001) and can be extended to multi-label segmentation (Boykov, Y. *et al.,* 2001). The data is handled as a structure of graph with edges along with vertices in the graph-cut method. Each pixel is represented by a vertex and a weighted edge connects the neighbouring pixels according to their similarity. The cases in which multi-label image segmentation is involved, every single label also contains a special vertex, named as terminal. Vertices of the pixels are connected to all terminals, here the weighted edges find out the likelihood of label assignment. Achieving the segmentation at least amount of energy will give solutions to determine cuts on a graph at low cost. Min-cut or max-flow algorithms can fix this problem (Greig, D. M. *et al.,* 1989). After cutting, each vertex remains linked to an individual terminal, which shows that the label is given in accordance with the related pixel. This research also uses a graph-cut segmentation method. In these processes user inputs are needed in the form of clues, so they are classified as supervised methods. Many graph-cut approaches are considered to process data of any dimension, but these are inapplicable for high dimensional data for example video footage (Boykov, Y. *et al.,* 2001). Video data contains an irregular structure along the time axis far from 3D volume data. If the irregular neighbour relationships of the data are considered accurately, it can improve the segmentation approaches. Like Nagahashi, T. *et al.,* (2009) defined the temporal neighbour relationships that are corresponding pixels of neighboring frames; this resulted in improving the video segmentation accuracy. 4D light field data and video data both have the same problem of complex redundancy in a light field. This research suggests the use of a graph-cut approach to focus on the 4D light field segmentation for the very first time in the image segmentation field. Although some unsupervised, methods are also applicable for 4D light segmentation or multi-view images. Berent, J. and Dragotti, P. L. *et al.,* (2007) suggested another 4D light field segmentation method that was based on a level set method, given by (Osher, S., & Sethian, J. A., 1988), which applies an active contour method for segmenting a 4D hyper volume. Kolmogorov, V. and Zabih,R. (2009) suggested a depth labelling approach for multi-view images based on that foreground objects cannot be obstructed by deeper objects. Kowdle, A. *et al.,* (2012) proposed an automatic method of object extraction from multi-view images was proposed while utilizing disparity cues.

Light Field Segmentation

The main purpose of this research is to assign each ray a label. To formulate the light field segmentation problem as a problem of energy minimization, some assumptions are made that are based on light field structures. According to Levoy, M. and Hanrahan, P., (1996), 4D light fields can be represented in various ways.

Figure 2. Complete flow of light field segmentation

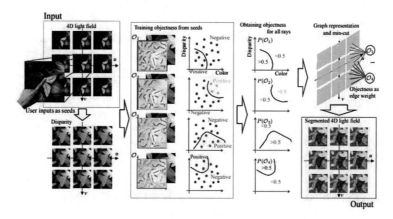

In figure.8, the 4D light field is the input and some seeds are specified in the centre viewpoint. The colour and estimated disparity distribution give SVMs for each label. The distance among every single decision plane helps in obtaining objectness. Then the 4D light field segmentation takes place that is based on graph-cut (S. Saeed *et al.*,2021).

To model rays in 3D space, we have applied a Lumi-graph method given by (Gortler, S. J. *et al.*, 1996). In this method, we define a ray by two intersection points with u–v and x–y planes in the 3D coordinate as shown in figure 2.10 (a). In the 4D space, a ray is shown as a point p = (u, v, x, y) and Ip represents the intensity of p. Lumi-graph representation is then converted into a multi-view representation given by (Levoy, M., and Hanrahan. P., 1996) that has two planes, an image and a viewpoint plane as given in figure 2.10 (b) and contrary. Here x–y and u–v planes correspond to image and viewpoint planes respectively (S. Saeed *et al.*,2021).

Figure 3. Types of 4D light field representation.

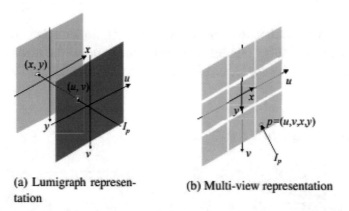

(a) Lumigraph represen-   (b) Multi-view representation
tation

The light field can be represented as:

1. Lumi-graph light field representation (Gortler, S. J *et al.*, 1996).
2. Multi-view light field representation

   Both of these light field representations are essentially equal given by (Levoy, M. and Hanrahan. P., 1996). The author in this research adopts a multi-view light field representation.

R5: What is key factor of Fourier and Laplace transform with medical images transformation to identifying the missing data in MRI images?

Fourier Transform Method

A numerical method used to transform a time function, x (t), into frequency function, X (ω) is called the Fourier Transform method. It is similar to the Fourier series. When the time interval, T→∞ for a function in the Fourier series, its Fourier Transform can be derived. For the derivation, we start with the following Fourier series synthesis equation:

$$x\left(t\right) = \sum_{n=-\infty}^{+\infty} c_n e^{jn\omega_0 t}$$

Here c_n can be determined by using the following Fourier Series analysis equation,

$$c_n = \frac{1}{T}\int_T x\left(t\right) e^{-jn\omega_0 t} dt$$

This can be rewritten as,

$$Tc_n = \int_T x\left(t\right)e^{-jn\omega_0 t}dt$$

When T→∞ the fundamental frequency that is given by $\omega_0 = 2\pi/T$ turns out to be too small and $n\omega_0$ turns into a continuous quantity, which may use any value as n has a wide set of ±∞. Therefore, one can evaluate a new variable $\omega = n\omega_0$; it is assumed that X (ω) =Tc_n. By substituting these values in the above expression, we can get the analysis equation for the Fourier Transform that is named as the Forward Fourier Transform.

$$X\left(\omega\right) = \int_{-\infty}^{+\infty} x\left(t\right)e^{-j\omega t}dt$$

Similarly, the synthesis equation, which is known as the Inverse Fourier Transform, can be obtained by beginning with the synthesis equation for the Fourier series then multiplying and dividing it by T.

$$x\left(t\right) = \sum_{n=-\infty}^{+\infty} c_n e^{jn\omega_0 t} = \sum_{n=-\infty}^{+\infty} Tc_n e^{jn\omega_0 t}\frac{1}{T}$$

When T→∞, $1/T = \omega 0/2\pi$. Here ω_0 is very small and if T increases, we will replace it with the quantity dω. We know that $\omega = n\omega 0$ and X (ω) =Tc_n. A few steps along with the replacement of the sum by an integral will give the synthesis equation of the Fourier Transform.

$$x\left(t\right) = \sum_{n=-\infty}^{+\infty} X\left(\omega\right)e^{j\omega t}\frac{d\omega}{2\pi} = \frac{1}{2\pi}\int_{-\infty}^{+\infty} X\left(\omega\right)e^{j\omega t}dw$$

Laplace Transformation

To solve the ordinary differential equations (ODEs) easily, these equations are transformed into algebraic equations, this transformation is called Laplace Transform. Zhang, S. *et al.*, (2018) noted an example-driven k-parameter computation in which several k values for various test samples are determined in prediction applications of kNN like regression, imputation of missing data, and classification. For this, a sparse coefficient matrix is rebuilt between test samples and training data. To produce an element wise sparsity coefficient matrix a $\ell 1-$norm regularization is applied and to preserve the local data structures Locality Preserving Projection (LPP) regularization is employed in the reconstruction process to obtain efficiency. Moreover, we apply the kNN approach for regression, imputation of missing data, and classification using the gained k value. The explanation of this method contains 20 real datasets which proved that the suggested algorithm gives more accurate results than the traditional kNN algorithms especially in data mining tasks like regression, imputation of missing data, and classification (Zhang, S. et al.,2018).

SAMPLING TECHNIQUES

Sampling strategies are typically obtained from accessible data sources applicable to brain cancer in terms of Low-Grade tumor, ranging from numerical data on CSF fluid leak as well, MRI images, image segmentation method, Supervised machine leaning method, 4DLFT applications/method, Fourier transformation and Laplace transformation for identifying the tumor or fluid through multiple techniques of segmentation. These results are useful for scientific purposes to connect the potential and strength of medical imaging (MR) to help the doctors and common man also to understand the terminology of MRI and CT scan etc (S. Saeed *et al.*,2017).

Sampling proof is based on human brain MRI images and sign of leakage of CSF fluid. The pattern length is extra than 10,000 target population for the harm due to the cases of low grade tumor or CSF fluid leak and the human sample collection experimental results. The records can analysis through machine learning algorithm(MLA) and supervised machine learning method. Most of them had been satisfied with the detecting tumor or range of fluid in brain through segmentation and other related to MLA techniques. The key regions of attention had been the importance of statistical facts, time manipulate and recognition of the primary area of affected the human brain (S. Saeed *et al.*,2017).

Hypothesis

R1: What is the common symptom of CSF Fluid leak in the brain and Brain Tumor?

R2: How can be investigation of Brian Tumor and CSF fluid leak through segmentation method? **R3:** How can we utilize the Supervised Segmentation Methods for detecting the brain tumor in MRI images?

R4: How can we investigate the Detection of tumor or CSF fluid through Hidden Markov model and Grab Cut algorithm in 4D Light field segmentation?

R5: What is key factor of Fourier and Laplace transform with medical images transformation to identifying the missing data in MRI images?

RESEARCH METHODOLOGY

The advantages of theoretical mapping are fundamental. It is a theoretically based technique for defining, comparing, and interpreting all data related to a specific study topic, target area, or other segmentation phenomenon. Systematic mapping is a well-established method for researching and synthesising scientific data about a methodology or procedure, identifying relevant regions and discrepancies in current studies, and providing specific information to researchers or clinicians to support a new investigation approach. A comprehensive mapping analysis differs from a standard literature review in that it requires more time and effort, but it also provides a broader understanding of the subject and a solid foundation for generating data on issues related to the studies reviewed. As illustrated in Fig. 1, this systematic mapping procedure consists of several steps. A comprehensive mapping process was coordinated, including details from all MRI images experimental records. Here's a quick rundown of the primary steps (S. Saeed *et al.*,2019) Convey research questions

1.   Explain the search engine with sequence

2. Explain the selection process, including inclusion and exclusion criteria
3. Data extraction and mapping with specific research questions
4. Analyse data and extract results

Figure 4. Systematic mapping study

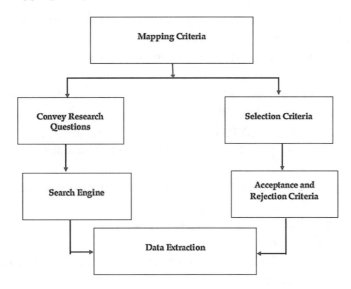

Academic Databases

Following many iterations and reviews, the following research series was completed to study these maps: The segmentation or brain tumor or CSF fluid or Fourier Transform and (Laplace Transform associated with brain cancer research series in the following digital libraries were finally used) The search string has also been modified in accordance with the search mechanism provided by these libraries:

1. IEEE Explore
2. IEEE Transaction
3. Direct science
4. SAGE
5. Springer Link

The five sites above were chosen because they are common locations for publishing low-grade tumor and CSF Fluid leak detecting papers. These databases have also been used by other scholars in their SLR reports as well.

Publication Selection

This section contains information on the inclusion and exclusion criteria used to select publications, as well as the process used to select relevant articles based on the study questions. Subsequent inclusion criteria were developed:

   The study period spanned nearly a decade of publication, with articles published between 2005 and 2021. The start date was chosen because the lowest grade tumours were first reported in 2005. However, because the studies were conducted in early 2012, the most recent publication corresponding to the end of 2012 was taken into account within the systematic mapping to look at:

1.   Experimental studies of detecting the low-grade tumor and CSF fluid identifying in MRI image through multiple segmentation techniques
2.   Studies that focused on providing implementation results for brain tumors detection in brain, and locate symptoms of cerebrospinal fluid (CSF). The following exclusion criteria were used:

   Studies that do not provide detailed information on the low-grade tumor and CSF fluid leak are:

1.   Duplicate studies, only the most recent ones were selected.
2.   Out of field provide discussion.
3.   Articles that only provide guidelines, recommendations, or descriptions of low-grade tumor.
4.   Introductory articles to workshops, special publications, and books.
5.   Chapters from books.
6.   Papers that is not accessed.

Table 1. Study selection

Source	Retrieved	Initial Selection	Final Selection
IEEE	209	70	40
IEEE Transactions	95	50	20
Science Direct	80	45	20
Springer Link	30	25	12
SAGE	40	30	14
Total	454	220	106

   Table 1 depicts the selection criteria for articles in the recognised indexing services' publishing databases. We can see how the information from the retrieved manuscripts is distributed, as well as the initial and final selection of the manuscripts that are targeted by gathering detailed information about low-grade tumor and CSF fluid.

Table 2. Publication venues with more than one selected study

Library	Type	Frequency
Science Direct	Journal	6
IEEE	Journal	5
IEEE Transaction	Journal	2
SAGE	Journal	1
Springer	Journal	1

Table 2 displayed information from the Libraries such as IEEE, IEEE Transactions, and Springer, as well as an excerpt for courses related to the evolving field of testing that had been published in journals. Among these three libraries, the frequency of articles on IEEE increased, accounting for 25% of the collection's articles. Springer and IEEE Transactions are ranked second and third in the group, respectively. Table 3 shows the unusual peaks for the first study with two or more repeats. According to the findings, the majority of articles are published in journals. The journal Appropriateness IEEE and IEEE transaction has the best articles (106 out of 220), although Information Science via Science Direct ranks second with 20 articles out of 106.

GENERAL DISCUSSION

R1: What is the common symptom of CSF Fluid leak in the brain and Brain Tumor?

Brain Tumor With MRI

The use of magnetic resonance imaging is expanding in the medical field. Several techniques are obtained to extract and make up meaningful and complete information from medical data. Brain tumor segmentation is an important task that, extracts details from the complex brain MRI images significantly. These days diagnostic imaging serves as a helpful instrument in medical data analysis. MRI, CT, digital mammography, along with several processes of imaging are effective modalities in the diagnosis of various diseases. The procedure of automated detection possesses improved and complete details of all the disease examinations for medical research. As the figure of patients is increasing, these automated detection methodologies serve a significant role in their diagnosis and treatments (Selvy, P. T. *et al.*, 2011). Segmentation has extensive applications in the medical imaging field. Automated delineation of various image factors is utilized to examine MRI of the brain, anatomical structures, and pathological areas like cancer and to split up a whole image into sub-regions like white matter (WM), grey matter (GM) along CSF spaces of the brain. In studying the brain, MRI is used mostly due to its outstanding contrast of soft tissues, non-invasive feature, and higher resolution. Segmentation of brain image helps significantly in the field of MRI as it partitions a portion into a pooped area in such a way that every area is spatially contiguous and has homogeneous pixels concerning pre-set basis. Texture, color, surface normal, surface curvatures, range, and concentration values are included in homogeneity conditions. Many kinds of research are made in the brain tumor segmentation domain but still, there is a high scope for research analysis in this field. To diagnose a brain tumor, imaging, and biopsy, in which a small quantity of the brain tissue is taken for the microscopic examination, studies are quite significant. Initially, X-rays and CT can help in the diagnosis. Nevertheless, MRI is considered more significant as it gives complete detail about the position, size, and kind of the tumor. Therefore, MRI is assigned for the diagnostic process, then for surgeries, and to monitor results of the treatment (Clarke, L. P. *et al.*, 1998). This is the reason to give a brief account of a brain tumours, MRI, and automated systems. Powerful magnets are used in MRI scanners or devices that polarize and excites the hydrogen nuclei to force the proton in human tissues for uniform alignment. It generates encoded signal that yield body images (Tzika, A. A. *et al.*, 2011). Following three electromagnetic fields are used in MRI .

1. Static field, which is a very strong field so that the hydrogen nuclei are polarized.
2. Gradient field, which is a weaker time fluctuating field in which spatial encoding occurs.
3. Radiofrequency field, which is a weak one in which manipulation of hydrogen nuclei happens, the signals produced are obtained through RF antenna.

The different behaviour of protons within variable tissues result in a variance in the appearance of the tissues. Figure 2.1 shows the brain MRI with T1 and T2 weights taken at various positions from the same patients.

Figure 5. Brain MRI
(Tzika, A. A. et al., 2011)

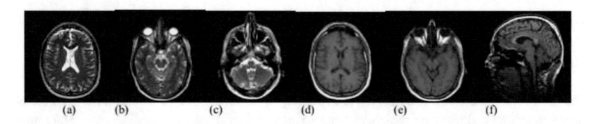

In this figure, T2 weighted MRI of (a) the brain, which shows the lateral ventricle, cortex, and cerebral flax; (b) the brain, which shows the eyeballs as well as the optic nerve, vermis, medulla, and temporal lobes with hippocampal regions; and (c) the head, which shows the maxillary sinus, cloves, nasal septum, inner ear, medulla, and cerebellum. T1 weighted MRI of (d) brain reveals cortex, third and lateral ventricles, putamen, white and grey matter, frontal and superior sagittal sinus, (e) brain reveals eyeballs as well as optic nerve, medulla, vermis, and temporal lobes with hippocampal regions, and (f) brain reveals cortex, lateral ventricle, corpus callosum, thalamus, pons, and cerebellum.

R2: How can be investigation of Brian Tumor and CSF fluid leak through segmentation method?

3-Dimensional (3D) Image Segmentation

Khalil, H. A. *et al.,* (2020) suggested that 3D- MRI is a very important technique of brain segmentation accurately for identifying and disease therapy planning. The changes in the size, composition, and type of the tumor lead to key challenges in brain segmentation. Errors and the number of iterations are reduced by selecting the accurate initial contour points. In this analysis, a two-step dragonfly algorithm (DA) clustering technique is suggested so that this problem will be resolved. In the pre-processing step, the brain is extracted from the head. Then, a two-step DA technique is used to obtain tumor edges, which are utilized as initial contour points (S. Saeed *et al.*,2019). Finally, a level set segmentation method is applied to drag the tumor region from all volume slices. The outcomes resulted by applying these techniques on 3D-MRI from the multimodal brain tumor segmentation challenge (BRATS) 2017 dataset reveal that the suggested technique is relative to the advanced methods (Khalil, H. A. *et al.,* 2020).

Brain image segmentation and biopsy are widely used to diagnose the tumor along with its causes (Lu, C. Y. *et al.*, 2019). Open biopsies are quite risky as a small hole is drilled in the skull to extract a tiny tissue piece for analysing the form, type, and cause of the tumor under a microscope. These imaging techniques are improving and revolutionizing medical diagnosis and prognosis. In figure 2.2, the left image is a brain tumor image and the right image shows the biopsy process. MRI scans enable us,

1. To know the accurate position, type, composition, and size of the tumor,
2. To differentiate soft tissues,
3. To determine small changes in the tissue density and physiological mutations. (Bauer, S *et al.,* 2013).

Another benefit of an MRI scanner is that it does not depend on the use of ionization radiations (Hansson Mild, K. *et al.*, 2019). A brain MRI has 3D scans of the brain or a sample of brain structure as illustrated in figure 2.3. Distinct labelling of MRI image pixels desired for MRI segmentation accurately so that it can help in treatment and radiation therapy. To diagnose the tumor tissues image segmentation modalities are applied (Zhuge, Y. *et al.*, 2017).

Investigation in image segmentation in the medical imaging domain has a very outstanding scope. Research usually concentrates on automated contouring rather than manual contouring because manual contouring requires too much time. In the segmentation process, the position of the concerned object is achieved by contouring that object. If there are visibility variations in the object of interest, the quantity of irregular boundaries increases that lead to problems in the segmentation process. According to previous researches, the intensity rate of healthy and unhealthy tissues usually overlaps. 3D image shows complete information in all dimensions whereas a 2D image shows a single view, so a 3D image is useful and better than a 2D image (Banerjee, S. and Mitra, S. *et al.*, 2020). As tumor diagnosis is not easy because of the intensity overlapping between normal and tumor tissues, therefore, the neighbouring healthy tissues are deformed and massive heterogeneity in shape, size, position, and appearance of tumors emerges (Popoola, J.J. *et al.*, 2019). 3D segmentation is progressing day today but there are still various challenges and unsolved problems that need to be tackled. Substantial memory space and computational resources are required for high-resolution MRI scanning due to the size of its huge data are one of the 3D segmentation issues (Angulakshmi, M. and Lakshmi Priya, G. G. *et al.*, 2017). Various methods are employed to overcome the issues of brain tumor segmentation of 3D MRI. To deal with the volumetric input, two methods are formulated in this research. In the first method, natural image segmentation is used in which 3D volume is cut into 2D slices, and then each slice is individually and sequentially processed by a 2D network. In the second method, volume is cut into patches, and then a 3D network processes these patches. In the next step, a sliding window is used by both methods to test the original volume. Both methods possess benefits along with drawbacks (Shirly, S. and Ramesh, K.

et al., 2019). The resolutions in the 3D MRI vary because of which these images are transformed into 2D slices. In the second method, level set-based segmentation is broadly applied which gives a direct way for measuring geometric properties of the progressing structures (Sajid, S. *et al.*, 2019). Figure 2.4 shows segmentation of brain tumor employing level set segmentation after adjusting the initial contour technique (Wang, D., 2019). One of the advantages to use this technique is its capability of illustrating contours of complex topology along with organizing the changes like splitting and merging efficiently and naturally. Another efficient procedure within the level set technique is gradient descent, which solves the optimization problem. Nevertheless, slow convergence and sensitivity to local optima are considered as their key disadvantages.

Figure 6. Segmentation of brain tumor with the level set method
(Wang, D., 2019)

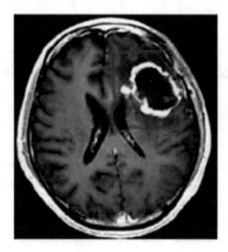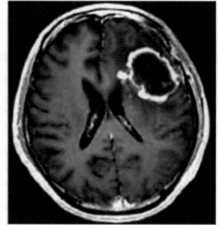

Rahman, C. M., and Rashid, T. M. *et al.*, (2019) suggested one of the most nature-inspired umbrella deployment of swarm algorithms for medical imaging applications as the dragonfly algorithm (DA). It is proved to be very effective in delivering optimal solutions. During the optimization process, it is necessary to ensure convergence. For this, dragonflies should properly adjust their weights so that they can be transformed into diversification from intensification. When the optimization process progresses, the neighbourhood region is expanded so that the flying path will be adjusted. Then, the swarm is strengthened in a group so that it can provide ideal outcomes at the final stage of the optimization process (Mirjalili, S *et al.*, 2016). The best result in DA will illustrate food and the worst will show the enemy. DA is easy to merge and a stable technique, which proves that it, is better than all other swarm algorithms. Convergence can expect to local optimum in the absence of internal memory. A difficulty that the user can face is a lack of correlation between the updating position and the centroid of the algorithm. This can force DA to converge to a local optimum and leads to optimal solution failure (KS, S. R. and Murugan, S. *et al.*, 2017).

4D MR Images Segmentation

The size of the tumor needs to be measured consistently to observe the significance of anticancer agents. Therapy responses may be classified as a partial response, complete response, progressive and stable diseases. The tumor variation with respect to time and location, are not expressed in this scheme, although many techniques do not require temporal information. In this research, an automated method applying probabilistic reasoning over time and position is introduced for brain tumor segmenting from 4D spatial-temporal MRI data. Using the hidden Markov model the 3D EM algorithm is extended so that the classification of tumor works out according to the earlier and following results. The 3D spatial model includes spatial coherence through a Markov Random Field. To analyse this method, we have used simulated and patient images from three independent references. Using spatial or temporal methods solitary cannot enhance the sensitivity and explicitness of tumor segmentation as the combined Spatio-temporal model modifies (S. Saeed *et al.*,2017).

The decrease in the size of the tumour evaluates that the good anticancer agent is effective. MRI with contrast enhancement portrays the accurate details of brain tumors that is why it is used frequently for diagnosing the stage and tracing the development of brain tumors (Haney, S. M. *et al.*, 2001). Figure 2.5 shows a T1-weighted, gadolinium-enhanced MRI that shows a brain tumor with irregular shape. Measuring the tumor size at baseline is basis for the patients' care and clinical trials for investigation as well. By performing consecutive MRIs, it can be defined whether the tumor is accepting the therapy and decreasing or it is progressing and increasing. Therefore, it is necessary to specify the reaction and progression of the tumor accurately. Methods that track the progression of tumors lay stress on the convenience and benefits in clinical practice. Rustin, G. J. *et al.*, (2004) suggested using simple linear measurements of the greatest diameter. In this approach, the greatest diameter is multiplied by the greatest perpendicular diameter of the selected MR section even if the tumor is not elliptical (Sattar, S. *et al.*, 2019). As the position of the head in the scanner differs in every trial, therefore 2D measurements are not duplicable and are always invariant. For achieving volumetric measure, a manual method called planimetry is used in which all the tumor enclosing MRI sections are tracked and added up. During tracing the tumor manually, borders of the tumour are required to be shown more accurately than the diameter measurements (Bohlen, M. *et al.*, 2019). However, this technique is too time-consuming, which is why it is not usually employed in clinical practice. Hu, C. *et al.*, (2018) suggested the technique of spatial resolution is also which, enhances the spatial resolution of the MRI system and produces more sections for analysis. This technique also reduces the use of manual tracing in clinical practices. To classify the brain tissues, several research articles have been published that emphasize automated segmentation for brain tissues. Various methods have centralized on EM approaches along with the Gaussian mixture model (Jafri, M. Z. M. *et al.*, 2017).

Figure 7. A gadolinium-enhanced T1-weighted MRI
(Jafri, M. Z. M. et al., 2017)

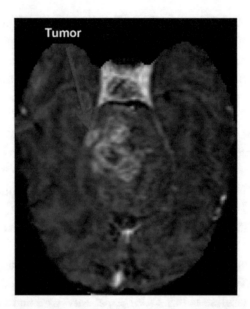

Kaur, A. *et al.*, (2021) described the analysis of detecting lesions with the optical flow or image subtraction approach in their research. The described temporal technique for brain lesions segmentation may have two prime drawbacks. First, the variation in shape or intensity is required to be detected (Cerri, S. *et al.*, 2020). However, if the change is minimal then lesions will not be detected and second, shape and intensity changes can be complicated. Therefore, these two measures are identical. The main objective of this research is to present a method, which employs the promising 3D spatial and unique temporal techniques for segmentation of brain tumors in MRI. This merged approach will utilize the earlier and subsequent segmentation techniques and provide a satisfactory brain tumor segmentation by optimizing it. This 4D segmentation does not need a vital change in the size of the tumor for observation thus, it proves to be a modification over 3D spatial or change detection techniques. Moreover, false-positive findings from iso-intense normal tissues are vastly minimized (Cerri, S. *et al.*, 2020).

R3: How can we utilize the Supervised Segmentation Methods for detecting the brain tumor in MRI images?

K-NN Missing Imputation

When we work with medical or biometric data sets usually, the problem of missing value imputation occurs. These problems must be eliminated on a prior basis. This is possible by imputing values for missing data but keeping in mind that such values must not influence data or change the balance of the class. A method is presented in the research that solves this problem for classification in the training data. To impute missing values, we have used an innovative method, k-NN classifier on separate features. This method allows us to use data from incomplete vectors for the imputation process. Conversely, in the conventional methods, only complete vectors can be utilized to impute vectors. This research also presents a test protocol, in which we use a Cross-Validation with a Set Substitution method like an explanation tool to achieve methods of missing value imputation (Orczyk, T. et al., 2021).

Pre-processing is considered as one of the essential processes in data mining, this process normalizes the data, removes noise, handle missing values and so on. This research aims to focus on tackling missing values while employing unsupervised machine learning techniques. For this purpose, flexible computational techniques and clustering techniques are combined to produce a novel method that can cope with the problems of inconsistency by handling the missing values. The suggested method is a rough K-means centroid-based imputation method that is further compared with other centroid-based imputation methods and parameter-based imputation methods. This approach gives promising results and proves the potency of various datasets as well (Raja, P. S., and Thangavel, K., 2020)

Support Vector Machine (SVM)

SVM method, being a potent approach, gives generalization and working especially in a very high dimension of the feature space. The concept used by it is that through some non-linear mapping it maps the input vector x into a feature space Z of high-dimension that is selected as a priori (Logeswari, T., and Karnan, M., 2010). SVM gained popularity when it utilized images as input and provided results that are more accurate. Object detection & recognition, biometrics, speech and text recognition, content-based image retrieval frequently use the SVM method (Lee, C. H. *et al.*, 2005). Support Vectors (SVs) are the training points for which the equality in the separating plan is satisfied the points (i.e. yi (xi. w + b) -1 ≥0, ∀i), that wind up lying on one of the hyperplanes H1, H2) and by elimination of which could alter the found results.

Support Vector Machine (SVM) serves as a famous tool to classify independent and identically distributed data (Ruan, S. *et al.*, 2007). It maximizes the margin between classes like in this research it uses simple linear feature space xi ·xj, by determining the best values in the Quadratic Programming problem that is given below in the dual Lagrangian form here the constant C bounds the misclassification error. Moreover, it uses T1-weighted and contrasts-enhanced T1- weighted images to categorize the brain as the brain tumor or non-tumor classes. To remove the miscalculations in classification, some morphological operations are suggested to use (Zhou, J *et al.*, 2006). Patient-specific training is used by this system and two SVM methods namely, the recent 1-class method and the standard 2-class method, are compared (Zhang, J. et *al.*, 2004). As the training examples for the tumor are required, only that is why a one-class method is used because the removal occurs in the manual time that is required to work out patient-specific training.

Figure 8. Segmentation output of brain tumor of two different patients with the matching ground truths(GT)
(Zhou, J. et al., 2006).

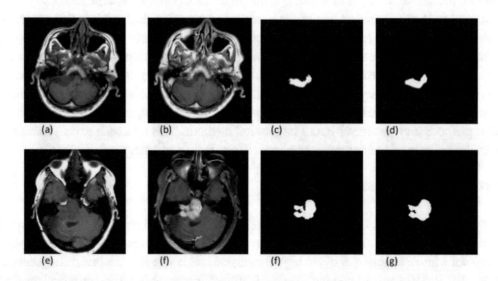

In figure.6 (a) and (e) are original T1weighted MR images that are taken before, (b) and (f) are images taken after enhancing contrast, (c) and (f) shows outcomes of segmentation employing the one-class SVM method and (d) shows GT given by expert radiologist.

High generalization and performance in feature space of high dimension are the main advantages of SVM method, so it is assumed that there are identical and independent data, which is not applicable for tasks like segmentation in the medical image that contains noise and inhomogeneity. To resolve this problem of spatial information SVM must be combined with other methods and must possess the advantages of such classifiers which do not depend on the dimensionality of the feature space and give accurate results, although the training time is relatively long The disadvantage of SVM-based methods include storage and patient-specific learning problems. It is also observed that the negative information in the regular one-class SVMs is not considered because of which it cannot understand the feedback sufficiently.

R4: How can we investigate the Detection of tumor or CSF fluid through Hidden Markov model and Grab Cut algorithm in 4D Light field segmentation?

Hidden Markov Model

Figure 9. A dynamic Bayesian network

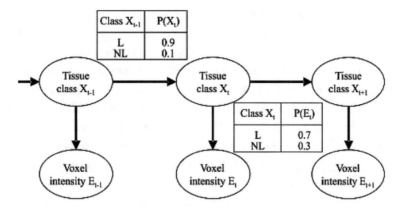

The above Figure 9 shows the graphical representation of this model giving the state of voxel i in the form of its tissue class. Here at time t, tissue class for voxel i is dependent on its class at time t − 1 through a transition matrix, and voxel intensity Ei is dependent on the tissue class at time t through a sensor model. For this case, classifying the voxel as a lesion says for example tumor at time t − 1, 0.9 is the probability that it will be a tumor at time t. As it is classified as a tumor so the probability of the voxel intensity Ei is 0.7. To provide models that are more significant rather than these popular models we develop improved sensor and transition models, which are as follows. Filtering is an HMM process, in which posterior distribution over the current state is computed but provided all evidence to date P (Xt|E1:t). If in this, state Xt is considered equivalent to lesion or non-lesion and Et is considered equivalent to intensity of pixel then the tissue classification, given the intensity values of the pixel, is provided by P(Xt|E1:t). For estimating the state of a pixel at time t+1 a recursive formula is developed while using Bayes' rule which is given below in Eq. (3).

$$P\left(X_{t+1} \mid E_{1:t+1}\right) = \alpha P\left(E_{t+1} \mid X_{t+1}\right) \sum_{x_t} P\left(X_{t+1} \mid X_t\right) p\left(X_t \mid E_{1:t}\right) \tag{3}$$

A normalizing constant is represented by this term, which adds all the probabilities equal to 1. Using the transition matrix, the present state is brought forward to t+1 from t, then it is updated with the new evidence ET+1 while employing the sensor model. Smoothing is also an HMM process that is utilized in computing the previous states, provided evidence until the current. It means that if one has estimated up to time point 5, then he can re-calculate the previous state at 1-4 time points. By using more collected information, the estimates of these states will be improved theoretically by this (Ibrahim, W. A., & Morcos, M. M, 2002).

Grab Cut Algorithm in 4D

In this method, the likelihood of foreground objects in multi-view images can be achieved by using disparity cues and appearance. The proposal of Xu, Y. *et al.*, (2019) uses an unsupervised method that can confine transparent object regions in a light field image. In this, a binary graph-cut segmentation method along with a light field distortion feature by (Maeno, K. *et al.*, 2013), shows the likelihood of pixel belonging to transparent object region. As the regions of interest are different for different users, therefore, these unsupervised methods, although being effective, are not appropriate for region selection for light field editing. Wanner, S.*et al.*, (2013) proposed a supervised approach for image segmentation in the 4D light field using appearance and disparity cues same as (Kowdle *et al.*, 2012). To deal with such inherently various information types, these researchers trained a random forest classifier that integrates appearance and disparity cues so that a single likelihood can be obtained for each label. This approach resulted in efficacy but gives output segmentation results only on the centre of the 2D image. The GCDL given by Wanner, S. *et al.*, (2013) was used in this research that exploit disparity from light field data and use this disparity and appearance so that the possibility of each region can be defined for each ray. In this research, support vector machines (SVMs) is used that integrates the likelihoods into a graph-cut algorithm.

4D Light Field Segmentation

Bishop, T. E., & Favaro, P., (2011) suggested supervised graph-cut algorithm technique in the four-dimensional (4D) light field segmentation method. 4D light field data is different from simple 4D hyper-volume as it has implicit depth information and holds redundancy. Spatial and angular neighbouring rays are specified to take care of redundancy in light field data. Along with this, we formulate a learning-based likelihood known as objectness that uses appearance and disparity cues to achieve higher segmentation accuracy. The efficacy of our method is presented through numerical interpretation and a few light field-editing applications utilizing both light fields, real-world and synthetic. Lumsdaine, A., & Georgiev, T., (2009) proposed that the current progress in the light field acquisition systems results in the wide use of light field imaging and the conventional digital cameras are going to be replaced by light-field cameras in the coming days (Ng, R. *et al.*, 2005). The improvement in the popularity of light field photography is gaining the needs for editing methods, tools, and products for example Photoshop R is a commonly used image-editing tool. Horn, D. R., & Chen, B., (2007) suggested a system that enables to utilize, combine, and provide many light fields. Jarabo, A. *et al.*, (2014) proposed that light field editing is still considered a challenge due to the reasons given below:

1.   Today many of the input and display devices are constructed for 2D structures and contents only; these do not apply to the 4D data light field.
2.   As light field holds redundancy, so any local edit is required to be propagated coherently to preserve redundancy.
3.   The depth information provided in a light field is not encoded explicitly.

The editing tool for the light field is considered to be effective if it has similar functions as Photoshop R, among which region selection is the most fundamental function. To obtain an efficient method for selecting region in a 4D light field, framework that is composed of multi-label segmentation is proposed in this research, which can cope with all the above-stated problems. In figure.9, each ray is assigned a proper label based on the geometrical composition of a light field.

Figure 10. Label assigning to every single ray according to the geometrical composition of a light field

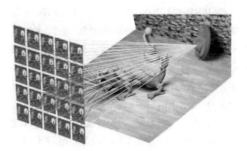

It is assumed in this framework that a user selects a portion, of the regions from the 4D light field data, through a 2D input tool. A functional user interface (UI) is suggested but the problem for the users to select all the regions in 4D space manually stays there (Jarabo, A. *et al.*, 2014). In our proposed method, it is required for the users to give cues for assigning a region of interest by labelling a portion of that region. Like, by using brush strokes the user can input a label on the centre viewpoint image that is a light field data subspace, for specifying the target object that is to be edited. Then this algorithm specifies the appropriate regions in the 4D light field based on the given inputs. It can be considered that by employing a 2D image segmentation method to each viewpoint image, results for a 4D light field segmentation can be achieved but with no assurance of the redundancy perseverance. The reason for this is the neighbouring relationships in the 4D light field data are not as simple as of a regular 3D volume grid, as the 4D light field contains redundancy difficulties. We use disparities in the 4D light field for defining appropriate neighbouring relationships so that the redundancies can be preserved. Moreover, these neighbouring relationships are defined among the rays in the 4D light field data so that the regions of interest can be estimated coherently. Some methods are suggested for exploiting the disparities in the light field data, as it contains no explicit depth information (Wanner, S., & Goldluecke, B., 2012). In this framework, regions are estimated appropriately by using colour and disparity details. To approximate the regions of interest, integrating disparity and colour details is a complicated task because both are inherently distinct. A learning-based approach is applied to integrate these colours and disparity cues so that we can find that all the rays are covered or not in a selected region.

R5: What is key factor of Fourier and Laplace transform with medical images transformation to identifying the missing data in MRI images?

Fourier Transform With Medical Images Transformation

For supporting the process of identifying medical images through Fourier transformation, we applied the selected methods of image processing. One of the famous and widely applied tools is Fourier transform that is used for various applications in image processing in various fields of science, technology, and medicine. Spatial frequencies are the main parts of the image processing study of Fourier transforms in medical images. These images form the basis and Fourier transformation is the appropriate tool to study skin lesions. It helps to study the distributions of selected colors in images obtained after applying Fourier transform (Sokołowski, A. and Pardela, T., 2014).

The problem of missing values in mass spectroscopy metabolomics datasets can be generated for various reasons, maybe technical or biological, and occurs frequently. Very brief information is available regarding their distributions across datasets, the requirement to include them in the data processing or not, the optimal way that provides those values according to analysis of univariate or multivariate data. By employing direct infusion, Fourier transforms ion cyclotron resonance mass spectrometry data we can overcome all the stated problems. As it is addressed missing data occurs frequently and systematically, it will calculate 20% of data and influence 80% of all variables and that missing data. It is shown that the results of data analysis face prime consequences of missing data estimation algorithms when the differences between the biological sample groups, which are included by t-test, ANOVA, and principal component analysis, are compared (Hrydziuszko, O. and Viant. M. R., 2012).

Moreover, we assessed the performance of eight algorithms to impute missing entries and found significant differences in results. Based on our findings we observed that the optimal approach for estimating missing values for our direct infusion mass spectrometry datasets is the k-nearest neighbor imputation method. However, more distinction of this analysis is to bring out the significance of missing metabolite levels in the data processing schedule and to suggest a technique or method that can determine optimal ways to treat missing data in metabolomics experiments (Hrydziuszko, O. and Viant. M. R., 2012).

Laplace Transformation

Zhang, S. et al., (2017) suggested that due to easy implementation and defined performance kNN is commonly used in various applications of data mining and machine learning. In the real applications suggesting the same k value to all the test data in the old kNN methods are verified of being ineffective. This research suggests a Correlation Matrix kNN (CM-kNN) classification in which test data points are reconstructed by training data so that several k values will be assigned to various test data points. We employ the least-squares loss function so that the reconstruction error will be minimized in reconstructing test data points by training data points. In the reconstruction process, a graph Laplacian regularizer is applied that keeps the structure of the nearest neighbours of the data save. To estimate several k values for various test data and to have low sparsity in the results by removing redundancy or noise from the reconstruction process, we employ a ℓ1-norm regularizer and a ℓ2, 1-norm regularizer. All the kNN techniques including our suggested CM-kNN method are used for not only classification purposes but also for missing data imputation and regression purposes as well. We did various investigations to show the efficacy and the outcomes proved that this method is additional efficient and accurate as compared to the previous ones in various data-mining applications like regression, imputation of missing data, and classification (Zhang, S. et al., 2017).

CONCLUSION

This chapter explains the systematic mapping of the study those are relates to the image segmentation method from several research studies. It includes the details of determining problems that delay the abilities of review this research technique. The 4D LFT segmentation of MRI images is still a challenging method because in the 4D space users still face difficulties in the manual selection of a complete region, the functional user interfaces therefore these are highly focused in the research. This study focuses on how to refine the 4D LFT segmentation method and cope with the difficulties generate during the application of this method. Literature on Fourier transformation and Laplace transformation is also a part of this section to construct the images and image processing segmentation techniques are also evaluated in this chapter.

k-NN algorithm is another part of this research is also evaluated in this literature to solves the problem of classification in the training data. This includes the K-NN algorithm imputation problem for missing data, k-means parameter-based imputation method, fuzzy C-means parameter-based imputation method, and so on. A detailed systematic review of the Hidden Markov Model (HMM) is also presented according to various research areas. This follows the detailed discussion of findings of issues and problems of identifying the images and reconstruct the images through probability calculation of reviewed techniques. Although, HMM still faces the challenges like evaluation, decoding and learning to find most likelihood classification, and these are still important research focus as evident from the literature. Further reconstruction of medical MRI images and it challenges to solve the identifying and reconstruction the images especially finding the CSF tissues/Fluid will be the focus of this study.

REFERENCES

Abbott, N. J., Pizzo, M. E., Preston, J. E., Janigro, D., & Thorne, R. G. (2018). The role of brain barriers in fluid movement in the CNS: Is there a 'glymphatic' system? *Acta Neuropathologica*, *135*(3), 387–407. doi:10.100700401-018-1812-4 PMID:29428972

Ahmed, M. M., & Mohamad, D. B. (2008). Segmentation of brain MR images for tumor extraction by combining kmeans clustering and perona-malik anisotropic diffusion model. *International Journal of Image Processing*, *2*(1), 27–34.

Al-Amri, S. S., & Kalyankar, N. V. (2010). *Image segmentation by using threshold techniques.* arXiv preprint arXiv:1005.4020.

Angulakshmi, M., & Lakshmi Priya, G. G. (2017). Automated brain tumour segmentation techniques—A review. *International Journal of Imaging Systems and Technology*, *27*(1), 66–77. doi:10.1002/ima.22211

Banerjee, S., & Mitra, S. (2020). Novel volumetric sub-region segmentation in brain tumors. *Frontiers in Computational Neuroscience*, *14*, 3. doi:10.3389/fncom.2020.00003 PMID:32038216

Bauer, S., Wiest, R., Nolte, L. P., & Reyes, M. (2013). A survey of MRI-based medical image analysis for brain tumor studies. *Physics in Medicine and Biology*, *58*(13), R97–R129. doi:10.1088/0031-9155/58/13/R97 PMID:23743802

Beevi, S. Z., Sathik, M. M., & Senthamaraikannan, K. (2010). *A robust fuzzy clustering technique with spatial neighborhood information for effective medical image segmentation.* arXiv preprint arXiv:1004.1679.

Berent, J., & Dragotti, P. L. (2007, September). Unsupervised Extraction of Coherent Regions for Image Based Rendering, In BMVC (pp. 1-10). doi:10.5244/C.21.28

Beretta, L., & Santaniello, A. (2016). Nearest neighbor imputation algorithms: A critical evaluation. *BMC Medical Informatics and Decision Making*, *16*(3), 197–208. doi:10.118612911-016-0318-z PMID:27454392

Bhide, A. S., Patil, P., & Dhande, S. (2012). Brain Segmentation using Fuzzy C means clustering to detect tumour Region. *International Journal of Advanced Research in Computer Science and Electronics Engineering*, *1*(2), 85–90.

Bishop, T. E., & Favaro, P. (2011). The light field camera: Extended depth of field, aliasing, and super-resolution. *IEEE Transactions on Pattern Analysis and Machine Intelligence*, *34*(5), 972–986. doi:10.1109/TPAMI.2011.168 PMID:21844629

Blanchet, L., Krooshof, P. W. T., Postma, G. J., Idema, A. J., Goraj, B., Heerschap, A., & Buydens, L. M. C. (2011). Discrimination between metastasis and glioblastoma multiforme based on morphometric analysis of MR images. *AJNR. American Journal of Neuroradiology*, *32*(1), 67–73. doi:10.3174/ajnr. A2269 PMID:21051512

Blumenfeld, H. (2010). *Neuroanatomy through clinical cases*. Sinauer Associates.

Bohlen, M., Busch, C. J., Sehner, S., Forterre, F., Bier, J., Berliner, C., Bußmann, L., & Münscher, A. (2019). Tumor volume as a predictive parameter in the sequential therapy (induction chemotherapy) of head and neck squamous cell carcinomas. *European Archives of Oto-Rhino-Laryngology*, *276*(4), 1183–1189. doi:10.100700405-019-05323-w PMID:30725209

Boykov, Y., & Kolmogorov, V. (2004). An experimental comparison of min-cut/max-flow algorithms for energy minimization in vision. *IEEE Transactions on Pattern Analysis and Machine Intelligence*, *26*(9), 1124–1137. doi:10.1109/TPAMI.2004.60 PMID:15742889

Boykov, Y., Veksler, O., & Zabih, R. (2001). Fast approximate energy minimization via graph cuts. *IEEE Transactions on Pattern Analysis and Machine Intelligence*, *23*(11), 1222–1239. doi:10.1109/34.969114

Boykov, Y. Y., & Jolly, M. P. (2001, July). Interactive graph cuts for optimal boundary & region segmentation of objects in ND images. *Proceedings eighth IEEE international conference on computer vision. ICCV 2001*, 105-112. 10.1109/ICCV.2001.937505

Brinker, T., Stopa, E., Morrison, J., & Klinge, P. (2014). A new look at cerebrospinal fluid circulation. *Fluids and Barriers of the CNS*, *11*(1), 1–16. doi:10.1186/2045-8118-11-10 PMID:24817998

Bzdok, D., Krzywinski, M., & Altman, N. (2018). Machine learning: Supervised methods. *Nature Methods*, *15*(1), 5–6. doi:10.1038/nmeth.4551 PMID:30100821

Calabrese, C., Poppleton, H., Kocak, M., Hogg, T. L., Fuller, C., Hamner, B., Oh, E. Y., Gaber, M. W., Finklestein, D., Allen, M., Frank, A., Bayazitov, I. T., Zakharenko, S. S., Gajjar, A., Davidoff, A., & Gilbertson, R. J. (2007). A perivascular niche for brain tumor stem cells. *Cancer Cell*, *11*(1), 69–82. doi:10.1016/j.ccr.2006.11.020 PMID:17222791

Cerri, S., Hoopes, A., Greve, D. N., Mühlau, M., & Van Leemput, K. (2020). A longitudinal method for simultaneous whole-brain and lesion segmentation in multiple sclerosis. In *Machine Learning in Clinical Neuroimaging and Radiogenomics in Neuro-oncology* (pp. 119–128). Springer. doi:10.1007/978-3-030-66843-3_12

Chang, M. M., Sezan, M. I., Tekalp, A. M., & Berg, M. J. (1996). Bayesian segmentation of multislice brain magnetic resonance imaging using three-dimensional Gibbsian priors. *Optical Engineering (Redondo Beach, Calif.)*, *35*(11), 3206–3221. doi:10.1117/1.601059

Christ, M. J., & Parvathi, R. M. S. (2012). Segmentation of medical image using K-means clustering and marker controlled watershed algorithm. *European Journal of Scientific Research*, *71*(2), 190–194.

Clarke, L. P., Velthuizen, R. P., Clark, M., Gaviria, J., Hall, L., Goldgof, D., Murtagh, R., Phuphanich, S., & Brem, S. (1998). MRI measurement of brain tumor response: Comparison of visual metric and automatic segmentation. *Magnetic Resonance Imaging*, *16*(3), 271–279. doi:10.1016/S0730-725X(97)00302-0 PMID:9621968

Das, D., Nayak, M., & Pani, S. K. (2019). Missing Value Imputation-. *RE:view*.

Dong, L., Ogunbona, P., Li, W., Yu, G., Fan, L., & Zheng, G. (2006, August). A fast algorithm for color image segmentation. *First International Conference on Innovative Computing, Information and Control-Volume I (ICICIC'06)*, 685-688. 10.1109/ICICIC.2006.192

Fang, Z., Tian, R., Jia, Y. T., Xu, T. T., & Liu, Y. (2017). Treatment of cerebrospinal fluid leak after spine surgery. *Chinese Journal of Traumatology*, *20*(2), 81–83. doi:10.1016/j.cjtee.2016.12.002 PMID:28336418

Gortler, S. J., Grzeszczuk, R., Szeliski, R., & Cohen, M. F. (1996, August). The lumigraph. *Proceedings of the 23rd annual conference on Computer graphics and interactive techniques*, 43-54.

Greig, D. M., Porteous, B. T., & Seheult, A. H. (1989). Exact maximum a posteriori estimation for binary images. *Journal of the Royal Statistical Society. Series B. Methodological*, *51*(2), 271–279. doi:10.1111/j.2517-6161.1989.tb01764.x

Guo, G., Wang, H., Bell, D., Bi, Y., & Greer, K. (2003, November). KNN model-based approach in classification. *OTM Confederated International Conferences On the Move to Meaningful Internet Systems*, 986-996. 10.1007/978-3-540-39964-3_62

Haney, S. M., Thompson, P. M., Cloughesy, T. F., Alger, J. R., & Toga, A. W. (2001). Tracking tumor growth rates in patients with malignant gliomas: A test of two algorithms. *AJNR. American Journal of Neuroradiology*, *22*(1), 73–82. PMID:11158891

Hansson Mild, K., Lundström, R., & Wilén, J. (2019). Non-Ionizing radiation in Swedish health care—Exposure and safety aspects. *International Journal of Environmental Research and Public Health*, *16*(7), 1186. doi:10.3390/ijerph16071186 PMID:30987016

Horn, D. R., & Chen, B. (2007, April). Lightshop: interactive light field manipulation and rendering. *Proceedings of the 2007 symposium on Interactive 3D graphics and games*, 121-128. 10.1145/1230100.1230121

Hrydziuszko, O., & Viant, M. R. (2012). Missing values in mass spectrometry based metabolomics: An undervalued step in the data processing pipeline. *Metabolomics*, *8*(1), 161–174. doi:10.100711306-011-0366-4

Hu, C., Song, L., Liu, M., Wang, J., & Zhang, L. (2018, October). A Novel Multi-Atlas and Multi-Channel (MAMC) Approach for Multiple Sclerosis Lesion Segmentation in Brain MRI. *Proceedings of the 2nd International Symposium on Image Computing and Digital Medicine*, 106-112. 10.1145/3285996.3286019

Ibrahim, W. A., & Morcos, M. M. (2002). Artificial intelligence and advanced mathematical tools for power quality applications: A survey. *IEEE Transactions on Power Delivery*, *17*(2), 668–673. doi:10.1109/61.997958

Jafri, M. Z. M., Abdulbaqi, H. S., Mutter, K. N., Mustapha, I. S., & Omar, A. F. (2017, June). Measuring the volume of brain tumour and determining its location in T2-weighted MRI images using hidden Markov random field: expectation maximization algorithm. In Digital Optical Technologies. International Society for Optics and Photonics.

Jarabo, A., Masia, B., Bousseau, A., Pellacini, F., & Gutierrez, D. (2014). How do people edit light fields? *ACM Transactions on Graphics*, *33*(4), 4. doi:10.1145/2601097.2601125

Kanungo, T., Mount, D. M., Netanyahu, N. S., Piatko, C. D., Silverman, R., & Wu, A. Y. (2002). An efficient k-means clustering algorithm: Analysis and implementation. *IEEE Transactions on Pattern Analysis and Machine Intelligence*, *24*(7), 881–892. doi:10.1109/TPAMI.2002.1017616

Kaur, A., Kaur, L., & Singh, A. (2021). State-of-the-art segmentation techniques and future directions for multiple sclerosis brain lesions. *Archives of Computational Methods in Engineering*, *28*(3), 951–977. doi:10.100711831-020-09403-7

Khalil, H. A., Darwish, S., Ibrahim, Y. M., & Hassan, O. F. (2020). 3D-MRI brain tumor detection model using modified version of level set segmentation based on dragonfly algorithm. *Symmetry*, *12*(8), 1256. doi:10.3390ym12081256

Khan, M. A., Lali, I. U., Rehman, A., Ishaq, M., Sharif, M., Saba, T., Zahoor, S., & Akram, T. (2019). Brain tumor detection and classification: A framework of marker-based watershed algorithm and multilevel priority features selection. *Microscopy Research and Technique*, *82*(6), 909–922. doi:10.1002/jemt.23238 PMID:30801840

Kharrat, A., Benamrane, N., Messaoud, M. B., & Abid, M. (2009, November). Detection of brain tumor in medical images. In *2009 3rd International conference on signals, circuits and systems (SCS)*. IEEE. 10.1109/ICSCS.2009.5412577

Kolmogorov, V., & Zabih, R. (2002, May). Multi-camera scene reconstruction via graph cuts. In *European conference on computer vision*. Springer.

Kowdle, A., Sinha, S. N., & Szeliski, R. (2012, October). Multiple view object cosegmentation using appearance and stereo cues. In *European Conference on Computer Vision*. Springer. 10.1007/978-3-642-33715-4_57

KS, S. R., & Murugan, S. (2017). Memory based hybrid dragonfly algorithm for numerical optimization problems. *Expert Systems with Applications*, *83*, 63–78. doi:10.1016/j.eswa.2017.04.033

Lavanyadevi, R., Machakowsalya, M., Nivethitha, J., & Kumar, A. N. (2017, April). Brain tumor classification and segmentation in MRI images using PNN. *2017 IEEE International Conference on Electrical, Instrumentation and Communication Engineering (ICEICE)*, 1-6. 10.1109/ICEICE.2017.8191888

Lee, C. H., Schmidt, M., Murtha, A., Bistritz, A., Sander, J., & Greiner, R. (2005, October). Segmenting brain tumors with conditional random fields and support vector machines. In *International Workshop on Computer Vision for Biomedical Image Applications*. Springer. 10.1007/11569541_47

Levoy, M., & Hanrahan, P. (1996, August). Light field rendering. *Proceedings of the 23rd annual conference on Computer graphics and interactive techniques*, 31-42.

Li, G., Citrin, D., Camphausen, K., Mueller, B., Burman, C., Mychalczak, B., Miller, R. W., & Song, Y. (2008). Advances in 4D medical imaging and 4D radiation therapy. *Technology in Cancer Research & Treatment*, *7*(1), 67–81. doi:10.1177/153303460800700109 PMID:18198927

Logeswari, T., & Karnan, M. (2010, February). An improved implementation of brain tumor detection using soft computing. *2010 Second International Conference on Communication Software and Networks*, 147-151. 10.1109/ICCSN.2010.10

Lu, C. Y., Xu, Z. S., & Ye, X. (2019). Evaluation of intraoperative MRI-assisted stereotactic brain tissue biopsy: A single-center experience in China. *Chinese Neurosurgical Journal*, *5*(1), 1–8. doi:10.118641016-019-0152-0 PMID:32922904

Lumsdaine, A., & Georgiev, T. (2009, April). The focused plenoptic camera. *2009 IEEE International Conference on Computational Photography (ICCP*1-8.

Luo, M., Ma, Y. F., & Zhang, H. J. (2003, December). A spatial constrained k-means approach to image segmentation. *Fourth International Conference on Information, Communications and Signal Processing, 2003 and the Fourth Pacific Rim Conference on Multimedia. Proceedings of the 2003 Joint*, 738-742.

Maeno, K., Nagahara, H., Shimada, A., & Taniguchi, R. I. (2013). Light field distortion feature for transparent object recognition. *Proceedings of the IEEE Conference on Computer Vision and Pattern Recognition*, 2786-2793. 10.1109/CVPR.2013.359

Mihara, H., Funatomi, T., Tanaka, K., Kubo, H., Mukaigawa, Y., & Nagahara, H. (2016, May). 4D light field segmentation with spatial and angular consistencies. *2016 IEEE International Conference on Computational Photography (ICCP)*, 1-8. 10.1109/ICCPHOT.2016.7492872

Mirjalili, S. (2016). Dragonfly algorithm: A new meta-heuristic optimization technique for solving single-objective, discrete, and multi-objective problems. *Neural Computing & Applications*, *27*(4), 1053–1073. doi:10.100700521-015-1920-1

Mustaqeem, A., Javed, A., & Fatima, T. (2012). An efficient brain tumor detection algorithm using watershed & thresholding based segmentation. *International Journal of Image, Graphics and Signal Processing*, *4*(10), 34–39. doi:10.5815/ijigsp.2012.10.05

Nagahashi, T., Fujiyoshi, H., & Kanade, T. (2009, September). Video segmentation using iterated graph cuts based on spatio-temporal volumes. In *Asian Conference on Computer Vision*. Springer.

Natarajan, P., Krishnan, N., Kenkre, N. S., Nancy, S., & Singh, B. P. (2012, December). *Tumor detection using threshold operation in MRI brain images. In 2012 IEEE international conference on computational intelligence and computing research*. IEEE.

Ng, R., Levoy, M., Brédif, M., Duval, G., Horowitz, M., & Hanrahan, P. (2005). *Light field photography with a hand-held plenoptic camera* (Doctoral dissertation). Stanford University.

Orczyk, T., Doroz, R., & Porwik, P. (2021, June). Missing Value Imputation Method Using Separate Features Nearest Neighbors Algorithm. *International Conference on Computational Science*, 128-141. 10.1007/978-3-030-77967-2_12

Osher, S., & Sethian, J. A. (1988). Fronts propagating with curvature-dependent speed: Algorithms based on Hamilton-Jacobi formulations. *Journal of Computational Physics*, *79*(1), 12–49. doi:10.1016/0021-9991(88)90002-2

Pan, W., Gu, W., Nagpal, S., Gephart, M. H., & Quake, S. R. (2015). Brain tumor mutations detected in cerebral spinal fluid. *Clinical Chemistry*, *61*(3), 514–522. doi:10.1373/clinchem.2014.235457 PMID:25605683

Pascal, N. E., Pierre, E., & Emmanuel, T. (2014). Hybrid Method Segmentation for Medical Image Based on DWT, FCM and HMRF-EM. *International Journal of Computer and Information Technology*.

Popoola, J. J., Godson, T. E., Olasoji, Y. O., & Adu, M. R. (2019). Study on capabilities of different segmentation algorithms in detecting and reducing brain tumor size in magnetic resonance imaging for effective telemedicine services. *European Journal of Engineering and Technology Research*, *4*(2), 23–29. doi:10.24018/ejers.2019.4.2.1142

Pradhan, S. (2010). *Development of Unsupervised Image Segmentation Schemes for Brain MRI using HMRF model* (Doctoral dissertation).

Prastawa, M., Bullitt, E., Moon, N., Van Leemput, K., & Gerig, G. (2003). Automatic brain tumor segmentation by subject specific modification of atlas priors1. *Academic Radiology*, *10*(12), 1341–1348. doi:10.1016/S1076-6332(03)00506-3 PMID:14697002

Rahman, C. M., & Rashid, T. A. (2019). Dragonfly algorithm and its applications in applied science survey. *Computational Intelligence and Neuroscience*, *2019*, 1–21. doi:10.1155/2019/9293617 PMID:31885533

Rahman, S. A., Huang, Y., Claassen, J., Heintzman, N., & Kleinberg, S. (2015). Combining Fourier and lagged k-nearest neighbor imputation for biomedical time series data. *Journal of Biomedical Informatics*, *58*, 198–207. doi:10.1016/j.jbi.2015.10.004 PMID:26477633

Raja, P. S., & Thangavel, K. (2020). Missing value imputation using unsupervised machine learning techniques. *Soft Computing*, *24*(6), 4361–4392. doi:10.100700500-019-04199-6

Rajalakshmi, N., & Prabha, V. L. (2012). Brain tumor detection of mr images based on color-converted hybrid pso+ k-means clustering segmentation. *European Journal of Scientific Research*, 5-14.

Rajasekaran, K. A., & Gounder, C. C. (2018). Advanced Brain Tumour Segmentation from MRI Images. *Basic Physical Principles and Clinical Applications, High-Resolution Neuroimaging*, 83-108.

Ray, S., & Turi, R. H. (1999, December). Determination of number of clusters in k-means clustering and application in colour image segmentation. *Proceedings of the 4th international conference on advances in pattern recognition and digital techniques*, 137-143.

Rother, C., Kolmogorov, V., & Blake, A. (2004). GrabCut" interactive foreground extraction using iterated graph cuts. *ACM Transactions on Graphics*, *23*(3), 309–314. doi:10.1145/1015706.1015720

Roy, S., Nag, S., Maitra, I. K., & Bandyopadhyay, S. K. (2013). *A review on automated brain tumor detection and segmentation from MRI of brain*. arXiv preprint arXiv:1312.6150.

Ruan, S., Lebonvallet, S., Merabet, A., & Constans, J. M. (2007, April). Tumor segmentation from a multispectral MRI images by using support vector machine classification. *2007 4th IEEE International Symposium on Biomedical Imaging: From Nano to Macro*, 1236-1239. 10.1109/ISBI.2007.357082

Rustin, G. J., Quinn, M., Thigpen, T., Du Bois, A., Pujade-Lauraine, E., Jakobsen, A., Eisenhauer, E., Sagae, S., Greven, K., Vergote, I., Cervantes, A., & Vermorken, J. (2004). Re: New guidelines to evaluate the response to treatment in solid tumors (ovarian cancer). *Journal of the National Cancer Institute*, *96*(6), 487–488. doi:10.1093/jnci/djh081 PMID:15026475

Saeed & Abdullah. (2021). Performance analysis of machine learning algorithm for health care tools with High Dimension Segmentation. *Machine learning healthcare: Handling and managing data, 1*(1), 1-30.

Saeed & Abdullah. (2021). Statistical Analysis the Pre and Post-Surgery of health care sector using High Dimension Segmentation. *Machine learning healthcare: Handling and managing data, 1*(1), 1-25.

Saeed & Abdullah. (2021). Combination of Brain Cancer with Hybrid K-NN Algorithm using statistical Analysis of Cerebrospinal Fluid (CSF) Surgery. *International Journal of Computer Science and Network Security, 21*(2), 120-130.

Saeed & Naqvi. (2019). Implementation of Fourier transformation. *Indian Journal of Science & Technology, 12*(37), 1-16.

Saeed, S., Abdullah, A., & Jhanjhi, N. (2019). Investigation of a Brain Cancer with Interfacing of 3-Dimensional Image Processing. *Indian Journal of Science and Technology*, *12*(34), 1–12. doi:10.17485/ijst/2019/v12i34/146150

Saeed, S., & Naqvi, M. (2017). Implementation of Failure Enterprise Systems in Organizational Perspective Framework. *International Journal of Advanced Computer Science and Applications*, *8*(5), 54–63. doi:10.14569/IJACSA.2017.080508

Saeed & Naqvi. (n.d.). Assessment of Brain Tumor Due to the Usage of MATLAB Performance. *Journal of Medical Imaging and Health Informatics*, *7*(6), 1454–1460. doi:10.1166/jmihi.2017.2187

Sajid, S., Hussain, S., & Sarwar, A. (2019). Brain tumor detection and segmentation in MR images using deep learning. *Arabian Journal for Science and Engineering*, *44*(11), 9249–9261. doi:10.100713369-019-03967-8

Sakka, L., Coll, G., & Chazal, J. (2011). Anatomy and physiology of cerebrospinal fluid. *European Annals of Otorhinolaryngology, Head and Neck Diseases*, *128*(6), 309–316. doi:10.1016/j.anorl.2011.03.002 PMID:22100360

Sattar, S., Alibhai, S. M., Spoelstra, S. L., & Puts, M. T. (2019). The assessment, management, and reporting of falls, and the impact of falls on cancer treatment in community-dwelling older patients receiving cancer treatment: Results from a mixed-methods study. *Journal of Geriatric Oncology*, *10*(1), 98–104. doi:10.1016/j.jgo.2018.08.006 PMID:30174258

Selvy, P. T., Palanisamy, V., & Purusothaman, T. (2011). Performance analysis of clustering algorithms in brain tumor detection of MR images. *European Journal of Scientific Research*, *62*(3), 321–330.

Shen, S., Sandham, W. A., & Granat, M. H. (2003, April). Preprocessing and segmentation of brain magnetic resonance images. *4th International IEEE EMBS Special Topic Conference on Information Technology Applications in Biomedicine*, 149-152. 10.1109/ITAB.2003.1222495

Shirly, S., & Ramesh, K. (2019). Review on 2D and 3D MRI image segmentation techniques. *Current Medical Imaging*, *15*(2), 150–160. doi:10.2174/1573405613666171123160609 PMID:31975661

Shokouhifar, M., & Abkenar, G. S. (2011). An artificial bee colony optimization for mri fuzzy segmentation of brain tissue. *2011 International Conference on Management and Artificial Intelligence IPEDR*.

Sokołowski, A., & Pardela, T. (2014). Application of Fourier transforms in classification of medical images. In *Human-computer systems interaction: backgrounds and applications* (Vol. 3, pp. 193–200). Springer.

Spector, R., Snodgrass, S. R., & Johanson, C. E. (2015). A balanced view of the cerebrospinal fluid composition and functions: Focus on adult humans. *Experimental Neurology*, *273*, 57–68. doi:10.1016/j.expneurol.2015.07.027 PMID:26247808

Sultan, H. H., Salem, N. M., & Al-Atabany, W. (2019). Multi-classification of brain tumor images using deep neural network. *IEEE Access: Practical Innovations, Open Solutions*, *7*, 69215–69225. doi:10.1109/ACCESS.2019.2919122

Taheri, S., Ong, S. H., & Chong, V. F. H. (2010). Level-set segmentation of brain tumors using a threshold-based speed function. *Image and Vision Computing*, *28*(1), 26–37. doi:10.1016/j.imavis.2009.04.005

Tatiraju, S., & Mehta, A. (2008). Image Segmentation using k-means clustering, EM and Normalized Cuts. *Department of EECS*, *1*, 1–7.

Telano, L. N., & Baker, S. (2020). *Physiology, Cerebral Spinal Fluid (CSF)*. StatPearls.

Tzika, A. A., Astrakas, L., & Zarifi, M. (2011). Pediatric Brain Tumors: Magnetic Resonance Spectroscopic Imaging. *Diagnostic Techniques and Surgical Management of Brain Tumors*, 205.

Van Leemput, K., Maes, F., Vandermeulen, D., & Suetens, P. (1998, October). Automatic segmentation of brain tissues and MR bias field correction using a digital brain atlas. In *International Conference on Medical Image Computing and Computer-Assisted. Intervention*. Springer. 10.1007/BFb0056312

Vasuda, P., & Satheesh, S. (2010). Improved fuzzy C-means algorithm for MR brain image segmentation. *International Journal on Computer Science and Engineering*, 2(5).

Wang, D. (2019). Efficient level-set segmentation model driven by the local GMM and split Bregman method. *IET Image Processing*, 13(5), 761–770. doi:10.1049/iet-ipr.2018.6216

Wang, L. (2019, December). Research and Implementation of Machine Learning Classifier Based on KNN. In *IOP Conference Series: Materials Science and Engineering*. IOP Publishing. 10.1088/1757-899X/677/5/052038

Wanner, S., & Goldluecke, B. (2012, June). Globally consistent depth labeling of 4D light fields. In *2012 IEEE Conference on Computer Vision and Pattern Recognition*. IEEE. 10.1109/CVPR.2012.6247656

Wanner, S., Straehle, C., & Goldluecke, B. (2013). Globally consistent multi-label assignment on the ray space of 4d light fields. *Proceedings of the IEEE Conference on Computer Vision and Pattern Recognition*, 1011-1018. 10.1109/CVPR.2013.135

Xu, Y., Nagahara, H., Shimada, A., & Taniguchi, R. I. (2019). TransCut2: Transparent Object Segmentation From a Light-Field Image. *IEEE Transactions on Computational Imaging*, 5(3), 465–477. doi:10.1109/TCI.2019.2893820

Zhang, D. Q., & Chen, S. C. (2004). A novel kernelized fuzzy c-means algorithm with application in medical image segmentation. *Artificial Intelligence in Medicine*, 32(1), 37–50. doi:10.1016/j.artmed.2004.01.012 PMID:15350623

Zhang, J., Ma, K. K., Er, M. H., & Chong, V. (2004, January). Tumor segmentation from magnetic resonance imaging by learning via one-class support vector machine. *International Workshop on Advanced Image Technology (IWAIT'04)*, 207-211.

Zhang, S., Cheng, D., Deng, Z., Zong, M., & Deng, X. (2018). A novel kNN algorithm with data-driven k parameter computation. *Pattern Recognition Letters*, 109, 44–54. doi:10.1016/j.patrec.2017.09.036

Zhang, S., Li, X., Zong, M., Zhu, X., & Cheng, D. (2017). Learning k for knn classification. *ACM Transactions on Intelligent Systems and Technology*, 8(3), 1–19.

Zhang, Y., Brady, M., & Smith, S. (2001). Segmentation of brain MR images through a hidden Markov field model and the expectation-maximization algorithm. *IEEE Transactions on Medical Imaging*, 20(1), 45–57. doi:10.1109/42.906424 PMID:11293691

Zhou, J., Chan, K. L., Chong, V. F. H., & Krishnan, S. M. (2006, January). Extraction of brain tumor from MR images using one-class support vector machine. *2005 IEEE Engineering in Medicine and Biology 27th Annual Conference*, 6411-6414.

Zhuge, Y., Krauze, A. V., Ning, H., Cheng, J. Y., Arora, B. C., Camphausen, K., & Miller, R. W. (2017). Brain tumor segmentation using holistically nested neural networks in MRI images. *Medical Physics*, 44(10), 5234–5243. doi:10.1002/mp.12481 PMID:28736864

Chapter 8
Optimized Hybrid Prediction Method for Lung Metastases

Soobia Saeed

Department of Software Engineering,
UniversitiTeknologi Malaysia, Malaysia

Afnizanfaizal Abdullah

UniversitiTeknologi Malaysia, Malaysia

Noor Zaman Jhanjhi

ⓘ https://orcid.org/0000-0001-8116-4733

Taylor's University, Malaysia

Mehmood Naqvi

Mohwak College, Canada

Muneer Ahmad

National University of Science and Technology,
Pakistan

ABSTRACT

Brain metastases are the most prevalent intracranial neoplasm that causes excessive morbidity and mortality in most cancer patients. The current medical model for brain metastases is focused on the physical condition of the affected individual, the anatomy of the main tumor, and the number and proximity of brain lesions. In this paper, a new hybrid Metastases Fast Fourier Transformation with SVM (MFFT-SVM) method is proposed that can classify high dimensional magnetic resonance imaging as tumor and predicts lung cancer from given protein primary sequences. The goal is to address the associated issues stated with the treatment targeted at unique molecular pathways to the tumor, together with those involved in crossing the blood-brain barrier and migrating cells to the lungs. The proposed method identifies the place of the lung damage by the Fast Fourier Technique (FFT). FFT is the principal statistical approach for frequency analysis which has many engineering and scientific uses. Moreover, Differential Fourier Transformation (DFT) is considered for focusing the brain metastases that migrate into the lungs and create non-small lungs cancer. However, Support Vector Machine (SVM) is used to measure the accuracy of control patient's datasets of sensitivity and specificity. The simulation results verified the performance of the proposed method is improved by 92.8% sensitivity, of 93.2% specificity and 95.5% accuracy respectively.

DOI: 10.4018/978-1-7998-8929-8.ch008

INTRODUCTION

Brain tumor is one of the most dangerous tumors especially in a couple of tissues within the skull and secondary tumors inside the cranium (cerebrum tumor) that migrate from other areas of the body. Furthermore, intracranial tumors are on frequent in lung cancer patients. The mechanisms for lung cancers that have progressed to the brain are complicated. They are inspired by a number of reasons. The discovery of receptors for lung cancers with brain metastases may have far-reaching implications for clinical pharmacology studies as well as improved first-class lives for patients. The lung can range from other primary places, making clinical care more difficult. Despite continuous advancements in science in recent years, survival rates remain low (Hazra et al., 2017). Furthermore, lung tumors, breast cancers, and malignant melanoma are the leading causes of brain metastases. To penetrate the brain, metastatic parenchymal cells must travel through the endothelial cell layer of cerebral capillaries, which forms the morphological base of the Blood-Brain Barrier (BBB).

BBB plays dual function within the improvement of brain metastases and paperwork near a membrane that forestalls the valuable nervous device from penetrating most cancers cells, but is also strongly worried with shielding metastatic cells all through brain leakage and proliferation. The mechanisms of contact among cancer cells and brain endothelial cells are largely uncharacterized. Metastatic cells are furnished; the brain rain metastases are a widespread therapeutic mission; it's far essential to recall the pathways of maximum cancer cells that communicate with BBB to find goals to deter brain metastases from growing (Bhowmik et al., 2015). However, there are two forms of lung cancer, consisting of small cellular lung cancers, which accounts for approximately 10 to fifteen percent of all lung cancers, and non-small cell lung cancers, which debts for approximately eighty to 85% of all lung cancers. Lung cancers typically spread to other areas of the body by lymphatic channels and blood vessels. While lung cancer is quicker to spread via the lymph arteries, it usually takes longer for secondary metastatic cancer to spread. For blood vessels, it is more difficult to reach cancer. However, it spreads relatively easily once. In general, metastases through blood cells are worse in the short term, and metastases through lymphocytes are worse in the long term (Bhowmik et al., 2015).

More specifically, the project seeks to provide a systematic approach to the quantitative study of motion and kinematics in {x, y, z, t} microscopic world recordings. Although the study of digital 2D and 3D images has been very good, many research issues remain totally open in the study of 4D phenomena. 4D Image Processing is an important next step in keeping with the aspects of what is physical reality. By comparison, 2D and 3D-Image processing through microscopy is essentially a reduction in the physical world by projection or time fixation (Bolourian & Mojtahedi, 2017). Fourier series provides an alternative technique for representing the information marker of different frequencies rather than representing the limit of the signal as a component of time. Fourier analysis allows us to isolate specific combinations of repeats. This investigation describes part of the basic ideas of Fourier order and demonstrates how this examination can be performed through software modeling. This research aims to build a research framework that can quantify or quantify the area of damage in BBB and the migration of cancer cells from the cell membrane using Fourier transform. Another research instrument, focused on the Fourier transform, is the primary statistical approach for event analysis and has a wide range of scientific and technical applications. DFT is a ubiquitous method, and is defined as "there was a wide-range observation of high-ways for the DFT account and active investigation has constant". DFT is also a method for computing DFT that is widely studied and active research continues. The DFT segmentation method provides several fast algorithms. To test DFT's results, we equipped it with two fast-acting algorithms in this article. Because of the 4D images and Fourier transformations, this analysis assists in the identification of brain metastases (Barrow & Colonna, 2017). Another main concept of the SVM is to establish a hyper-chromic level that optimally distinguishes examples of data belonging to two groups such that the minimum distance between the nodes and the hyperboloid is improved. It is best to generalize uncertain examples in this manner. SVM mitigates systemic risks and obtains zero training errors thus reducing model complexity. In certain cases, where linear differentiation is not feasible as SVMs decrease the number of misclassified instances in the training set by adding slack variables and control variations (Ali et al., 2013). Nowadays, the observations of biological processes are mostly performed by the collection, processing and study of 4D time-lapse images. The multiple configurations of the body can be studied concurrently by the acquisition of multi-channel imagery data sets. This paper provides a programming paradigm that aims to facilitate the management of this type of multi-dimensional image, the creation and validation of new image processing algorithms, and the image segmentation using different visualization techniques. We describe a real scenario in which the system was used to discover and segment biological cell membranes and picture nucleus. 4D imaging aims to develop an integrated approach for the quantitative visualization and analysis of spatial processes in cells and tissues. This includes designing new illumination sensors, marking procedures, and developing new approaches to imaging, visualization and image estimation. A novel methodology addresses two basic biomedical/biomedical problems such as the structure of the mammalian dynamic interphase nucleus in relation to gene expression and the dynamics of cell interaction and cytoskeletal matrix. The development of new approaches for processing, quantitative analysis and visualization of 4D images, that is, time series of 3D images, using confocal scanning microscopy (Bolourian & Mojtahedi, 2017).

To best our knowledge, this research is the first attempt to propose a Fast Fourier Transformation method to identify brain metastases for cell metastases for lung cancer. The biggest issue in the MRI imaging is the lack of freely accessible data sets. While certain data sets are accessible on the Internet, the amount of images devoted to our issue is much smaller. We therefore, use extensive data expansion by optimizing data with different parameters and techniques to fill the data gap and perform system transformation. The technical contribution of this paper is presented as follows.

1. A new hybrid Metastases Fast Fourier Transformation with SVM (MFFT-SVM) method is anticipated that can predict lung cancer from given protein main sequences with respect to prediction enactment and computational research.
2. Furthermost discriminant features are predictable for the prediction of human lungs and non-small lungs cancer.

The rest of the paper is organized as follows: Section 2 presents the related work that explains the past history of associated articles. In Section 3, the proposed hybrid method (MFFT-SVM) based on the detection of brain metastases and lung cancer is described through MRI-4D interface images. Section 4 represents the details of findings and discussions, with consequences and new achievements. Finally, the conclusion is given with the future research directions in Section 5.

RELATED WORK

In order to be successful in the treatment of blood-borne cancer, a large amount of cancer cells cross the wall of the blood vessel and the resistance of the nearby microenvironment must be overcome around most cancer cells and brain metastases. This study reveals the Blood-Brain Barrier (BBB) cell and molecular additives, a specialized neurovascular unit designed to hold brain homeostasis (Hazra et al., 2017). Tumors are assumed to jeopardize the integrity of the BBB, which happens inside the improvement of blood vessels called the Blood Test Barrier (BTB), that are especially heterogeneous and characterized by a spread of great features, inclusive of atypical permeability and lively molecular go with the flow (Bhowmik et al., 2015; Bolourian & Mojtahedi, 2017). The look explores the requirements of BBB and BTB distribution for drug transmission, how multi-cells sort dictate BBB characteristics, and the feature of BTB inside the production and treatment of sicknesses. Finally, this observation sheds mild on novel biochemical, cell and physical strategies to improving drug shipping in BBB and BTB and explores their effect at the development of traditional and new healing alternatives, alongside novel immune barrier inhibitors and T-cells (Barrow & Colonna, 2017). The increased knowledge of BBB and BTB through the introduction of single-cell imaging and sequencing strategies and the establishment of biomarkers for BBB integrity in conjunction with biosynthesis strategies could allow new techniques explicitly designed for the correction of primary brain and brain metastases for tumors (Ali et al., 2013; Dohm et al., 2018).

Natural Killer (NK) cells murder cells that lower MHC-I in full tumors, close to those in immune-privileged areas where the environment is isolated from peripheral blood. NK cells are said to be quantitatively and qualitatively amazing from the cytotoxic cells of the blood on immune-privileged pages. This research indicates that cytotoxic and extended NK cells developed in most of the people of cancer sufferers may turn out to be pathogenic in the event that they result in immune-privileged microenvironments in prone people, consisting of those with most brain cancers or blood-brain barrier illness (Arvanitis et al., 2020; Krafft, Shapoval, Sobottka, Geiger et al, 2006; Salman et al., 2015).

Brain metastases occur as most cancer cells migrate to the mind from their preliminary vicinity. Any cancer can spread to the mind; however, the shape maximum probably to encourage mind metastases is lung, breast, colon, kidney, pore, and pores and skin most cancers. Brain metastases, or additional mind tumors, develop in 10% to 30% of human beings with the general public of cancers. As metastatic brain tumors develop, they cause pressure and change the characteristics of the underlying brain tissue. Brain metastases should be seen with certain signs and symptoms. Typically, surgery, radiation therapy, or each medication is used by people whose brain most tumors have spread. Chemotherapy and immunotherapy are beneficial in some situations. Treatment also relies on the elimination of pain and signs due to most cancers. Brain metastases occur as cancer cells migrate from the initial tumor via the bloodstream or lymphatic device and propagate (metastasize) to the brain (Krafft, Shapoval, Sobottka, Schackert et al, 2006). They continue to multiply and Metastatic most cancers that have spread from the initial web page are known as primary cancers. For example, the majority of cancers that have spread from the breast to the brain are classified as metastatic breast cancers, not the majority of cancers in the brain. There are several hypotheses on why some types of cancer propagate and why some type of most cancers metastasizes to the brain. Brain metastases from lung cancer are also seen early in the disease and the bulk of breast metastases increase the number of cancers that have been delayed (Nieder, Guckenberger, Gaspar et al, 2019).

To take a look at our neuropsychiatric signs and symptoms and signs and symptoms, remedy and effects in lung cancer patients with Brain Metastases (BM), with the goal of reaching early detection of these signs and their well-timed remedy. Lung most cancers are the maximum commonplace malignancy in the global. It can without issues spread to the brain, bones, liver, lymph, and different organs / tissues. The ailment develops swiftly after metastases, and the survival price of the inflamed person is drastically decreased. In truth, the prevalence of mind metastases (BM) is better in patients with lung cancer sufferers with cancer, breast cancer, prostate cancer, numerous colorectal cancers and numerous common tumors such as a) The maximum uncommon number one tumors that spread to the brain were Non-Small Cell Lung Cancers (NSCLCs) and Small Cell Lung Cancers (SCLCs) 34.5% and 21.4% respectively, and b) Often, everyday runs, dizziness, nausea, and headache are ordinary signs and symptoms/symptoms and symptoms in sufferers without maximum cancers and accordingly also do now not suggest BM. As a result, early diagnosis of BM because of lung cancer is complicated. Conditions also are worse than maximum cases when human beings with lung cancer have neuropsychiatric symptoms and symptoms. When someone with lung cancers indicates neuropsychiatric signs and symptoms, maximum lung cancers ought to be taken into consideration without hesitation. Early analysis will bring about valuable time for therapy as BM of lung most cancers has finally been shown in all sufferers (Guillerey et al., 2016). Fig.1 shows the intense kingdom of lungs cancer metastases represents a sophisticated level of metastases and is the leading reason for cancers-related mortality. Metastases are a multi-step procedure that consists of the migration and invasion of maximum cancer cells which might be the hallmarks of malignancy. These tactics include the involvement of a vast variety of mobile pathways guided by cytoskeletal dynamics, in addition to molecular changes which include the expression of proteolytic enzymes and adhesion.

Figure 1. Cancer spread from another part of the body.

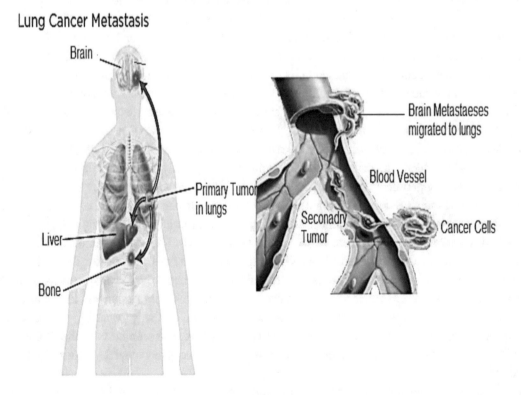

Cell migration itself is a well-included method that calls for the production of cytoplasmic distension, attachment and traction. Additional secondary variations related to mobile migration and invasion encompass the advent of Reactive Oxygen Species (ROS), the enhancement of chemical-resistant cancer stem cells, the boom of mutations in DeoxyriboNucleic acid(DNA) damage repair genes, and the contribution of microRiboNucleic Acid (miRNA) (Krafft, Shapoval, Sobottka, Schackert et al, 2006). The cell release of exosomes and their involvement in cell conduct alternate is an interesting new observation. This studies, primarily based on molecular modulation of cancer cellular proliferation, invasion, and metastases, one of the different studies checked out the binding partner of AG73, a lamina chain peptide, in breast maximum cancer cells that mediate most cancers development (Nieder, Haukland, Mannsåker et al, 2019). The Consequences confirmed an intrinsic interplay among AG73 and syndecanes that mediate adhesion and invasion of most cancers cells. This research looked at the expression of syndecans, especially in carcinoid cells, lobular breast cancer and ductal breast most cancers. Surgical Day Care changed into 90% cancer epithelium of each histological type. It was additionally expressed more frequently inside the tumor-associated stroma. In metastatic epithelium, Surgical Day Care changed into negatively associated with patient age and Estrogen Receptor (ER) and Progesterone Receptor (PR) status in primary tumors, while metastatic stroma confirmed a fantastic affiliation with range of foci in primary tumors and a terrible association with RP in number one tumors. One study observed a function for syndecan-2 in the migration of colon and rectal cancer cells. This finding can also be useful resource expertise of oncology biology and advocate that syndecan-2 can be used as a target for both treatment and diagnosis (Kaznowska et al., 2017; Kaznowska et al., 2018).

The inspection of patients with NSCLCs is alarming. However, some findings display that at the time of preliminary screening, sufferers with brain metastases had a higher positive survival burden than people with superior NSCLC without brain metastases. This research assisted the detection of behavioral metastases in patients with early brain metastases and in patients with brain metastases in a retrospective cohort of all new lung cancers seen by the majority of patients at Canadian Tertiary level between July 2005 and June 2007. It unfolds at a later date (Belykh et al., 2020). During the 2-365 days' period, 91 of the 878 patients (10.4%) had superior brain metastases. The common age in this community has risen to 64 years. At 45, brain metastases have been present inside the early diagnosis, and at forty-six, mind metastases stepped forward later within the ailment. The median survival of the complete populace turned into 7.8 months. Survival considering the fact that prognosis with brain metastases has stepped forward to plenty as patients of prognosis with brain metastases and in the end sickness (4.8 months' vs 3.7 months, P = 0.53) (Großerueschkamp et al., 2015; Putz et al., 2020). As a result, patients who had cerebral metastases later had an extended normal lifespan than human beings with cerebral metastases at analysis (9.8 months as opposed to 4.8 months). For patient's present process chemotherapy, the survival charge of patients with mind metastases has modified to terrible analysis (6.2 months). This look indicates the decreased survival of patients with NSCLC brain metastases and that a cautious selection of sufferers for an extra extensive treatment approach is critical (Klingemann, 2013; Zhao et al., 2016).

This research uses Infrared Radiation (IR) spectroscopy to differentiate ordinary mental tissue from mental metastases and to identify primary tumors from four different brain metastases, in particular most lung cancers, most colorectal cancers, and highest breast and renal cell carcinoma. Often, standard strategies do not measure the production of psychiatric metastases. Since metastatic cells combine molecular knowledge from primary tissue cells and infrared spectroscopy from cytoskeletal fingerprinting studies, infrared spectroscopy approaches provide a novel technique for the identification of mental metastatic tumors. The infrared spectral image was captured with a macro digital pattern Fourier Transformation

Infrared Radiation (FTIR) spectrometer coupled to a focal plane collection detector. Unsupervised group investigation of the infrared image found copies within each sample and between samples of the same tissue type. Infrared spectra have been selected based on the common behavior of tissue instructions with recognized diagnostics to build a scale of 8 parameters. This expertise furnished a supervised class version based completely on a linear discriminant evaluation that became used to stumble on the place to begin of 20 freezing strategies, alongside brain metastases of an undisclosed primary tumor (Aoyama et al., 2007). The ability to rapidly diagnose the majority of high-sensitivity and specific cancers is crucial in order to build on advances in modern therapies and produce dramatic decreases in mortality and morbidity. Current cancer diagnostic tests that analyze the shape of the tissues and the expression of specific proteins for specific forms of most cancers have inter-observer diversity, negative detection loads, and arise when an affected person has symptoms. New method for cancer detection the use of 1-ll human serum, susceptible basic inversion: Fourier infrared spectrum evaluation and sample recognition algorithms were said using a dataset of 433 patients (3,897 spectra) (Hands et al., 2016; Yao et al., 2014). This research offers the largest examination of medium infrared spectroscopy in blood for cancer research. This research investigated the sensitivities and premier residences using help support vector machine the radial base function among 8.0 and 100% for all layers and recognized the principle spectral residences, and as a result, the Biochemical additives, chargeable for the discrimination inside every layer (Engh et al., 2007) research tested the SVM study on the basis of cancer features relative to non-cancer carcinogens and performed 91.5%, 80% and 3.0% sensitivity and precision, respectively. This work illustrates the use of infrared light to provide a spectral fingerprint of human serum in order to locate cancerous and non-cancer metastases for the first time as opposed to small tissues, the magnitude of brain cancer, and the same organ sample as metastatic disease and Enable category review on the basis of the necessary science advice (Depciuch et al., 2017).

These studies addressed a medical research at the 3-D Magnetic Resonance Imaging (MRI) collection of the brain and its use in the coaching of brain metastases radiotherapy. The scale collection Magnetization Prepared Rapid Acquisition with Gradient Echo sequence (MPRAGE) calls for one hundred-80 diploma inversible pulses intended for magnetization, followed by low-level pulses of excitation and gradient imaging echoes. Following 0.1 mmol/kg bw, the T1-weighted MPRAGE images were compared to the 2-dimensional (2D) T1-weighted Spin-Echo (SE) image. Diethylenetriamine Penta-Acetic Acid (Gd-DTPA) was administered to ten patients with predictable brain metastases. Authentic or re-formatted multi-floor images from a dataset of 128 parts of 3-D MPRAGE sequences provided a pleasing analysis, close to the 2D SE shot (Dong et al., 2019; Su & Lee, 2020). Gd-DTPA enhancement and lesion targeting were similar in most sufferers with SE and MPRAGE images. During imaging and recuperation, the injured person's head becomes immobilized in a stereotactic displacement tool that can be visible in MRIs and linear accelerator centers. The measurement of the radiosurgery planning dose was largely based on 3-D MRI records, suggesting that the homogeneous attenuation expense inside the head was adequate to measure the correct dose, as the heterogeneity of the tissues was not sufficient. They significantly have an effect on the proportional form of dose distribution, specifically for brain radiosurgery. In this example, the dose calculation can best be primarily based on the 3-D geometry of the patient's head. An easy set of rules may be used to plan treatment if the MRI facts are unfastened from engineering anomalies (Schouten et al., 2002). The definition of the goal point, outer head circumference and essential structures may be precisely defined in MPRAGE 3-D images that offer vital benefits (for instance, advanced spatial decision, reconfigurable photos, rapid 3D pictures, brief experiment time and mask fixation, resulting in expanded Patient consolation, progressed profile, reduced results of vascular pulsation, better soft tissue choice and variable contrast because of crucial section coding association, and extra particular low absorption rate) on traditional 2D SE images. In addition, target volume, computed dose distribution and critical structures can be provided as 3-D shaded structures for higher evaluation of purpose volume matching and dose distribution (Campana et al., 2008; Leber & Efferth, 2009; Niemiec et al., 2011; Schad et al., 1994; Tahtamouni et al., 2019). These outcomes, in conjunction with exclusive benefits of 3-D imaging, propose that MPRAGE sequencing may offer a possibility to 2D T1-weighted SE imaging in planning radio-surgical remedy of brain metastases (Anzalone et al., 2013; Bergner et al., 2013; Brown et al., 2018). The aim of this statement is to investigate, for the first time, the optical Spatial Frequency Spectroscopy Acid (SFSA) combined with the Raman spectroscopy approach to discern human brain metastases from adenomas in most carcinomas. Lung Carcinomas (LC) and Squamous Cell Carcinomas (SCC) are two types of tissue cancers. A total of 31 unmarked micrographs of brain tissue kinds were gathered using a confocal micro-Raman spectroscopy gadget. The Raman spectroscopy variety of the corresponding samples changed into synchronously pooled the use of an excitation wavelength of 532 nm on the equal tissue locations (Lewis et al., 2010; Martinive & Houtte, 2018; Ostrom et al., 2019; Saeed & Abdullah, 2021a; Saeed & Abdullah, 2021b; Saeed & Abdullah, 2021c; Saeed & Abdullah, 2021d; Saeed & Afnizanfaizal, 2019; Saeed & Naqvi, 2017; Saeed & Naqvi, 2017; Taylor et al., 2019). Using the SFSA manner, the spontaneous differentiation of spatial frequency structures became studied the usage of the Gaussian feature in a micrograph (Jiang et al., 2015; Saeed et al., 2019; Zhou, Liu, Pu et al, 2019; Zhou, Zhang, Wu et al, 2019; Zhou et al., 2020).

METHODS

Datasets

This segment addresses the analysis of data sets in depth. Rich and high quality data is used to a successful Multi-image segmentation method to increase the resolution of medical image dataset display. The dataset for lung cancer consists of several contrast-enhanced MRI images from 200 patient's data from the UK's National Cancer Research Institute (NCRI). The resolution of these images is 514 x 514 with a pixel dimension 0.49 x 0.49 mm. The distance between the slides is 1mm and the width of the slide is 6mm. Statistics for this dataset is seen in Table 3. The accuracy obtained from the original data sets increased following the introduction of various FFT techniques to the data as defined in section 3.2.5.

Proposed Framework

The proposed method will be based on brain metastases and their calculations, which are calculated using CT / MRI scans. In this proposed exploration, we exclude brain metastases and its specific developmental dimension and quantify regions of a local fraction by selecting different dimensions associated with cancer. These steps suggested that the dimension or area present to move the cell to migrate from one place to another and determine the age of the cancer, that people do throughout their lives with development and they measure the damaged area of the brain to determine the metastases in the brain (cancer) due to using artificial intelligence software (MATLAB simulation). The main goal of our work is to develop a method that can detect the migration of Brain metastases and the lungs and breast area or that can separate patients with tumors. Initially, the input MRI image is a 4D (light field tool) to divide the image for the rest of the frame. The basis of this study is the detection of Brain metastases due to the interface of 4D images. The researcher analyzes the damaged Brain metastases due to brain cell abnormalities. It is a qualitative research study. The proposed method is based on two parts such as (i) FFT and combination of 4D images to detect the migration of cells from lungs cancer to metastases in the brain and (ii) detection of brain metastases due to the interface of MRI- HD images with SVM classification of datasets of lungs cancer. The existing clinical diagnostic methods of Lungs cancer critically diagnose through medical checkup and identify the cell migration cell inside of lungs from brain metastases. This procedure shows the availability of cancer cells in lungs and which type of Lungs cancer is available in the body as shown in Fig. 2. Moreover, the proposed method is divided into five phases which are given in the following subsections. In addition, Algorithm 1 describes the entire procedure of the proposed method.

Figure 2. Proposed clinical diagnostic methods of Lungs cancer

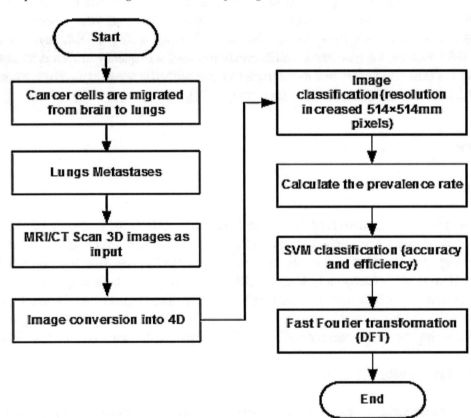

Image Conversion

The classification issue discussed in this article lacks a satisfactory amount of data to help the deep learning architecture and to achieve the necessary precision. Therefore, in order to obtain the desired precision, we expand the current data using the FFT using 4D MRI images as shown in Table 3(a-b). In this investigation, we are focusing on lungs cancer for migration brain metastases. To transform 3D images to 4D, we use the 4d movie collection SPM program to achieve the difference in input data needed for SPM, which targets my computing flow, and FSL. Specifically, this disparity allowed the data played from NIFTI 3D files to be transferred to a single 4D NIFTI format. FSL has a utility for this (fslmerge) that is included in the backend image that transforms the script by combining an image by (simulation) program. The graphical user interface of the image can be found in the SPM>Util batch editor menu, and by default, the selected 3D NIFTI images are stored in a single 4D NIFTI image in the same directory.

This research contributes the 4D images for lungs cancer as these images represent the signaling lungs cancer can reduce precision by combining anatomical and functional representations from multimodal structures. It may complicate the capture of minor accidents and lead to a sharp decline in activity. The strategies proposed to date include simultaneous anatomical and functional respiration acquisitions. In order to improve the signal-to-noise ratio of concurrent PET images, methods of non-flexible transformation have been proposed during the reconstitution process. In several of these methods, 4Dimages is used to extract the necessary deformation matrices. However, variations between the 4D PET/CT/ MRI scan acquired and the corresponding CT/MRI image sequence were identified due to differences in lungs conditions during PET acquisitions. In addition, the radiation exposure weight of receiving 4D CT will not be justified for all patients.

Image Classification of Lungs Cancer

Lung cancers are usually divided into two types: Small Cell Lung Cancer (SCLC) and Non-Small Cell Lung Cancer (NSCLC) (NSCLC). The designation is based on the appearance of cancer cells under the microscope. Lungs cancer can be identified by imaging scans, such as a CT scan of the lungs, which gives a more accurate view. This investigation provides a method for producing dynamic CT images from a mixture of reference CT image and distortion matrices derived from 4D PET image recordings that have not been corrected for decline. Our method reduces the need for dynamic computed tomography. On the one side, it also guarantees strong continuity between CT and PET images, allowing for precise attenuation correction of simultaneous PET acquisition processes. The suggested method implements datasets of lungs cancer samples (simulated datasets) on 4D CT images with corresponding actual CT images. Various levels of statistical accuracy of the PET/MRI image were considered to investigate the influence of image noise on the 4D CT array. Our findings suggest that clinically appropriate PET-CT acquisition times can be used to incorporate such an approach, rendering this option more appealing provided the lack of additional dose received from the acquisition of normal 4D CT. In addition, this method can extend to other multimedia devices such as PET/MRI.

Prevalence Rate of Lungs Cancer

The prevalence rate of any disease can be measured via sensitivity and specificity. Sensitivity and specificity are statistical results for the achievement of the binary classification which might be normally utilized in medication. The concept of sensitivity and specificity are defined as follows:

Sensitivity measures the true positive ratio that has been correctly identified (for example, the percentage of persons who already have a disease (affected).

Specificity measures the percentage of true negatives (for example, the proportion of individuals who do not actually have the disease (unaffected).

Sensitivity is an indicator of the precision of the test to detect the true positive of the diagnostic test and can also be referred to as regeneration/infection rate/true positive rate. This is the proportion, or ratio, of the true positive of all disease tests (true positives and false negatives). The accuracy of the test will help to show how well the samples are labeled with this condition. Higher sensitivity means that one procedure clearly classifies a sample with a more positive condition than another with a lower sensitivity. The accuracy of the diagnostic test is an indicator of the efficacy of the test to detect true negatives. Specificity is also referred to as selectivity or true negative number, and is the proportion or ratio of true negatives in all non-disorder samples (true negatives and false positives). The higher-precision test indicates that more samples are explicitly labeled as non-conditional than the lower-consistency test as formulated in following equations.

True Positive Rate (TPR):

$$\text{TPR} = \frac{TP}{T} = \frac{TP}{TP+FN} = 1\text{-FNR} \tag{1}$$

False positive rate (FPR):

$$\text{FPR} = \frac{FP}{N}\frac{FP}{FP+TN} = 1\text{-TPR} \tag{2}$$

Positive Predictive Value (PPV):

$$\text{PPV} = \frac{TP}{N}\frac{TP}{TP+FP} = 1\text{-FDR} \tag{3}$$

Negative Predictive Value (NPV):

$$\text{NPV} = \frac{TN}{TN+FN} = 1\text{-FOR} \tag{4}$$

Whereas,

TP= True Positive and True **positive:** Patients correctly recognized as sick, and **True negative:** Healthy people correctly recognized as healthy
TPR= True positive rate and False **positive:** Healthy people have been incorrectly recognized as sick
FPR = False positive rate and **False negative:** Patients were incorrectly recognized as healthy
FDR= false discovery rate
FOR= false omission rate

Since collecting the numbers of true positive, false positive, true negative and false negative, the accuracy and precision of the test can be measured. If the sensitivity turns out to be high, then the test rate as positive is likely to be accurate. On the other hand, if the precision is high, then someone who finds it to be a true negative is likely to be a true negative.

Potential Clinical Validation of SVM Classification

The proposed method considers SVM to predict disease status for 100 patients who were enrolled as part of a possible clinical validation trial from 200 datasets of lung cancer images. This method incorporates the imaging result before the algorithm was developed in terms of datasets training and testing using SVM classification. The reported sensitivity of 93.2% and the specificity of 92.8% showed a substantial decrease comparative to results from patient's data for brain metastases migration of lung cancer. This can initially suggest a reduced capability to identify cancer patients.

Fast Fourier Transformation

In this phase, FFT is used with 4D images to increase the incidence rate with image resolution and detect lung cancer symptoms to perform an image classification task reconstruction. In addition, FFT and DFT are used to sequence a periodic function cycle; DFT sets all non-zero values for the DFT loop. The DFT is the most important single transformation used to perform the Fourier analysis in a variety of functional applications for the probabilistic family partners.

EXPERIMENTAL RESULTS

This section explains the simulation results including all the acquired results. Typically, in lungs tumor cell metastases reside in the Central Nervous System (CNS). However, this work focuses on pathways behind brain metastases in non-small cell lung cancer; there are a variety of possible methods that may be used to improve targeting metastases (disorder) form of cancer cells. Consequently, lead towards the accelerated transition of FFT in order to recognize the frequency signal ratio, detection of brain metastases and lungs cancer. Referring to Figure 3 (a-g), the images are processed by FTT method to highlight the targeted area of the cancer cell in brain metastases migrated to lungs due to the use of frequency signal power and also increase the intensity by its values.

Pseudo Code of Hybrid Fast Fourier Transformation Method

The pseudo code of *Hybrid Fast Fourier Transformation* algorithm is given below:

```
1. Input: (A, B);
2. Output: Images
3. Upload Images I1 (Image.1)
4. Get Image (AxB)
5. Initialize Display Images I1 (fig.1);
6. Get Image (Gray Image);
7. Originate
8. Initialize Display Images I1 (fig.2);
```

```
9. Get Fourier Transform of an image
10. Get F=fft2 (imdata)
11.  Initialize Display Images I1 (fig.3);
12. Get centered spectrum
13. Get Fsh=fftshift(F);
14. Display Images I1 (fig.4);
15. While Apply log transform
16. While A³B; do; S1=log (1+abs (Fsh));
17. Initialize Display Images I1 (fig.5);
18. Get reconstructs the Image // for attributes function
19. Get F=ifftshift(Fsh);
20. Get f=ifft2 (F);
21. Display Images I1 (fig. 6);
22. Get reconstructed Image     // for attributes function
and;
23. While Apply Fs=1000 for selection occurrence // 24. for objective function
25. Get Ts=1/Fs for selection period of time phase
26. While Ts³0; do;
27. CALCULATE the variance dt=0; Ts=5-Ts;
28. %signal duration
 29. Else;
30. Load f1=10;
31. Load f2=70;
32. Load f3=100;
33. While Apply Formula Y =Asin(2*pift+theta);
34. CALCULATE the variance Y1=10*sin (2*pi*f1*dt);
35. CALCULATE the variance Y2=10*sin (2*pi*f2*dt);
36. CALCULATE the variance Y3=10*sin (2*pi*f3*dt);
37. CALCULATE the scheming of Y4=Y1+Y2+Y3;
38. APPLY nfft=length (Y4); % length of time domain signal
39. APPLY nfft2=2^nextpow2 (nfft); %length of signal in power of 2
40. While fft³Y4; do;
41. GET ff=fft (Y4, nfft2);
42. GET fff=ff (1: nfft2/2);
43. Display the outcome of  fft=Fs*(10: nfft2/2-1)/nff2);
44. APPLY Ylabel Amplitude (Y)
45. Display the outcome of  Period Territory Indication
46. APPLY XlabelFrquency(Xs)
47. APPLY YlabelNormaized Amplitude
48. SHOW the result of  Occurrence Territory Indication
49. Compute SVM classifier
50. Else,
51. Generate zero or empty results
52.  Train a classifier
```

```
53. Compute Classification SVM
(a) Compute cross-validation
(b) Compute validation predictions
 (c)Compute validation accuracy
54. end while
55. end if
56. end procedure
57. End
```

Calculation of the Prediction Method

This section presents the results obtained by combining lung cancer images of Fourier transform extraction method with machine learning detection technique. Moreover, FFT plays a vital role for detecting the cancer cell indication of the body due to the using of FTIR spectroscopy as a screening device and clinical resection in terms of Patient-Controlled Analgesia (PCA) examination as a new screening instrument for lung cancer. Table 1 presents the comparison of the proposed work with the most relevant research articles as FFT in the search for frequency band and power signals and the number of samples examined in this dataset illustrates cancer (pathology), whereas Table 2 identifies the existing potential threats of lung cancer. The selection of MRI images can significantly affect the outcomes of prediction method using SVM classification and calculates the estimated values of brain metastases to lungs cancer cell are given in Fig.4.

Figure 4. The prediction method shows that calculation of a sensitivity and specificity ratio of lungs cancer through brain metastases by the acquired values of truth positive and false positive rates in terms of accuracy and efficiency.

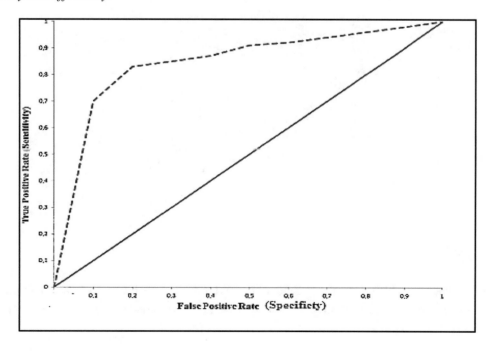

Figure 5. The accuracy of the entire predictive method is shown by which the positive and negative predictive class values indicate the symptoms of brain metastases

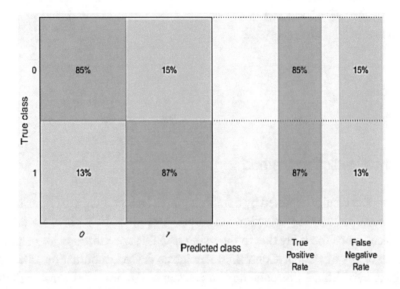

Figure 6. The expected category of each row and column is calculated as the accurate values of non-small cancer cells

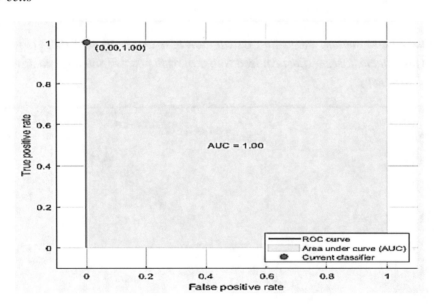

CONCLUSION

Various approaches have been reported in State of the Art, but they are based on customization and can deal with a specific problem. However, a general approach is still needed that can solve many problems and can be applied in different situations. Several investigators have dealt with the detection issue, especially the cell migration cases, efficiently based on the capabilities of their images. There is a least amount of past literature. We proposed a lung cancer localization method to predict the accuracy and efficiency of the images. In MRI images, the tumor volume is focused via FFT and SVM classification method. The DFT partitioning and SVM methods are used to measure the performance of the control patient datasets with 92.8% sensitivity, 93.2% specificity and 95.5% accuracy respectively. This investigation demonstrates brain metastases using severe lung cancer images between the MRI images and illustrates the consequences of our most recent proposed estimates.

In the future, we are planning to incorporate the multiple techniques of FFT with FTIR in brain metastases images which relies upon personalized medication that objectives specific tumor molecular pathways, such as the ones concerned in crossing the blood-brain barrier and cell migration. Furthermore, to improve the layout of the images with different FFT strategies such as Extreme Learning Machine (ELM) set of rules and its versions, and the application of clustering strategies. In addition, the combination of extraordinary types of features extracted from lungs cancer ultrasound images and the migration of cells to another other part of the body.

REFERENCES

Ali, A., Goffin, J. R., Arnold, A., & Ellis, P. M. (2013). Survival of patients with non-small-cell lung cancer after a diagnosis of brain metastases. *Current Oncology (Toronto, Ont.)*, *20*(4), 300–306. doi:10.3747/co.20.1481 PMID:23904768

Anzalone, N., Essig, M., Lee, S. K., Dörfler, A., Ganslandt, O., Combs, S. E., & Picozzi, P. (2013). Optimizing contrast-enhanced magnetic resonance imaging characterization of brain metastases: Relevance to stereotactic radiosurgery. *Neurosurgery*, *72*(5), 691–701. doi:10.1227/NEU.0b013e3182889ddf PMID:23381488

Aoyama, H., Tago, M., Kato, N., Toyoda, T., Kenjyo, M., Hirota, S., Shioura, H., Inomata, T., Kunieda, E., Hayakawa, K., Nakagawa, K., Kobashi, G., & Shirato, H. (2007). Neurocognitive function of patients with brain metastasis who received whole brain radiotherapy plus stereotactic radiosurgery or radiosurgery alone. *International Journal of Radiation Oncology, Biology, Physics*, *68*(5), 1388–1395. doi:10.1016/j.ijrobp.2007.03.048 PMID:17674975

Arvanitis, C. D., Ferraro, G. B., & Jain, R. K. (2020). The blood–brain barrier and blood–tumour barrier in brain tumours and metastases. *Nature Reviews. Cancer*, *20*(12), 26–41. doi:10.103841568-019-0205-x PMID:31601988

Barrow, A. D., & Colonna, M. (2017). Tailoring Natural Killer cell immunotherapy to the tumour microenvironment. Seminars in Immunology, 31, 30-36. doi:10.1016/j.smim.2017.09.001

Belykh, E., Shaffer, K. V., Lin, C., Byvaltsev, V. A., Preul, M. C., & Chen, L. (2020). Blood-Brain Barrier, Blood-Brain Tumor Barrier, and Fluorescence-Guided Neurosurgical Oncology: Delivering Optical Labels to Brain Tumors. *Frontiers in Oncology*, *10*, 739. doi:10.3389/fonc.2020.00739 PMID:32582530

Bergner, N., Romeike, B. F. M., Reichart, R., Kalff, R., Krafft, C., & Popp, J. (2013). Tumor margin identification and prediction of the primary tumor from brain metastases using FTIR imaging and support vector machines. *Analyst (London)*, *13*(14), 3983–3990. doi:10.1039/c3an00326d PMID:23563220

Bhowmik, A., Khan, R., & Ghosh, M. K. (2015). *Blood brain barrier: a challenge for effectual therapy of brain tumors*. BioMed.

Bolourian, A., & Mojtahedi, Z. (2017). Possible damage to immune-privileged sites in natural killer cell therapy in cancer patients: Side effects of natural killer cell therapy. *Immunotherapy*, *9*(3), 281–288. doi:10.2217/imt-2016-0137 PMID:28231718

Brown, N. M. O., Pfau, S. J., & Gu, C. (2018). Bridging barriers: A comparative look at the blood–brain barrier across organisms. *Genes & Development*, *32*(7-8), 466–478. doi:10.1101/gad.309823.117 PMID:29692355

Campana, M., Rizzi, B., & Melani, C. (2008). A Framework for 4-D Biomedical Image Processing, Visualization and Analysis. GRAPP, 403-408.

Depciuch, J., Kaznowska, E., Koziorowska, A., & Cebulski, J. (2017). Verification of the effectiveness of the Fourier transform infrared spectroscopy computational model for colorectal cancer. *Journal of Pharmaceutical and Biomedical Analysis*, *145*(1), 611–615. doi:10.1016/j.jpba.2017.07.026 PMID:28793272

Dohm, A., McTyre, E. R., Okoukoni, C., Henson, A., Cramer, C. K., LeCompte, M. C., Ruiz, J., Munley, M. T., Qasem, S., Lo, H.-W., Xing, F., Watabe, K., Laxton, A. W., Tatter, S. B., & Chan, M. D. (2018). Staged stereotactic radiosurgery for large brain metastases: Local control and clinical outcomes of a one-two punch technique. *Neurosurgery*, *83*(1), 114–121. doi:10.1093/neuros/nyx355 PMID:28973432

Dong, K., Liu, L., Yu, Z., & Di Wu, Q. Z. (2019). Brain metastases from lung cancer with neuropsychiatric symptoms as the first symptoms. *Translational Lung Cancer Research*, *8*(5), 682–691. doi:10.21037/tlcr.2019.10.02 PMID:31737504

Engh, J. A., Flickinger, J. C., Niranjan, A., Amin, D. V., Kondziolka, D. S., & Lunsford, L. D. (2007). Optimizing intracranial metastasis detection for stereotactic radiosurgery. *Stereotactic and Functional Neurosurgery*, *85*(4), 162–168. doi:10.1159/000099075 PMID:17259753

Großerueschkamp, F., Thieltges, A. K., Behrens, T., Brüning, T., Altmayer, M., & .... (2015). Marker-free automated histopathological annotation of lung tumour subtypes by FTIR imaging. *Analyst (London)*, *140*(7), 2114–2120. doi:10.1039/C4AN01978D PMID:25529256

Guillerey, C., Huntington, N. D., & Smyth, M. J. (2016). Targeting natural killer cells in cancer immunotherapy. *Nature Immunology*, *17*(9), 1025–1036. doi:10.1038/ni.3518 PMID:27540992

Hands, J. R., Clemens, G., Stables, R., Ashton, K., Brodbelt, A., Davis, C., Dawson, T. P., Jenkinson, M. D., Lea, R. W., Walker, C., & Baker, M. J. (2016). Brain tumour differentiation: Rapid stratified serum diagnostics via attenuated total reflection Fourier-transform infrared spectroscopy. *Journal of Neuro-Oncology*, *127*(3), 463–472. doi:10.100711060-016-2060-x PMID:26874961

Hazra, A., Bera, N., & Mandal, A. (2017). Predicting lung cancer survivability using SVM and logistic regression algorithms. *International Journal of Computers and Applications*, *17*(2), 1–12.

Jiang, W. G., Sanders, A. J., Katoh, M., Ungefroren, H., Gieseler, F., Prince, M., Thompson, S. K., Zollo, M., Spano, D., Dhawan, P., Sliva, D., Subbarayan, P. R., Sarkar, M., Honoki, K., Fujii, H., Georgakilas, A. G., Amedei, A., Niccolai, E., Amin, A., ... Santini, D. (2015). Tissue invasion and metastasis: Molecular, biological and clinical perspectives. *Seminars in Cancer Biology*, *35*, 244–275. doi:10.1016/j. semcancer.2015.03.008 PMID:25865774

Kaznowska, E., Depciuch, J., Szmuc, K., & Cebulski, J. (2017). Use of FTIR spectroscopy and PCA-LDC analysis to identify cancerous lesions within the human colon. *Journal of Pharmaceutical and Biomedical Analysis*, *134*(1), 259–268. doi:10.1016/j.jpba.2016.11.047 PMID:27930993

Kaznowska, E., Łach, K., Depciuch, J., Chaber, R., Koziorowska, A., Slobodian, S., Kiper, K., Chlebus, A., & Cebulski, J. (2018). Application of infrared spectroscopy for the identification of squamous cell carcinoma (lung cancer), Preliminary study. *Infrared Physics & Technology*, *89*(2), 282–290. doi:10.1016/j. infrared.2018.01.021

Klingemann, H. G. (2013). Cellular therapy of cancer with natural killer cells—Where do we stand? *Cytotherapy*, *15*(10), 1185–1194. doi:10.1016/j.jcyt.2013.03.011 PMID:23768925

Krafft, C., Shapoval, L., Sobottka, S. B., Geiger, K. D., Schackert, G., & Salzer, R. (2006). Identification of primary tumors of brain metastases by SIMCA classification of IR spectroscopic images. *Biochimica Biophysica Acta (BBA)- Biomembranes*, *1758*(7), 883–891. doi:10.1016/j.bbamem.2006.05.001 PMID:16787638

Krafft, C., Shapoval, L., Sobottka, S. B., Schackert, G., & Salzer, R. (2006). Identification of primary tumors of brain metastases by infrared spectroscopic imaging and linear discriminant analysis. *Technology in Cancer Research & Treatment*, *5*(3), 291–298. doi:10.1177/153303460600500311 PMID:16700626

Leber, M. F., & Efferth, T. (2009). Molecular principles of cancer invasion and metastasis. *International Journal of Oncology*, *34*(4), 881–895. PMID:19287945

Lewis, P. D., Lewis, K. E., Ghosal, R., Bayliss, S., Lloyd, A. J., Wills, J., Godfrey, R., Kloer, P., & Mur, L. A. J. (2010). Evaluation of FTIR spectroscopy as a diagnostic tool for lung cancer using sputum. *BMC Cancer*, *10*(1), 640. doi:10.1186/1471-2407-10-640 PMID:21092279

Martinive, P., & Houtte, P. V. (2018). The challenge of brain metastases from non-small cell lung cancer is not only an economical issue. *Annals of Palliative Medicine*, *8*(2), 203–206. doi:10.21037/ apm.2018.12.05 PMID:30691276

Nieder, Haukland, Mannsåker, Pawinski, & Yobuta. (2019). *Presence of Brain Metastases at Initial Diagnosis of Cancer: Patient Characteristics and Outcome.* Academic Press.

Nieder, C., Guckenberger, M., Gaspar, L. E., Rusthoven, C. G., Ruysscher, D. D., & ... . (2019). Management of patients with brain metastases from non-small cell lung cancer and adverse prognostic features: Multi-national radiation treatment recommendations are heterogeneous. *Radiation Oncology (London, England)*, *14*(1), 33. doi:10.118613014-019-1237-9 PMID:30770745

Niemiec, M., Głogowski, M., Tyc-Szczepaniak, D., Wierzchowski, M., & Kępka, L. (2011). Characteristics of long-term survivors of brain metastases from lung cancer. *Reports of Practical Oncology and Radiotherapy: Journal of Greatpoland Cancer Center in Poznan and Polish Society of Radiation Oncology, 16*(2), 49–53. doi:10.1016/j.rpor.2011.01.002 PMID:24376956

Ostrom, Q. T., Cioffi, G., Gittleman, H., Patil, N., Waite, K., Kruchko, C., & Barnholtz-Sloan, J. S. (2019). Cbtrus statistical report: Primary brain and other central nervous system tumors diagnosed in the United States in 2012-2016. *Neuro-Oncology, 21*(Supplement_5), 100. doi:10.1093/neuonc/noz150 PMID:31675094

Putz, F., Mengling, V., Perrin, R., Masitho, S., Weissmann, T., Rösch, J., Bäuerle, T., Janka, R., Cavallaro, A., Uder, M., Amarteifio, P., Doussin, S., Schmidt, M. A., Dörfler, A., Semrau, S., Lettmaier, S., Fietkau, R., & Bert, C. (2020). Magnetic resonance imaging for brain stereotactic radiotherapy. *Strahlentherapie und Onkologie, 196*(5), 1–13. doi:10.100700066-020-01604-0 PMID:32206842

Saeed & Abdullah. (2021a). Performance analysis of machine learning algorithm for health care tools with High Dimension Segmentation. *Machine learning healthcare: Handling and managing data, 1*(1), 1-30.

Saeed & Abdullah. (2021b). Comparison analysis of medical health care information of Graph Cutting using Multi Dimension Segmentation. *Machine learning healthcare: Handling and managing data, 1*(1), 1-23.

Saeed & Abdullah. (2021c). Statistical Analysis the Pre and Post-Surgery of health care sector using High Dimension Segmentation. *Machine learning healthcare: Handling and managing data, 1*(1), 1-25.

Saeed & Abdullah. (2021d). Combination of Brain Cancer with Hybrid K-NN Algorithm using statistical Analysis of Cerebrospinal Fluid (CSF) Surgery. *International Journal of Computer Science and Network Security, 21*(2), 120-130.

Saeed & Afnizanfaizal. (2019). Implementation of Fourier transformation. *Indian Journal of Science & Technology, 12*(37), 1-16.

Saeed, S., Abdullah, A., & Jhanjhi, N. (2019). Investigation of a Brain Cancer with Interfacing of 3-Dimensional Image Processing. *Indian Journal of Science and Technology, 12*(34), 1–12. doi:10.17485/ijst/2019/v12i34/146150

Saeed, S., & Naqvi, M. (2017). Implementation of Failure Enterprise Systems in Organizational Perspective Framework. *International Journal of Advance Computer Science and Application, 8*(5), 54–63. doi:10.14569/IJACSA.2017.080508

Saeed, S., & Naqvi, S. M. (2017). Assessment of Brain Tumor Due to the Usage of MATLAB Performance. *Journal of Medical Imaging and Health Informatics, 7*(6), 1454–1460. doi:10.1166/jmihi.2017.2187

Salman, A., Sebbag, G., Argov, S., Mordechai, S., & Sahu, R. K. (2015). Early detection of colorectal cancer relapses by infrared spectroscopy in normal anastomosis tissue. *Journal of Biomedical Optics, 20*(7), 75–107. doi:10.1117/1.JBO.20.7.075007 PMID:26178200

Schad, L. R., Blüml, S., Hawighorst, H., Wenz, F., & Lorenz, W. J. (1994). Radiosurgical treatment planning of brain metastases based on a fast, three-dimensional MR imaging technique. *Magnetic Resonance Imaging*, *12*(5), 811–819. doi:10.1016/0730-725X(94)92206-3 PMID:7934668

Schouten, L. J., Rutten, J., Huveneers, H. A. M., & Twijnstra, A. (2002). Incidence of brain metastases in a cohort of patients with carcinoma of the breast, colon, kidney, and lung and melanoma. *Cancer*, *94*(1), 2698–2705. doi:10.1002/cncr.10541 PMID:12173339

Su, K. Y., & Lee, W. L. (2020). Fourier Transform Infrared Spectroscopy as a Cancer Screening and Diagnostic Tool: A Review and Prospects. *Cancers (Basel)*, *12*(1), 115. doi:10.3390/cancers12010115 PMID:31906324

Tahtamouni, L., Ahram, M., Koblinski, J., & Rolfo, C. (2019). Molecular regulation of cancer cell migration, invasion, and metastasis. *Analytical Cellular Pathology (Amsterdam)*, *2019*, 1–2. doi:10.1155/2019/1356508 PMID:31218208

Taylor, O. G., Brzozowski, J. S., & Skelding, K. A. (2019). Glioblastoma multiforme: An overview of emerging therapeutic targets. *Frontiers in Oncology*, *9*, 963. doi:10.3389/fonc.2019.00963 PMID:31616641

Yao, H., Shi, X., & Zhang, Y. (2014). The use of FTIR-ATR spectrometry for evaluation of surgical resection margin in colorectal cancer: A pilot study of 56 samples. *Journal of Spectroscopy*, *2014*, 1–5. doi:10.1155/2014/213890

Zhao, H., Li, G., Yu, C., & An, Z. (2016). The proceedings of brain metastases from lung cancer. *Open Life Sciences*, *11*(1), 116–121. doi:10.1515/biol-2016-0016

Zhou, Y., Liu, C.-H., Pu, Y., Wu, B., Nguyen, T. A., Cheng, G., Zhou, L., Zhu, K., Chen, J., Li, Q., & Alfano, R. R. (2019). Combined spatial frequency spectroscopy analysis with visible resonance Raman for optical biopsy of human brain metastases of lung cancers. *Journal of Innovative Optical Health Sciences*, *12*(2), 1950010. doi:10.1142/S179354581950010X

Zhou, Y., Zhang, S., Wu, B., Yu, X., & Cheng, G. (2019). A portable visible resonance Raman analyzer with a handheld optical fiber probe for in vivo diagnosis of brain glioblastoma multiforme in an animal model. Proc. In Laser Science, 3-5. doi:10.1364/FIO.2019.JW3A.5

Zhou, Y., Zhang, S., Wu, B., Yu, X., & Cheng, G. (2020). Human glioma tumors detection by a portable visible resonance Raman analyzer with a hand-held optical fiber probe. *Biomedical Vibrational Spectroscopy, 11236*(1).

Chapter 9
Virtual Technical Aids to Help People With Dysgraphia

Navirah Kamal
Amity University, Noida, India

Pragati Sharma
Amity University, Noida, India

Rangana Das
Amity University, Noida, India

Vipul Goyal
Amity University, Noida, India

Richa Gupta
Amity University, Noida, India

ABSTRACT

In this chapter, a deep study of dysgraphia and its various available technical aids is discussed. A person suffering from dysgraphia struggles to carry out day-to-day activities like schoolwork, paperwork, and other writing activities. A suitable aid is required to overcome the hurdles due to the suffering. This literature establishes the various effects of dysgraphia in adults and children. An analysis of various effective tools is carried out in the study. Some tools are directly designed to tackle the inconveniences that come along with this disability; others provide a more general aid for writing. The literature also identifies the patterns and quirks commonly found in the handwriting. Algorithms for handwriting recognition is discussed to lay the foundation of aids present for dysgraphia. The objective of the chapter is to provide foundation work to create aids for dysgraphia by categorizing the various related key points.

DOI: 10.4018/978-1-7998-8929-8.ch009

INTRODUCTION

Communication through the means of writing is undoubtedly important, but it can prove to be quite challenging for people with dysgraphia (Hamstra-Bletz & Blöte, 1993). Dysgraphia is a learning disability that affects one's ability to write properly. This, in turn, affects many aspects of one's day-to-day life and therefore a need for a reliable solution is paramount. Before constructing an effective tool, an analysis of patterns and quirks found in the handwriting of those with dysgraphia is done. Some of the most prominent features of dysgraphia are the illegibility of the writing, the spacing between characters, and inconsistency. A popular writing aid is a Smartpen that is designed to provide a general solution for everyone. It can be quite useful for those with dysgraphia. Meanwhile, there are some mobile applications made to help by involving its users in some activities to better their ability to write properly. These are remedial solutions. Some assistive aids also exist that help those with dysgraphia to write correctly. It is evident that a solution is required that will be able to help tackle many aspects of this disability and provide assistance during everyday activities.

This paper aims to construct an appropriate solution for those dealing with this disability and provide the required details to understand the aids for writing. The existing literature takes a dive into the analysis of dysgraphia and attempts to provide a suitable solution. However, the literature review lacks to collectively presents all the related tools for writing and psychological point of view. In this study a foundation is laid that is required, to create an effective aid. Also, various aspects of dysgraphia are discussed. The works describes the conditions and its effects on someone. Finally, to gain insight into the aids already designed to help those with dysgraphia are stated and analyzed.

This literature review will attempt to provide an overall view of issues faced by those with dysgraphia and the helping aids that have immerged in the past years. It will not concentrate on how handwriting can be used to diagnose dysgraphia or explore possible ways to better someone's condition but be used to analyse and provide a suitable solution to those who will benefit from it.

The paper is organized as follows: First section discusses the background of dysgraphia and its effects; next handwriting recognition algorithms are described. Subsequent sections concentrate on dysgraphic handwriting and existing aids respectively, followed by results and discussion. Finally, future research directions are specified, followed by conclusion.

BACKGROUND

Dysgraphia is a written-language disorder that concerns mechanical writing skill. The effect of this disorder is prominent in school going children as it manifests itself in poor writing performance. These children are of at least average intelligence who do not have a distinct neurological disability and/or an overt perceptual-motor handicap. It can still be quite challenging for them to carry out activities at school with ease. Writing notes, recipes, prescriptions, messages, cheques, and filling out applications (Crouch & Jacubecy, 2007), all of these tasks demand proper writing abilities from the person, and hence, providing aid for it becomes a necessity.

Dysgraphia can be classified into four subtypes: phonological, surface, mixed, and semantic/syntactic dysgraphia (Crouch & Jacubecy, 2007). Students with phonological dysgraphia face difficulties in spelling a word by its sound and rely mostly on its orthographic representation. Spelling is a task that relies mostly on hearing, therefore, students with this subtype of dysgraphia do poorly at spelling tests.

Surface dysgraphia is the exact opposite. Students with this subtype have trouble with the visual aspects of a word and depend mostly on the sound of it. They usually form their letters poorly. The third subtype is mixed dysgraphia. It is a mix of the first two subtypes. Students mix up their spelling formations, struggle with spelling and they often get confused as there are so many rules when it comes to writing. Lastly, students with semantic dysgraphia face issues with grammar such as how words can be used together to make meaningful and complete (Crouch & Jacubecy, 2007).

Crouch & Jakubecy (2007) describe two different approaches to address dysgraphia. The remedial approach uses systematic techniques that improve functioning. Fine motor programs or direct instruction of handwriting are a few ways used to help improve handwriting. The use of Technology is another approach that comes under by-pass strategies. This is a way around the handwriting difficulties (Khan et al., 2017) mention prevention as another method that can be used to assist dysgraphia. Prevention is done by providing early training to grade one or kindergarten students. Drill and practice, building fine motor skills, and providing spelling assistance are some of the remedial approaches (Crouch & Jakubecy, 2007; Ediger, 2002). Word processors and oral answer facilities are two examples of the accommodation approach (Khan et al., 2017), but these do not cover the entirety of the problem and provide an effective solution.

Figure 1. Dysgraphia approaches

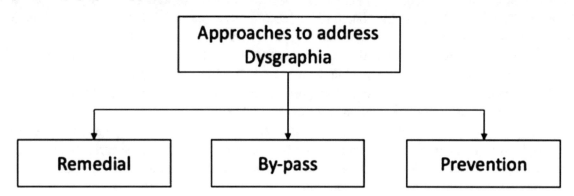

Impedovo and Pirlo (2018), in their paper, point out the most relevant research results related to the application of online handwriting analysis to the assessment of PD and AD disorders. The research is principally organized from a pattern recognition perspective, typically based on data acquisition, feature extraction, and data analysis and classification.

Another application of online handwriting analysis is introduced by Mucca et al. (2018) based on fractional derivatives applied in PD handwriting quantification. The proposed methodology was evaluated on a database that consists of 33 PD patients and 36 healthy controls who performed several handwriting tasks.

To explore the incidence of spelling deficits in patients with unilateral cortical lesions and validate the test in a population of lesioned patients, Baxter and Warrington (1994) describe the construction of a graded-difficulty spelling test for adults consisting of two alternative forms each containing 30 words (GDST, Forms A and B). The test was validated in a group of 26 patients with left hemisphere and 20 patients with right hemisphere lesions. Spelling was shown to be lateralized to the left hemisphere and there appeared to be a shift in scores of the left hemisphere group towards the lower quartile, with 65% of the left hemisphere group falling within this band.

Handwriting plays an important role while trying to formulate the possible solutions or aids that can be designed for those with dysgraphia. Hence, the study handwriting recognition and analysis of handwritten text are considered important aspects. The next section discusses the former.

PRELIMINARIES

In this section we talk about handwritten text recognition model for normal handwriting. Since Dysgraphia is closely related to one's handwriting, it is an important aspect of the solution. There exist various handwritten text recognition algorithms that have been used over the years.

Handwritten Text Recognition

On dividing handwriting recognition into two types, we get online recognition is the recognition of text in the course of its entering into the system, and offline recognition is the recognition of text already entered into the system as an image.

The approach presented by Scheidl & Harald et al. in the thesis (Scheidl et al., 2011) uses a popular machine learning tool in python known as TensorFlow to achieve quite accurate handwriting recognition. Here, with the use of the Neural Network (NN) model, the text that exists in the images is segmented into words. This particular trained model had an error rate of just 10% and can be made better.

Along with the decoders that come along with TensorFlow, word beam search (Scheidl et al., 2018) is used for decoding. This enables the model to constrain to only those words that exist in the dictionary but at the same time not ignore characters that are not letters like a full stop, exclamation mark, and numbers.

While exploring the overview of the handwritten text recognition system given in the figure below, it can be seen that a piece of handwritten text goes through CNN, i.e., convolutional neural network, with multiple layers, and an RNN, i.e., recurrent neural network, with multiple layers.

Figure 2. Neural network operations and data flow
Source: https://towardsdatascience.com/build-a-handwritten-text-recognition-system-using-tensorflow-2326a3487cd5

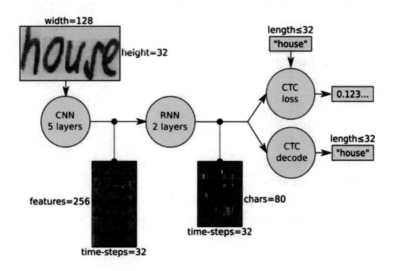

After discussing the background work for handwritten text recognition for normal handwriting it is required to understand the specific features found in dysgraphic handwriting.

DYSGRAPHIC HANDWRITING

There are certain distinct features that can be observed in the handwriting of those with dysgraphia. The handwritten documents written by someone with this learning disability may be illegible due to unclear letter formations or consist of other dynamic features that separate them from common handwritten texts.

Illegible Text

Most handwriting recognition uses classification or segmentation on given images. Generative Adversarial Networks (GAN) on the other hand uses text-image-to-text-image conversion (Karimi et al., 2020). This means that the original text gets converted to a message similar to machine print. This gives more accurate results as it can now be transcribed using OCR-like techniques. It does so by using two networks: a generator network that generates fake samples resembling the real ones, and a discriminator network that selects the real samples from the fake ones. The two networks compete with each other until an equilibrium is reached. There are some issues with this approach: non-convergence, mode collapse, and vanishing gradient problem. The paper focuses on a variant of GAN called Wasserstein GAN which addresses these issues. Instead of using Jensen-Shannon divergence between distributions, it uses the Wasserstein Distance.

The proposed method by Karimi et al. (2020) was HW2MP-GAN (handwritten to machine print). In this method, two discriminator networks are used instead of one. They are character level discriminator that generates characters and a word-level discriminator that generates words. The generator network uses U-Net architecture with 5 layers of encoder and decoder each. The loss function of GAN is normally,

$$\min_{G} \max_{D} \mathbb{E}_{x \sim \mathbb{P}_r} \left[\log\left(D\left(x\right)\right)\right] + \mathbb{E}_{\hat{x} \sim \mathbb{P}_g} \left[\log\left(1 - D\left(\hat{x}\right)\right)\right] \tag{1}$$

where G represents a generator, D represents a discriminator and x is the realization of true samples. Pr is the true data distribution and Pg denotes the generator's distribution that is modelled implicitly by $\tilde{x} \sim G(z)$ and $z \sim P(z)$ (the latent space or noise z is sampled usually from a uniform distribution or a spherical Gaussian distribution).

For the proposed method, the loss function is

$$L^{total} = L^{w} + \lambda_{char} L^{c} + \lambda_{recons} \mathbb{E}_{\substack{x \sim \mathbb{P}_r \\ x \sim \mathbb{P}_g}} \left\| \tilde{x} - x \right\|_1 \tag{2}$$

where λchar and λrecons are hyper-parameters for balancing between word-level loss, character-level loss and the reconstruction loss function.

It combines both character level and word level models. The HW2MP is used to reinforce handwriting recognition, that is, a joint attention model works with both handwritten images and HW2MP generated images. The baseline model CNN layers followed by bi-directional LSTM layers after which is the Connectionist Temporal Classification loss. For evaluation, the distance between the real images and the images generated by HW2MP GAN and the legibility of these images were measured. This was done by using a pre-trained handwriting recognition model to recognize the generated images. The model was compared with the state-of-the-art GANs such as DCGAN, LSGAN, WGAN, SWGAN, WGAN-GP, and Pix2Pix. The proposed model had the highest word accuracy, and the lowest Frechet Handwritten Distance and Levenshtein Distance (LD).

Another experiment was carried out in which the performance of handwriting recognition models trained by handwritten images, machine-generated print, and a combination of both was evaluated. It was found that the models trained by both machine-generated print and handwritten images had the lowest LD and highest word accuracy, slightly outperforming the ones trained by handwritten images. This shows the potential of using generated images as input for training models. Therefore, HW2MP can be used as a reinforcement for existing handwritten recognition models.

Handwriting Analysis

Usually, dysgraphic handwriting is assessed by the overall readability of the paragraph and characteristics that define readability such as degree of slant, letter formation, and word slant (Rosenblum et al., 2006). However, Rosenblum et al. (2006) pointed out, this method has low reliability, takes a long time to process, and has a major limitation: it does not consider the dynamic characteristics of a child's handwriting which can give an insight into their motor control.

For example, BHK has been the standard for evaluating dysgraphia (Asselhorn et al., 2020). However, it has its limitations. According to Asselborn et al. (2020), as a rule-based system, the rules are formulated by human experts based on their subjective knowledge of a very complex problem. Secondly, rule-based tests do not update themselves which is a severe limitation as the field of education is a constantly evolving one. Another limitation is that these tests aim to simplify the complex problem into "rules" (Asselhorn et al., 2020). On top of this, the BHK scale keeps on changing. 25% of the features used in the original BHK had to be discarded as they were not able to differentiate between dysgraphic and non-dysgraphic handwriting (Rosenblum et al., 2004).

Dynamic Features

DANKOVIČOV et al. (2019) collected 80 samples, out of which 39 are from dysgraphic patients and 41 are from healthy patients. They used Wacom Intuos Pro Large to collect the samples. They asked the participants to write repetitions of the letter 'l', syllable 'le', words 'leto' and 'hamolhen', and the sentence 'V lete bude taplo a sucho'. They then analyzed the samples using Python programming language. A decision tree was the chosen classification model using the CART algorithm. They used the Mann-Whitney U test, a non-parametric statistical test to compare the calculated parameters of the control with that of the tested subjects (those with dysgraphia) and see if there were any statistical differences between the features.

Rosenblum et al. (2006) conducted similar tests with children aged 8 to 9 years old with a gender ratio of 5 girls to 9 boys. The participants wrote in the Hebrew language. They used the Teacher's Questionnaire for Handwriting Proficiency and Hebrew Writing Evaluation to manually identify dysgraphic handwriting. They conducted the tests in environments similar to what the children would normally experience such as their school. They asked the children to copy a 107-character paragraph in Hebrew which includes all the letters of the language from the computer screen onto the A4 paper affixed to WACOM x-y Intuos II digitizing tablet. After data collection, they applied automatic segmentation to divide the data into segments based on the times when pen pressure dropped below or exceeded 4% of the maximum pen pressure. They then combined the segments into Hebrew letters. Both the individual segments and entire letters were analyzed by measuring their temporal and spatial kinematic parameters.

Asselhorn et al. (2020) selected 390 children aged 5 to 12 from 30 classes in 5 primary schools in Haute Savoire, France. 48 children with severe dysgraphia were recruited from therapy centers. These 448 children were asked to write the first five sentences on iPad. The iPad-based Dynamic application recorded the x and y coordinates, pressure, azimuth, and altitude angle of the pen. They formulated a Z-score to measure how different a feature of handwriting is from the mean for a child of the same age and gender. They used the PCA algorithm to determine the predictive importance of each feature based on the Z-score, that is, how much did it deviate from the mean.

$$Z\text{-}score = \frac{\left|feature - f_{mean}\left(age\right)\right|}{f_{std}\left(age\right)} \quad score = e^{-\alpha * Z\text{-}score^{\beta}} \tag{3}$$

where α and β are two positive parameters, f_{mean} f_{std} are the means and standard deviations of the features as a function of age and $Z\text{-}score$ denotes a score between 0 and 1 computed for each feature according to the deviation from the average.

DANKOVIČOV et al. (2019) found that the time parameters such as time over the tablet, writing time, and total time were statistically different whereas pen pressure parameters such as minimum, maximum, average, and median pressures were not statistically different. Furthermore, when they classified and created decision trees, the tree with only minimum speed as the parameter had the highest accuracy, sensitivity, and specificity. For the tree without minimum speed, the most dominant parameter was total writing time.

Rosenblum et al. (2006) discovered that there were instances where a letter written in one segment by proficient hand writers was written in six segments by dysgraphic hand writers. The number of raw segments and "direction reversal" (Rosenblum et al., 2006) segments were significantly less in proficient handwriting. The number of letters for the first minute and the number of letters per minute for the whole paragraph was significantly higher than dysgraphic handwriting. There was no significant difference in the distance between the letters in the x-direction among the two samples. The "In-Air" (Rosenblum et al., 2006) time between letters was significantly less in the proficient handwriting sample.

Through the paper (Asselhorn et al., 2020), it can be noticed that kinematic and pressure were best at predicting dysgraphia. They had the highest sensitivity and specificity. Among these categories, Entropy of Mean of Speed Frequencies, Distance of Mean of Speed Frequencies and In-Air-Time Ratio from kinematics, and Standard Deviation of Pressure, Nb of Peaks of Pressure Change per Second and Maximum Pressure from pressure showed the greatest variation from the mean value of all participants.

SOLUTIONS AND RECOMMENDATIONS

As explored earlier, writing cleanly can prove to be quite challenging for those who have dysgraphia. To provide some respite, various kinds of writing aids have immerged in the past years. Some of them may not exactly be designed for those with dysgraphia, but they're certainly designed to help with any kind of writing assignment. Along with issues related to the act of writing, jotting down correct information can also be one major source of inconvenience for those with dysgraphia. Spelling words correctly or framing grammatically correct sentences can be challenging.

Technology has played a very important role in providing aid to those with learning disabilities and has helped them improve the quality of their work (Ellis, 2016). The author of this thesis (Ellis, 2016) conducted a study that showed the positive reaction of students with learning disabilities towards the use of technology.

Writing Aids

Smartpens are designed to convert handwritten text to digital text. This technology isn't specifically designed for those with dysgraphia but can prove to be quite useful as it may allow conversion to legible text resulting in a quicker evaluation of the information that a person wishes to convey. In order to capture the handwritten text, these Smartpens use a tiny digital camera near to the tip of the pen. The dotted pattern in the paper helps to determine the exact location of the tip on the paper (Siddiqui & Muntjir, 2017).

Boyle and Joyce (2019) have succeeded in describing how Smartpens can be used to support the note-taking skills of students with learning disabilities. Through the use of recording abilities of a Smartpen, children with learning disabilities can effectively capture the essence of their lectures in their notes. The Livescribe Smartpen is a popular commercially available Smartpen. It is capable of creating audio files for what is written using it. According to the study conducted by the authors of (Ellis, 2016), users preferred the Livescribe Smartpen over audio recordings due to its non-linear playback functionality. The extent of the utility of a Smartpen is evident, but it must be noted that these devices are very expensive and hence cannot be affordable for all. Along with this, Smartpen technology does not provide any aid to alter the written text to make it meaningful and correct.

Mobile Applications

Some mobile applications have also been designed to help those with dysgraphia. DysgraphiCoach (Mohd Ariffin et al., 2018) is one such application. It has three interactive sections. One, to teach alphabet writing, another for number writing, and finally a section designed to improve short-term memory and speed recognition skills (Mohd Ariffin et al., 2018). DysgraphiCoach was made in Malaysia and currently has writing aid only for the Malay Language. Such applications are designed to help better one's ability to write and not to provide instant assistance.

Another application called 'THE CURE' (Avishka et al., 2018) focuses on detecting the severity level of dysgraphia as well as dyslexia in its users. It provides with an interactive interface that is designed to help those with these learning disabilities by offering them a place to practice reading and writing on their own. The two models described in the paper (Avishka et al., 2018) were trained on two different datasets. While of the models concentrates on the words spelled out by those with dyslexia, the other focuses on identifying written characters by those with dysgraphia. For character recognition, convolutional neural networks are used, and k-means clustering is used for severity prediction.

Spelling and Word Prediction

Khan et al. (2017) have provided an assistive solution for spelling using augmented reality. Many aids and IT assistance have been made available for students diagnosed with dysgraphia. They have expanded on the previously available solutions and introduced a model called the AR-based dysgraphia assistance writing environment (AR-DAWE) model. It uses the Google Cloud Speech to text API (Khan et al., 2017). It converts speech into 3D text and displays it on smart glasses or smartphones. On the flip side, this system might falter if the distance between the notebook and the phone is greater than one meter.

Quenneville (2001) mentions various ways in the article the technology which can be used to provide aid to those with learning disabilities. One of these methods is by using word predictors that predict the complete word as the user is typing each letter. It can also learn unusual words used by the user and add them to its dictionary, so that it can efficiently predict those words in the future. Another method mentioned is by using auditory feedback to reinforce the writing process (Quenneville, 2001). This is done by using talking word processors. Whatever is being written by the user can be read aloud simultaneously to ensure correctness of the content typed.

Digital Audio Voice Recorder

The process of notetaking by students is made easier by a digital audio voice recorder. The lectures can be recorded by the students with learning disabilities like dysgraphia to refer to or study from later. The 'set it and forget it' aspect of this by-pass approach makes it popular amongst its users (Ellis, 2016). However, it restricts one's ability to note down particular thoughts and does not provide a non-linear playback facility.

Figure 3. Existing solutions for dysgraphia

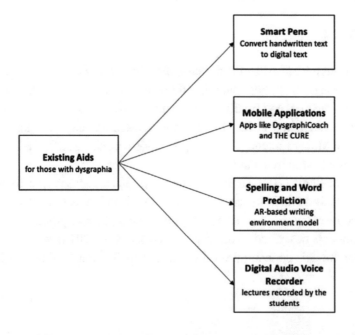

Table 1. Studies for Dysgraphia, its features and aids

Study	Features	Approach	Specification	Description
Hamstra-Bletz & Blote, 1993)	BHK scale	PRINCALS & Long matrix	Dysgraphia	An evaluation scale for children's handwriting (the BHK scale) was used for rating the scripts on 13 characteristics and for measuring the speed of writing.
(Baxter & Warrington, 1994)	Measuring dysgraphia	Graded difficulty spelling test (GDST)	Dysgraphia	To explore the incidence of spelling deficits in patients with unilateral cortical lesions and validate the test in a population of lesioned patients.
(Quenneville et al., 2001)	Tech Tools	Word predictors & auditory feedback	Learning disabilities	The paper presents various ways in which technology can be used to provide aid to those with learning disabilities.
(Ediger, 2002)	Assessing Handwriting Achievement.	Handwriting instruction	Handwriting	Handwriting achievement can be assessed in degrees from being legible to being illegible.
(Rosenblum et al., 2004)	Handwriting evaluation, Process versus product	Digitizing Tablet, Hebrew Handwriting Evaluation (HHE)	Dysgraphia	To compare the abilities of digitizer-based evaluation of the handwriting process and conventional evaluation of the handwriting product
(Rosenblum et al., 2006)	X–Y digitizing tablets	POET software (Penmanship Objective Evaluation Tool),	Dysgraphia	It is an online program that gives the writing prompt and collects and analyses data.
(Crouch & Jakubecy, 2007)	Dysgraphia and its effects	drill activities and fine motor activities,	Dysgraphia	To improve the handwriting of a student with dysgraphia.
(Scheidl, 2011)	Handwritten Text Recognition	Neural Network (NN) model, convolutional neural network (CNN), recurrent neural network (RNN)	handwriting recognition	The approach presented in the thesis uses a popular machine learning tool in python known as TensorFlow to achieve quite accurate handwriting recognition
(Ellis, 2016)	Accommodation approach	Livescribe smart pens, Digital Audio Voice Recorder	Students with disabilities	Livescribe pens are capable of creating audio files for what is written using it. The process of notetaking by students is made easier by a digital audio voice recorder.
(Khan et al., 2017)	AR-DAWE (Augmented Reality – Dysgraphia Assistive Writing Environment) model	Augmented Reality (AR)	Dysgraphia	It uses the Google Cloud Speech to text API. It converts speech into 3D text and displays it on smart glasses or the smartphones
(Siddiqui & Muntjir., 2017)	Pen and Paper learning	Smart pens and smart papers	Smart study	Pen Computing simply refers to a user-interface (UI) which works by using a pen, rather than traditional input devices such as a mouse or keyboard
(Avishka et al., 2018)	Mobile App (THE CURE)	Convolutional neural networks and k-means clustering	Dyslexia and Dysgraphia	It provides with an interactive interface that is designed to help those with these learning disabilities by offering them a place to practice reading and writing on their own
(Mohd Ariffin et al., 2018)	Mobile Application	DysgraphiCoach	Dysgraphia	It has three interactive sections. One, to teach alphabet writing, another for number writing, and finally a section designed to improve short-term memory and speed recognition skills.
(Mucha et al., 2018)	Parkinson's Diseases Dysgraphia Analysis	Fractional Derivatives (FDE)	Parkinson's Diseases	To proof the potential of FDE in PD dysgraphia quantification employing classification analysis

Continued on following page

Table 1. Continued

Study	Features	Approach	Specification	Description
(Scheidl et al., 2018)	Connectionist Temporal Classification (CTC) loss	Recurrent Neural Networks (RNNs)	Handwritten Text Recognition (HTR)	To propose word beam search decoding,
(Boyle & Joyce, 2019)	To Support Note-Taking Skills	Smartpens	Learning Disabilities	Smartpens use a tiny digital camera near to the tip of the pen to capture handwritten text. The dotted pattern in the paper helps to determine the exact location of the tip on the paper.
(DANKOVIČOV et al., 2019)	Extraction of parameters for CDSS (Clinical Decision support systems)	Machine learning methods, Decision tree methods, and python programming language	Dysgraphia	CDSS is used in healthcare. It aids clinicians in their decision making by processing, analyzing, and retrieving information from available sources.
(Impedovo & Pirlo, 2019)	Dynamic Handwriting Analysis	Pattern Recognition Perspective	Alzheimer's disease (AD) and Parkinson's disease (PD)	The aim is to develop research in the direction of a computer-aided diagnosis (CAD) system.
(Asselborn et al., 2020)	Estimating Handwriting Quality	BHK test (Concise Evaluation Scale for Children's Handwriting)	Dysgraphia	To evaluate handwriting difficulties in a modernized way.
(Karimi et al., 2020)	HW2MP-GAN (handwritten to machine print).	Generative Adversarial Networks (GAN)	Text recognition	In this method, two discriminator networks are used instead of one. They are character level discriminator that generates characters and a word-level discriminator that generates words.

RESULTS AND DISCUSSION

It can be noticed that majority of the works explored for dysgraphia were primarily divided into two-year segments, 1993-2007 and 2017-2020. Aids for which were more significantly seen in the second segment. From apps like DysgraphiCoach (Mohd Ariffin et al., 2018) and the CURE (Avishka et al., 2018) to handheld tools like the Smartpen (Ellis, 2016; Siddiqui & Muntjir, 2017; Boyle & Joyce, 2019) were worked on. An article by Quenneville (2001) is one of the earlier works that describe other aids used by children with learning disabilities like the use of digital audio recorder or word prediction softwares. Approaches taken by these solutions provided great insight into each of the approaches that can be used to address dysgraphia.

Analysis work for dysgraphia and dysgraphic handwriting can be observed to happen throughout the two-year segments. While earlier papers provided with thorough knowledge about the learning disability and the problems faced by those who are diagnosed with dysgraphia and those around them. Over the years different features of the dysgraphic handwriting were analysed. Features were observed to be dynamic. While comparing proficient handwriting with that of those with dysgraphia it was found that airtime was more, speed of writing was significantly slower, and more segments were taken while writing the same letter (Rosenblum et al., 2006) in the case of latter. Asselhorn et al. also discuss ratio with the airtime shows high variation (Asselhorn et al., 2020). DANKOVIČOV et al. (2019) also points that writing time and total time are statically different.

Through the years a variation on the approaches taken while addressing dysgraphia is significantly varied. Some attempt to use technology to predict if someone has dysgraphia or analyse the peculiarity found in dysgraphic handwriting, while others concentrate more on the various ways in which a remedial, accommodation or prevention aid can be provided.

FUTURE RESEARCH DIRECTIONS

Taking into considerations the various approaches and corresponding aids mentioned above, new solutions can be designed that provide effectiveness and usability. There is scope for creation under the accommodation approach since not many aids exist, and those that do exist might not tackle multiple problems faced by those diagnosed with a learning disability like dysgraphia. building upon the handwritten text recognition algorithm discussed, such an aid can be designed. Furthermore, in-depth analysis of the problems and available remedial aids has potential for building a helpful aid that can be used to improve one's condition.

CONCLUSION

There are various aspects to the issues faced by those with dysgraphia and different approaches that one can choose from while designing a suitable solution or aid. Performing simple tasks such as taking notes in a class, writing cheques, or filling forms can be challenging for those with this learning disability. Understanding the hindrances in one's ability to carry out day to day tasks is of importance. Another important aspect is one's handwriting and how it is different from that of those who do not have this learning disability. Few distinct features like the illegibility of the writing, the spacing between characters, and inconsistency can be noticed. There exist some aids designed to help better one's handwriting, while others provide assistance like spelling correction. Some solutions take an accommodation approach and provide a solution that does not concentrate on bettering one's condition but provide instant aid like Smartpens. An absence of an integrated system that can provide an effective by-pass solution is prominent and can be worked on. This can include various aspects of the problems faced by those with dysgraphia like bad handwriting and spelling or grammar difficulties.

REFERENCES

Asselborn, T., Chapatte, M., & Dillenbourg, P. (2020). Extending the Spectrum of Dysgraphia: A Data Driven Strategy to Estimate Handwriting Quality. *Scientific Reports*, *10*(1), 3140. Advance online publication. doi:10.103841598-020-60011-8 PMID:32081940

Avishka, I., Kumarawadu, K., Kudagama, A., Weerathunga, M., & Thelijjagoda, S. (2018). Mobile App to Support People with Dyslexia and Dysgraphia. *2018 IEEE International Conference on Information and Automation for Sustainability (ICIAfS)*. 10.1109/ICIAFS.2018.8913335

Baxter, D. M., & Warrington, E. K. (1994). Measuring Dysgraphia: A Graded-Difficulty Spelling Test. *Behavioural Neurology*, *7*(3–4), 107–116. doi:10.1155/1994/659593 PMID:24487323

Boyle, J. R., & Joyce, R. L. (2019). Using Smartpens to Support Note-Taking Skills of Students with Learning Disabilities. *Intervention in School and Clinic*, *55*(2), 86–93. doi:10.1177/1053451219837642

Crouch, A. L., & Jakubecy, J. J. (2007). Dysgraphia: How It Affects A Student's Performance and What Can Be Done About It. *Teaching Exceptional Children-Plus, 3.*

Dankovičová, Z., & Uchnár, M.Dankovičová. (2019). Extraction of parameters from dysgraphic handwriting for CDSS systems. *Acta Electrotechnica et Informatica*, *19*(1), 48–54. doi:10.15546/aeei-2019-0007

Ediger, M. (2002). Assessing handwriting achievement. *Reading Improvement*, *39*, 103–110.

Ellis, K. R. (2016). *Students with disabilities' perceptions of assistive technology, the livescribe smartpen, audio recording, and note-taking service accommodations* (M.A. thesis). California State University, Sacramento, CA, United States. Retrieved from https://scholarworks.calstate.edu/concern/theses/th83kz62t

Hamstra-Bletz, L., & Blöte, A. W. (1993). A Longitudinal Study on Dysgraphic Handwriting in Primary School. *Journal of Learning Disabilities*, *26*(10), 689–699. doi:10.1177/002221949302601007 PMID:8151209

Impedovo, D., & Pirlo, G. (2019). Dynamic Handwriting Analysis for the Assessment of Neurodegenerative Diseases: A Pattern Recognition Perspective. *IEEE Reviews in Biomedical Engineering*, *12*, 209–220. doi:10.1109/RBME.2018.2840679 PMID:29993722

Karimi, M., Veni, G., & Yu, Y. Y. (2020). Illegible Text to Readable Text: An Image-to-Image Transformation using Conditional Sliced Wasserstein Adversarial Networks. *2020 IEEE/CVF Conference on Computer Vision and Pattern Recognition Workshops (CVPRW)*. 10.1109/CVPRW50498.2020.00284

Khan, M., Hussain, M., Ahsan, K., Saeed, M., Nadeem, A., Ali, S., Mahmood, N., & Rizwan, K. (2017). Augmented Reality Based Spelling Assistance to Dysgraphia Students. *Journal of Basic and Applied Sciences*, *13*, 500–507. doi:10.6000/1927-5129.2017.13.82

Mohd Ariffin, M., Zarith Nabilah Tengku Othman, T., Shakirah Aziz, N., Mehat, M., & Izza Arshad, N. (2018). Dysgraphi Coach: Mobile Application for Dysgraphia Children in Malaysia. *International Journal of Engineering & Technology, 7*(4.36), 440. doi:10.14419/ijet.v7i4.36.23912

Mucha, J., Mekyska, J., Faundez-Zanuy, M., Lopez-De-Ipina, K., Zvoncak, V., Galaz, Z., Kiska, T., Smekal, Z., Brabenec, L., & Rektorova, I. (2018). Advanced Parkinson's Disease Dysgraphia Analysis Based on Fractional Derivatives of Online Handwriting. *2018 10th International Congress on Ultra Modern Telecommunications and Control Systems and Workshops (ICUMT)*. 10.1109/ICUMT.2018.8631265

Quenneville, J. (2001). Tech Tools for Students with Learning Disabilities: Infusion into Inclusive Classrooms. *Preventing School Failure*, *45*(4), 167–170. doi:10.1080/10459880109603332

Rosenblum, S., Dvorkin, A. Y., & Weiss, P. L. (2006). Automatic segmentation as a tool for examining the handwriting process of children with dysgraphic and proficient handwriting. *Human Movement Science*, *25*(4–5), 608–621. doi:10.1016/j.humov.2006.07.005 PMID:17011656

Rosenblum, S., Weiss, P. L., & Parush, S. (2004). Handwriting evaluation for developmental dysgraphia: Process versus product. *Reading and Writing, 17*(5), 433–458. doi:10.1023/B:READ.0000044596.91833.55

Scheidl, H. (2011). *Handwritten Text Recognition in Historical Documents* [Unpublished diploma thesis]. Technische Universität Wien, Austria.

Scheidl, H., Fiel, S., & Sablatnig, R. (2018). Word Beam Search: A Connectionist Temporal Classification Decoding Algorithm. *2018 16th International Conference on Frontiers in Handwriting Recognition (ICFHR)*. 10.1109/ICFHR-2018.2018.00052

Siddiqui, A. T., & Muntjir, M. (2017). An Approach to Smart Study using Pen and Paper Learning. *International Journal of Emerging Technologies in Learning, 12*(05), 117. doi:10.3991/ijet.v12i05.6798

Chapter 10
A Systematic Mapping Study of Low-Grade Tumor of Brain Cancer and CSF Fluid Detecting Approaches and Parameters

Soobia Saeed
Universiti Teknologi Malaysia, Malaysia

Habibullah Bin Haroon
Universiti Teknologi Malaysia, Malaysia

Mehmood Naqvi
Mohawk College, Canada

Noor Zaman Jhanjhi
(iD) https://orcid.org/0000-0001-8116-4733
Taylor's University, Malaysia

Muneer Ahmad
National University of Science and Technology, Pakistan

Loveleen Gaur
Amity University, Noida, India

ABSTRACT

Low-grade tumor or CSF fluid, the symptoms of brain tumor and CSF liquid, usually require image segmentation to evaluate tumor detection in brain images. This research uses systematic literature review (SLR) process for analysis of the different segmentation approach for detecting the low-grade tumor and CSF fluid presence in the brain. This research work investigated how to evaluate and detect the tumor and CSF fluid, improve segmentation method to detect tumor through graph cut hidden markov model of k-mean clustering algorithm (GCHMkC) techniques and parameters, extract the missing values in k-NN algorithm through correlation matrix of hybrid k-NN algorithm with time lag and discrete fourier transformation (DFT) techniques and parameters, and convert the non-linear data into linear transformation using LE-LPP and time complexity techniques and parameters.

DOI: 10.4018/978-1-7998-8929-8.ch010

INTRODUCTION

The motive of this chapter is to evaluate and use a proper scientific method of research methodology use in the research platform to solve the research problems in a systematic and organized body of knowledge. This chapter examines three multiple techniques use to explain the background of Hybrid GCHMkC, CM-DFT, and LE-LPP-TC techniques and multiple parameters details to use in segmentation method of MRI and research questions that are mentioned in details. Research methodology is an approach to scientifically find solutions to all the research questions. It is the skill of studying how research work is done systematically and finding the research problem together with the techniques or methods to be used. It is very important to know not just only the research methodology, but also the phases to follow in carrying out the research. This research explains the research methodology to be adopted in this research work. An overview of the phases of this research is to be explained and presented in this research.

Research Questions

R1: What is the concept of methodological framework use in the research platform to solve the research problems of missing imputation hybrid k-NN algorithm?

R2: How Operational Research Framework method implement in this research?

R3: What technique we use for Research Problem Formulation of missing imputation of hybrid k-NN algorithm and how it will solve the problem?

R4: What is the key factor of Implementation, Testing and Performance Evaluation and experimental setup of this research?

R5: What are parameters we use to solve the problem formulation of missing imputation hybrid k-NN algorithm in this research?

R1: What is the concept of methodological framework use in the research platform to solve the research problems of missing imputation hybrid k-NN algorithm?

Methodological Framework

The general research framework is divided into three main parts including Hybrid GCHMkC, CM-DFT, and LE-LPP-TC techniques. These main parts of the research have been clarified to set out the research questions of the problem as well as the research methodology utilized to accomplish research objectives. The performance measurement used is explained with the sole purpose of assuring the correctness of the achieved results. The first part introduces a Hybrid k-NN model by utilizing the novel technique of GCHMkC for segmenting and reconstructing the datasets of images to enhance the accuracy of the images and increase the efficiency of the k-NN algorithm. It begins with studying and planning, where the research problem is formulated. The process then proceeds to design, developed, simulate and evaluate the technique (S.Saeed *et al.*,2019).

The second section introduces the Correlation Matrix of Discrete Fourier Transform (CM-DFT) technique for correlation matrix to reconstruct test data points by training data to assign different k values of different test data points, referred to as the Correlation Matrix of k-NN (CM-kNN) classification, by improving performance in terms of the least-squares loss function is used to minimize the reconstruction error to reconstruct each test data point by all training data points. It also involves the experiment and running phase, in which the experiment setup, the dataset is explained.

The third part introduces a technique for minimizing the execution time of a hybrid k-NN model in medical images of datasets by combining the Laplace Transformation of Eigen maps with Locally Preserving Projection (LELPP) and Time complexity. The purpose of this technique is to minimize the execution computational time in the transformation of linear matrix by non-linear features in the datasets to become achieve better outcomes of optimizing solutions of the proposed method.

R2: How Operational Research Framework method implement in this research?

Operational Research Framework

The operational research framework consists of three main research phases illustrated in Figure 1. The first operational phase includes the background, analysis and problem formulation. The second operational phase integrates the design and development of improved hybrid *k*-NN model techniques of 4D images for the segmentation method. The third operational phase encompasses the details of implementation, testing and performance evaluation. Furthermore, the generated results are analyzed, evaluated, and comparatively discussed alongside results from existing techniques.

Background, Analysis and Planning

The background preparation, problem formulation and planning are performed through a detailed and extensive literature review of existing k-NN algorithms. The main focus of this phase of research is to highlight the current issues and problems for 4D medical MRI/CT scan images of proposed datasets in the hybrid k-NN model, for accuracy and efficiency (Wang, L, 2019). The merits and limitations of the existing k-NN algorithm, Graph Cut Hidden Markov of k-mean cluster(GCHMkC) technique, Correlation Matrix of Discrete Fourier Transformation (CM-DFT) and Laplace Transformation of Eigen maps with Locally Preserving Projection(LELPP) and Time complexity (TC) techniques are carefully and critically investigated with the planned framework design. In light of the highlighted limitations of the reviewed kinds of literature and techniques, the research problems are formulated (S.Saeed *et al.*,2019).

Figure 1. Operational research framework

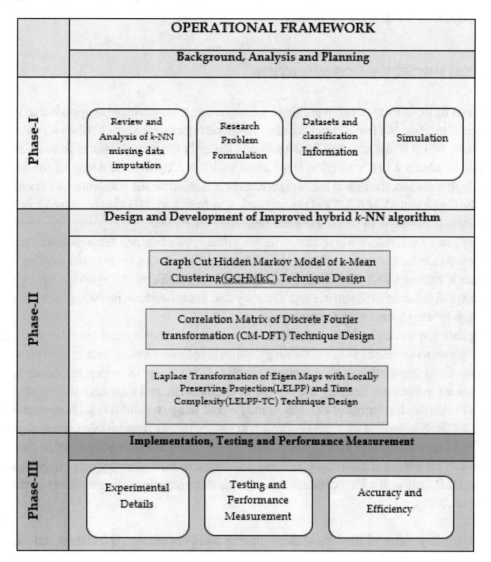

The Review and Analysis of 4DMRIs Images for CSF Fluid Leak and Low-Grade Tumor Images in Hybrid k-NN Model

A very wide critical literature review of hybrid k-NN algorithms with proposed medical datasets of 4D MRIs CSF fluid leak and low-grade tumor (initial growth of brain tumor) images are first conducted. Most of the state-of-the-art, different medical datasets and algorithms are extensively reviewed. The hybrid k-NN algorithms techniques are further classified and reviewed according to the parameter used in the evaluation of the performance and efficiency (Orczyk, T. et al., 2021). These state-of-the-art algorithms are illustrated and analyzed by pointing out critical loopholes and drawbacks in both their design and implementation. A comprehensive appraisal of hybrid k-NN algorithms for 4D images is also done with the help of a light field toolkit (Bohlen, M. *et al.*, 2019).

R3: What technique we use for Research Problem Formulation of missing imputation of hybrid k-NN model and how it will solve the problem?

RESEARCH PROBLEM FORMULATION

To present and formulate the research problem, a complete and comprehensive appraisal to improve the performance of medical MRI images of CSF and low-grade tumor (brain tumor) discovery at the specific site in the brain which is less effective for detection in the early stage until it stems from a sizeable apart in the brain. To obtain a better solution is achieved with the proposed technique of the hybrid k-NN algorithm. In this section, the hybrid k-NN algorithm is presented for the combination of two techniques including the Graph Cut SVM (GCSVM) hybridization technique and Hidden Markov Model of k-mean cluster(HMMkC) technique to become the one technique GCHMM.

Another phase of this research is related to missing data imputation problems and minimize the computational execution time is done in the hybrid k-NN algorithm. In this section, the missing imputation data problem is solving by CM-DFT and LE-LPP technique and TC in the hybrid k-NN algorithm. To obtain an optimal solution to the efficiency, accuracy and execution time problem, the system is represented by step-by-step formalizing the problem.

Missing data imputation in k-NN algorithm consignment of starting and completion times for the several operations to be executed. Like other imputation problems, missing data in k-NN is a procedure that appliesto the segmentation of the proposed GCHMkC technique to trained the datasets, generally refine the values in datasets, filtering the images in the datasets, and minimize the missing values to accomplish the demands of medical datasets in the field of image resolution and segmentation (Singh, A. P *et al.*, 2020). It is applied for HMM approach to ensure that the less visible values, object (sign of CSF fluid and tumor) detection in the images, and hidden information identify from the images in the given datasets This approach identifies CSF fluid and tumor in MRI at a very early stage It also makes sure that the HMM can deal with the hidden values, with these techniques by providing a better solution (S.Saeed *et al.*,2021).

R4: What is the key factor of Implementation, Testing and Performance Evaluation and experimental setup of this research?

Design and Development of Proposed Method

The design and development phase provides the segmented, planned, prepared, and executed proposed techniques according to the set objectives of this research. In the first subsection, a new technique known as Graph Cut Hidden Markov Model of k-mean cluster (GCHMkC) technique is designed and presented. This optimization technique tries to improve the performance of the hybrid k-NN algorithm by enhancing quality and accuracy. The next subsection presents the design and developmental components of a proposed Correlation Matrix of Discrete Fourier Transform (CMD-DFT) technique by reducing missing imputation and empty space convert to non-zero values in the same sequence using the Discrete Fourier transformation to enhance the efficiency of the data. While the last subsection presents the mechanisms of minimizing the time by Laplace Transformation of Eigen maps with Locally Preserving Projection

(LE-LPP) technique and Time complexity(TC) to improve the execution time strategies and achieve large distance margin values as a linear transformation with less consuming time.

Proposed Graph Cut Hidden Markov of K-Mean Cluster (GCHMkC) Technique Design

There are several techniques based on the classification of the hybrid k-NN algorithm to enhance the poor quality of MRI tumor images and create the efficient k-NN algorithm shown in Figure 2. There are some limitations for medical images datasets such as CSF Fluid and low-grade tumor to identify in MRI images to maintain the accuracy and quality of the images are given to this novel technique. The GCHMkC technique provides the complete comprehensive details of redundancy, accuracy and evaluates the images for reconstructing and refining procedure to avoid their limitations.

Figure 2. Composition of hybrid graph cut hidden Markov of k-mean cluster (GCHMkC) technique

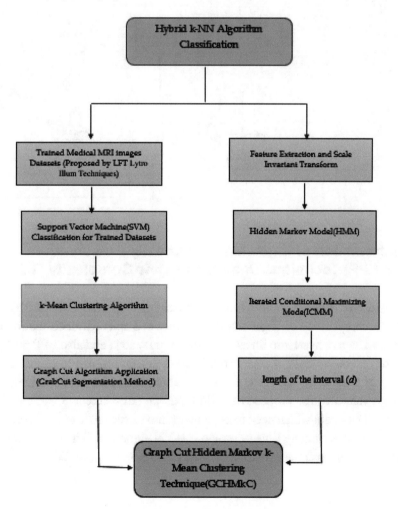

Proposed Correlation Matrix and Discrete Fourier Transform (CM-DFT) Technique Design

Figure 3 represents the working mechanism of the Correlation Matrix of Discrete Fourier transform (CM-DFT) technique for finding the missing imputation data. CM-DFT technique optimizes the missing data in the datasets of images simultaneously and achieve the results on accurate position of empty space and replace with numeric (non-empty space) values are produced in the images. The block diagram is illustrated in Figure 3show the complete details of working mechanism.

Figure 3. Block diagram of discrete fourier transformation missing data imputation

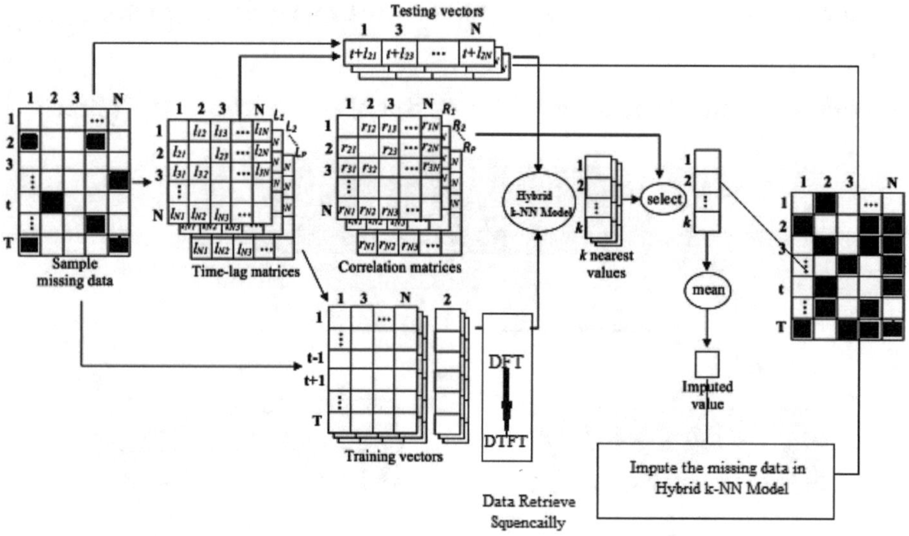

Laplace Transformation of Eigen Maps of Locally Preservation Projection (LE-LPP) Technique Design and Time Complexity (TC)

Laplace Transformation of Eigen maps with Locally Preserving Projection (LE-LPP) technique and Time complexity (TC) is a composition of Eigen mapping values of Laplace transformation for removing the non-linear feature and then convert into linear transformation matrix and also LPP preserves the original data during the conversion process of linear transformation to minimize the time and store the space in time complexity of time series data. The LE-LPP technique applies to minimize the execution time of the reconstructed values of the proposed hybrid k-NN model whereas, Gradient iterative approach check again the non-linear data which need to be convert into linear form and TC compare the proposed technique time with average running time of previous k-NN algorithm. The block diagram is illustrated in Figure 4 are show the linear transformation of MRI data (S.Saeed *et al.*,2021).

Figure 4. Linear transformation of the images by dimension reduction method of proposed technique

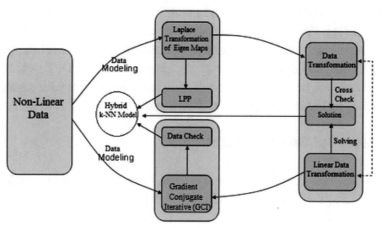

Implementation, Testing and Performance Evaluation

The implementation, testing and performance evaluation of the proposed techniques are the final phase of the operational research framework of this research. In the previous section, the design and development of the three proposed techniques have been presented for missing imputation data in the hybrid k-NN model. These include the GCHMkC technique, the CM-DFT technique and the LE-LPP technique with TC. In this section, the experimental setup, testing and evaluation are to be presented and discussed to the performance metrics and comparison with existing algorithms.

Experimental Setup

A feature and carefully implemented simulation is carried out for the proposed k-NN algorithm by using the trained datasets with the uses of LFT kit for enhancing the image quality. Many other tools are also available in LFT kit to enhance the quality of images which is utilize in the hybrid k-NN model that increase the efficiency of proposed hybrid k-NN model such as image filtering classification, object detection, diseases detection easily is preferred because it has support for the simulation of interactive processing of plenoptic images and improved calibration accuracy, efficiency and also functionalities to provide the rapid processing of raw light field images. In addition, its functionality for simulation of volumetric imaging of targeted brain regions, viewer location and orientation, CSF fluid, low grade tumors, targeted the flow of CSF liquid in the MRI images (S.Saeed *et al.*, 2021). The proposed model of hybrid k-NN algorithm is built on top of the higher resolution images and efficient techniques. Hybrid k-NN model use three different techniques to develop this improve hybrid model. Over the years several extensions have been introduced to the modified features of proposed k-NN model to enhance its functionalities. These include; improved metadata, colour correct vision, and improved rendering quality of images.

R5: What are parameters we use to solve the problem formulation of missing imputation hybrid k-NN model in this research?

The proposed three techniques parameters are used for evaluating the improvement of image quality by using the LFD, missing data imputation, and minimizing the execution time in hybrid k-NN algorithm (S.Saeed *et al.*,2021). These parameters are based on SVM classification, grabCut segmentation, Max-flow, Min- cut algorithm, scale invariant feature transform (SIFT) extraction, Iterative Conditional Maximizing Mode(ICMM) and statistical interval (d), Lagged time(Lp), DFT performance, and RMSE. This research study considers performance metrics in to two components with regarding to each objective, these performance metrics are discussed as follows (Ullah, A *et al.,* 2021):

Hybrid SVM Graph Cut Segmentation

The hybrid model is use to improve the quality of images, this section develops the hybrid model for the combination of SVM and graph cut algorithm into two phases.

SVM Classification

The SVM classification is utilized to improve quality of images with the help of k-mean algorithm. SVM draws a decision boundary which is a hyper plane between any two classes in order to separate them or classify them. SVM also used in Object Detection and image classification. To classify the brain or CSF MRI images is divided in to four categories such as white matter, gray matter, CSF matter, and background as an initial class label with the uses of k-mean algorithm to store the images data for classification (Ullah, A *et al.,* 2021). Extracting the feature is also a part of SVM which is applied in this technique for labeling the class of trained datasets and then applied the Gaussian kernel function for classification that can generate the two classes either positive and negative(Liu. J and Guo. L, 2015).

Graph Cuts for Image Segmentation

This study employs a segmentation technique that employs a graph to address the images and a Min-Cut/Max-Flow algorithm to segment the diagram. Nodes on the graph are used to address pixels in the images. The edge weights on the graph are defined by a cost function, which is defined by area and limit data from the image. By limiting the cost function, a Min-Cut/Max-Flow algorithm is used to segment the image. This strategy makes use of high-intensity images. (Marsh. *M et al.,*2006). Need to use latest reference

Li *et al.* (2004), present an interactive segmentation method based on graph minimization techniques. It consists of two significant stages. The first stage is the object marking stage, in which specific pixels are designated as either background or foreground. These are strict criteria that must be met during the segmentation process. Graph cuts are used in conjunction with an over segmentation result to significantly speed up segmentation and provide segmentation results to clients quickly. The next step is a limit editing step in which individual vertexes on the segmentation can be moved around until the client is satisfied (Vijayalakshmi, B *et al.,* 2021).

Detection Approach: Iterative Conditional Maximizing Mode (ICMM)

The iterated conditional maximizing mode (ICMM) algorithm is used in this study to obtain an arrangement of a neighborhood limit of the joint likelihood of a Markov random field. It accomplishes this by iteratively maximizing the likelihood of each factor based on the others. The Iterated Conditional Modes (ICM) algorithm was modified to address the issue of movement assessment in MRI image arrangements. Iterated contingent modes (ICM) sequentially amplify nearby preventive probabilities. In iterative local maximization, the ICMM algorithm employs the "greedy" procedure. The algorithm sequentially updates each into by maximizing the conditional (posterior) likelihood given the information "d" and different labels. The outcomes are represented on MRI image sequences (Magnetically Resonance depends on the properties of the images in the arrangement, these Imaging) (Sedghi A *et al.,*2021).

Time Lags

In this study, this section uses the time lag technique to test and prepare vectors, first determining which factors are correlated and at what time lags. This research use cross-correlation, which is a measure of similarity between two-time series as a function of a time delay applied to one of them (Chatfield. C and Xing. H, 2019), where T is the series length, x and y are the means of x and y separately, "d" ranges from – (D-1) to (D-1), and D is the maximum time delay. Because some x and y qualities may be missing, the instances are used only where both x and y are available in this estimation.

Matrices are created for each of the p lags, with correlations requested from 1... p in decreasing order of strength. As a result, for each pair of variables, L1 contains the lag, d, with the strongest correlation (max jrxyj) and Lp contains the lag with the weakest (max jrxyj). Each L is an N× N matrix with components that address the time lags for each correlation between the N variables. A component lxy can be either positive (values s of variable y have a delayed response unit lxy to values of x) or negative (values of variable x have a delayed response unit lxy for values of y), and lxy = - lyx. The diagonal components of the matrix are not processed because they provide the signal's auto-connection and are not used in this algorithm. The corresponding correlation values, jrxyj, for all lxy are stored in the matrices R1... Rp, which are used in the neighbor selection step (Chatfield. C and Xing. H, 2019).

Discrete Fourier Transformation (DFT)

The Discrete Fourier Transform (DFT) is used to test the Fourier transform of a periodic discrete time sequence. As a result, a link between the sampled Fourier transform and the DFT has already been established. When a signal is periodic in the time domain, it is possible to use discrete time Fourier series (DTFS) demonstration. The spectrum in that frequency domain will then be discrete and periodic. If the signal is non-periodic or of finite duration, but the frequency domain illustration is periodic and continuous. The finite duration sequence will be feasible to frequency domain by precisely utilizing the periodicity property of the DTFS illustration.

This is then referred to as a discrete Fourier transformation. This study employs DFT to shape a data segment with data from the beginning of the signal to the last non-missing data point. In variable structures, where values are available or imputed. This interaction occurs when DFT (the discrete Fourier transform) generates Fourier descriptors for a variable v and IDFT (converse DFT) regenerates a signal of length "T" from the Fourier descriptors "F" because the imputed data point focuses are close to the actual values. The proposed strategy entails determining the most precise value for each missing value based on the observed data (Rahman S. An *et al.,* 2015).

Iteration Method of Linear Transformation

This research use Iteration method for identifying the non-linear data. Iteration is the repetition of a process in order to generate an outcome. The sequence was approach some end point or end value. Each repetition of the process is a single iteration, and the outcome of each iteration is then the starting point of the next iteration. The iteration method is applied to check the non-linear data for the conversion of linear transformation until to complete the cross checking all the data during reconstruction of imputes missing data of k-NN algorithm.

Locally Preservation Projection (LPP)

This study employs Locality Preserving Projections (LPP) for linear projective maps that emerge from solving a variety problem that ideally preserves the neighborhood structure of the missing information of the k-NN algorithm through Laplace transformation. LPP should be considered as an alternative to Principal Component Analysis (PCA), a traditional linear strategy that projects data in the direction of maximum variation. The Locality Preserving Projections are obtained by finding the optimal linear approximations to the Eigen elements of the Laplace Transformation when the high dimensional data is lying on a low dimensional complex inserted in the surrounding space (Khairandish, M. O et al., 2021). As a result, LPP shares many of the data representation properties of nonlinear techniques, such as Laplacian Eigen maps. However, LPP is linear and, more importantly, is defined anywhere in the surrounding space rather than just on the training data points. LPP can be performed in either the first space or the repeating part Hilbert space into which data points are mapped. This results in kernel LPP. On real datasets, LPP produces better results, and experimental results show that the k-NN algorithm outperforms other learning algorithms such as classification, regression, and missing value imputation (Zhang.S et al.,2014).

Root Mean Square Error (RMSE) by Objective Testing of Missing Values

This research tool was used, and the root mean square error (RMSE) was calculated for imputed missing data over the specified time period. These procedures are useful measurement methods for analysing non-missing imputation data. The example standard deviation of the difference between actual and estimated values is addressed by RMSE as follows:

$$RMSE = \sqrt{\frac{\sum_{i=1}^{n}\left(x_i^{obs} - x_i^{imputed}\right)^2}{n}}$$

As a result, it is appropriate when penalizing large errors is desired. Where n denotes the number of test samples, Xi obs denotes the ith target value, and Xi imputed denotes the predicted value for the ith test sample. The RMSE value indicates how close the displayed and observed values. RMSE is calculated by taking the square root of the average square error and assigning a high weight to large errors. As a result, it is appropriate while penalizing large errors is attractive (Pazhoohesh. M et al., 2019).

246

HYPOTHESIS

R1: What is the method of research methodology use in the research platform to solve the research problems of hybrid k-NN algorithm?

R2: How Operational Research Framework method implement in this research?

R3: What technique we use for Research Problem Formulation and how it will solve the problem?

R4: What is the key factor of Implementation, Testing and Performance Evaluation and experimental setup of this research?

R5: What is parameters we use to solve the problem formulation of hybrid k-NN algorithm in this research?

Methodological Framework

Figure 5 illustrates the methodological framework used in this study. The framework starts with an initial stage of reviewing previous works. This stage aims to identify the present works on detecting the evidence of CSF leakage fluid and a low-grade brain tumor in MRI images. As is already mentioned in the previous section for finding the CSF fluid in MRI is difficult and fewer chances to identify in MRI images and also focus the proposed technique that is fulfilled the requirement of the proposed hybrid k-NN algorithm (S.Saeed *et al.*,2017). Furthermore, this is important to gain the knowledge of the involved data and to understand how to evaluate and implement in this research to become the improvement of the proposed method. This study is composed of three stages of contributions, namely the effectiveness of the proposed technique of GCHMkC; The improvement of missing imputation data due to CM-DFT technique to handling missing imputation data analysis, time-lagged delay and minimize the computational consuming time for the use of LE-LPP technique to generate the new values of proposed hybrid k-NN algorithm which make this method to become improve method compare than the previous method. Each contribution is explained in the following stage.

Figure.5 shows the proposed methodological structure as shown above to follow the direction of these step by step to the proposed significant framework.

In the first stage of the contribution, a comparative study is performed among the existing method and produce the new technique is to detect the CSF fluid and low-grade tumor in the images to the segmentation method to generate the high quality of the images with the help of GCHMkC technique of the given trained MRI datasets. This technique provides an easy platform for image processing, segmentation method and visualization field to identify the noisy and less visible data in the datasets. This research is practically conducted by human brain samples images in the University of Calgary, Canada from the Cuming School of Medicine Lab from the source of data gathered is https://cumming.ucalgary.ca/. Cuming School of Medicine Lab conducts the work on neuroscience and their related work. Their focus is based on solving the human brain diseases and also data gathered by various hospital sectors such as "National Cancer Care Institute(NMI)"https://www.ncci.org.pk/ and "Medicare hospital" in Pakistan, from the source of data gathered, is https://www.medicarehospital.pk/. This stage serves as an empirical analysis to evaluate the effectiveness of the proposed technique which is related to the main objective of the proposed method (S.Saeed *et al.*,2017).

For the next stage of this research, to reduce the missing imputation data and minimize the distance of long values as one of the motives of this research are to target the long-distance values of the proposed method. This research study introduces the new chronicle datasets of medical images and utilizes the proposed technique which is already mentioned in the previous section. Furthermore, this stage assists the empirical analysis to evaluate the efficiency of the proposed technique which is related to the second objective of the proposed technique.

Figure 5. Proposed methodological framework

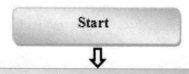

Start

Stage 1: Literature Study

Analyze previous works on the parameter of leakage of CSF and low-grade brain tumor images.

Stage 2: Graph Cut Hidden Markov Clustering (GCHMC) Technique
Contribution A new technique proposed based on GCHMkC is used to improve the quality of noisy or hidden information in images of MRI. The proposed technique finding some uniqueness of the images after reconstructing which provide the better achievements of the segmentation method.
Deliverable: To improve the quality of images using the Lytro tools kit which enhance the quantity as it is already mentioned in experimental results with the classification of GCSVM and HMM with k-mean cluster. These techniques improved CSF fluid images that can easily identify the liquid of fluid in MRI images.

Stage 3: Improved Missing Hybrid Algorithm and enhance the computational time
Contribution: A new hybrid k-NN method is proposed based on two techniques used in this stage of research. The proposed techniques are finding the solution to overcome the missing data and reduce the execution time delay which is addressed by the k-NN algorithm
Deliverable: To proposed an improved hybrid k-NN model using (CM-DFT) technique to overcome the missing imputation data and minimize the execution computational time with the help of the LELPP technique. These techniques made the improvement of Imputation data, convert linear transformation of the data, and less consuming time for reconstruction of the empty space by replacing the non-empty space.

Stage 4: Result and discussion

Contribution: Mentioned all experimental results with discussion outcomes. This stage aims to discuss the performance of the method in terms of computational time and overcome the empty values of *the hybrid k*-NN model.

Stage 5: Report Writing

- Documentation of outcome examines
- Writing for journal articles and thesis

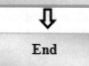

End

The last stage of this research is to minimize the execution computational time for the proposed k-NN algorithm and remove the non-linear transformation into linear transformation by Laplace Transformation of Eigen maps with Locally Preserving Projection (LE-LPP) and Time complexity (TC) technique. This stage aims to enhance the performance of the proposed model based on the analysis provided by the previous stage. The contribution of this stage is to design and develop the improved technique of less consuming time in the experiment and the training data are arising from the storage of datasets are linked with improving the calculated information mentioned in the previous section. The improved technique is to evaluate the duration of the current technique time and compare with the average time of execution to identify the proposed method improvement of minimizing the duration of time that become to maintain the efficiency of the proposed method. The last stage of the framework involves documentation of the work. This may include thesis writing and journal article publications.

Publication Selection

This section includes information on the inclusion and exclusion criteria used to select publications, as well as the process for selecting relevant articles based on the study questions. Following that, the following inclusion criteria were developed:

The research period spanned nearly a decade, with articles published between 2005 and 2021. Because the lowest grade tumors were first reported in 2005, the start date was chosen. However, because the studies were conducted in early 2012, the most recent publication corresponding to the end of 2018 was used in the systematic mapping to look at:

1. Experiments on detecting low-grade tumors and identifying CSF fluid in MRI images using various segmentation techniques.
2. Research aimed at providing implementation results for brain tumor detection in the brain, as well as locating symptoms of cerebrospinal fluid (CSF). We used the following exclusion criteria:

The following studies do not provide detailed information on the low-grade tumor and CSF fluid leak: There were duplicate studies, so only the most recent ones were chosen.

1. Provide discussion outside of the field.
2. Articles containing only guidelines, recommendations, or descriptions of low-grade tumors.
3. Workshop, special publication, and book introductory articles
4. Book chapters
5. Papers that is not accessible.

Table 1. Study selection

Source	Retrieved	Initial Selection	Final Selection
IEEE	96	40	08
IEEE Transactions	66	20	10
Science Direct	50	15	5
Springer Link	20	15	4
SAGE	10	10	2
Total	242	100	29

Table 1 depicts the selection criteria for articles in the publishing databases of recognized indexing services. We can see how the information from the retrieved manuscripts is distributed, as well as the preliminary and final selection of manuscripts that are targeted by gathering detailed information about low-grade tumor and CSF fluid.

GENERAL DISCUSSION

Testing and Performance Evaluation

In order to get more precise results, the experimental setup is classified into three phases. This classification will cover the three experimental phases of Graph Cut Hidden Markov of k-mean Cluster (GCHMkC) technique. The first phase SVM classification is used for evaluating the quality of medical images by SVM classification for maintain the accuracy, and clear vision to identify the object in the MRI images. The second phase cover the graph cut algorithm with minimum energy function, these parameters are based on GrabCut Segmentation, Feature Extraction and Scale Invariant Transform. In the end, the third phase is based on HMM parameters are used for diagnosing the CSF Fluid and tumor region in MRI.

Phase-I, Phase-II and Phase-III are used for evaluating the performance of GCHMkC technique. The measurement of improve quality, efficiency, and accuracy are shown in Table 2 to Table 7for Phase-I to III. These phases discussed above are implemented for simulation based on trained LFD MRI datasets. The proposed hybrid k-NN algorithm improves quality, accuracy, and efficiency due to the performance of this novel technique. The parameters setting of selected SVM classification variables and their values are shown in the given below:

Phase-I: SVM Classification

See Table 2.

Table 2. Simulation parameters setting of SVM hyperplane classification

Sr.No	Datasets	Parameter	Values
1	Datasets-I	Kernel Function	Linear
		Box Constraint Level	2
		Kernel Scale	0.7
		Multi-Class Method	One v/s All
		Standardize Data	True
		PCA Enable	No
2	Datasets-II	Kernel Function	Linear
		Box Constraint Level	1
		Kernel Scale	0.68
		Multi-Class Method	One v/s All
		Standardize Data	True
		PCA Enable	No
3	Datasets-III	Kernel Function	Linear
		Box Constraint Level	0.9
		Kernel Scale	0.658
		Multi-Class Method	One v/s All
		Standardize Data	True
		PCA Enable	No
4	Datasets-IV	Kernel Function	Linear
		Box Constraint Level	0.829
		Kernel Scale	0.678
		Multi-Class Method	One v/s All
		Standardize Data	True
		PCA Enable	No
5	Datasets-V	Kernel Function	Linear
		Box Constraint Level	0.88
		Kernel Scale	0.695
		Multi-Class Method	One v/s All
		Standardize Data	True
		PCA Enable	No

Phase-I(a): Graph Cut Algorithm

This research focuses on CSF fluid leak and low-grade tumor so the graph cut minimizing energy function is implement only three datasets: CSF fluid, low-grade tumor, and CSF with low-grade tumor. The parameters setting of selected graph cut algorithm to reduce the minimizing energy function values, grabcut segmentation method for reorganizing the both parameters of foreground and background values using gray level histogram method parameters values and Max-cut, Min flow algorithm values, and Scale Invariant Feature parameters values are shown in Table 3.

Table 3. Simulation parameters setting of graph cut algorithm

Algorithms	Parameters Values	
	Foreground Seed	**Background Seed**
GrabCut	150	180
	170	80
	200	40

Table 4. Simulation parameters setting of feature extraction and scale invariant featuretransform

Image	Octave Values	Scale Values	Sigma Values
D-I MRI Image	3	5	1.3
D-II MRI Image	3	5	1.4
D-III MRI Image	3	5	1.3

Phase-II: Hidden Markov Model

The Hidden Markov Model (HMM) is used to tracking the segmentation of brain tissue and CSF fluid over time in a given subject in phase-III, and the 4D segmentation process is repeated independently for each time point. Because this study focuses on CSF fluid leak and low-grade tumor, HMM only uses three datasets: CSF fluid, low-grade tumor, and CSF with low-grade tumor. The selected HMM parameters considered the state of each voxel in 4D MRI datasets to be tumor presence or CSF fluid leak, with possible values of presence and absence. Table 5 depicts the system state (presence / absence), which is represented in this model by two transition states with the settings parameters used to show the visible MR signal intensity at each voxel. The simulation results are indicating these parameters which are highlight the tumor and CSF fluid leakage presence in the MRI images.

Table 5. Simulation parameters setting of hidden Markov model (HMM)

Sr.No	Datasets	HMM Parameter	Value
1		C	2.5
		A1	5
		A2	15
	Datasets-I	$\mu1$	186
		$\mu2$	11
		$\sigma1$	3
		$\sigma2$	8
2		C	2.7
		A1	4.5
		A2	12
	Datasets-II	$\mu1$	255
		$\mu2$	11
		$\sigma1$	3
		$\sigma2$	8
3		C	2.8
	Datasets-III	A1	4.55
		A2	13.5
		$\mu1$	255
		$\mu2$	12
		$\sigma1$	3.25
		$\sigma2$	8

Table 6. Simulation parameters setting of iterative conditional maximizing mode(ICMM) over hidden Markov model (IIMM)

Sr.No	Datasets	ICMM parameter	Values
1	D-I MRI Images	Beta (β)	0.33
		Mu (μ)	0.20
		Variance (σ)	3
2	D-II MRI Images	Beta (β)	0.31
		Mu (μ)	0.22
		Variance (σ)	2.99
3	D-III MRI Images	Beta (β)	0.34
		Mu (μ)	0.20
		Variance (σ)	3.1

Performance Metrics of CM-DFT Technique Simulation

CM-DFT technique is used for reducing the missing data imputation in images. These parameters are used for the improvement of the missing data in images especially MRIs and CT scan in terms of time-lagged, Fourier descriptor, Discrete-Time of Fourier Transform matrix etc. This research study considers performance metrics into three groups of datasets with regarding each objective, these performance metrics are discussed as follows:

Table 7. Combination of CM-DFT parameters

Sr.No	Datasets	Hybrid k-NN Parameters	DFT Parameters
1	D-I-MRI Images	K=10	n=2 point
2	D-II-MRI Images	K=10	n=6 points
3	D-III-MRI Images	K=10	n= 8 points

Performance Metrics of Laplace Eigen Maps of Locally Preserving Projection (LE-LPP) and Time Complexity (TC) Techniques Simulation

LE-LPP technique and TC is used for minimizing the execution time with the conversation of non-linear transformation into linear transformation to become the long-distance values after maintaining the large margin values. These parameters are included Laplacian Eigen maps (LE) values, locally preserving projection tool, eigenvalue, Root Mean Square Error (RMSE), and computational complexity of time series function.

Table 8. Simulation parameters setting of Laplace Eigen maps of LPPfor datasets-I

Sr.No	Parameters	Assigned Values
1	X	K_i_j
2	Dimension (d)	4
3	k	10.41
4	σ	2.5
5	eig_impl	'Matlab';

Table 9. Simulation parameters setting of Laplace Eigen maps of LPP for datasets-II

Sr.No	Parameters	Assigned Values
1	X	**K_i_j**
2	Dimension (d)	4
3	k	10
4	σ	2.5
5	eig_impl	'Matlab';

Table 10. Simulation parameters setting of Laplace Eigen maps of LPP for datasets-IIII

Sr.No	Parameters	Assigned Values
1	X	**K_i_j**
2	Dimension (d)	4
3	k	10.41
4	σ	3.52
5	eig_impl	'Matlab';

CONCLUSION

This research presents the research methodology and proposed framework used for the design and development of missing imputation data using the improved hybrid k-NN model. The research operational and methodological framework is categorized into three main phases. In the first operational phase, the hybrid k-NN model improves the efficiency of trained MRI images datasets for use of the GCHMkC technique and 4D MRI images are highlighted and critically analyzed through available kinds of literature. The research problem is also formulated and the experimental datasets are explained. In the second phase of this research framework, the design and development of the reduced missing imputation data method for CM-DFT and LE-LPP techniques are presented. The proposed GCHMkC technique, CM-DFT and LE-LPP techniques are designed and developed in line with the research objectives. In the third and final phase of the operational framework, the experimental implementation, testing and performance evaluation are presented in detail. This final phase also explains the experimental setup, and performance metrics are mentioned and also show the methodological framework as a contribution of this proposed method.

REFERENCES

Ahmed, M. M., & Mohamad, D. B. (2008). Segmentation of brain MR images for tumor extraction by combining kmeans clustering and perona-malik anisotropic diffusion model. *International Journal of Image Processing*, 2(1), 27–34.

Banerjee, S., & Mitra, S. (2020). Novel volumetric sub-region segmentation in brain tumors. *Frontiers in Computational Neuroscience*, *14*, 3. doi:10.3389/fncom.2020.00003 PMID:32038216

Bohlen, M., Busch, C. J., Sehner, S., Forterre, F., Bier, J., Berliner, C., Bußmann, L., & Münscher, A. (2019). Tumor volume as a predictive parameter in the sequential therapy (induction chemotherapy) of head and neck squamous cell carcinomas. *European Archives of Oto-Rhino-Laryngology*, *276*(4), 1183–1189. doi:10.100700405-019-05323-w PMID:30725209

Boykov, Y., & Kolmogorov, V. (2004). An experimental comparison of min-cut/max-flow algorithms for energy minimization in vision. *IEEE Transactions on Pattern Analysis and Machine Intelligence*, *26*(9), 1124–1137. doi:10.1109/TPAMI.2004.60 PMID:15742889

Brinker, T., Stopa, E., Morrison, J., & Klinge, P. (2014). A new look at cerebrospinal fluid circulation. *Fluids and Barriers of the CNS*, *11*(1), 1–16. doi:10.1186/2045-8118-11-10 PMID:24817998

Chatfield, C., & Xing, H. (2019). *The analysis of time series: an introduction with R*. Chapman and Hall/ CRC. doi:10.1201/9781351259446

Greig, D. M., Porteous, B. T., & Seheult, A. H. (1989). Exact maximum a posteriori estimation for binary images. *Journal of the Royal Statistical Society. Series B. Methodological*, *51*(2), 271–279. doi:10.1111/j.2517-6161.1989.tb01764.x

Htun, S. N. N., Zin, T. T., & Tin, P. (2020). Image Processing Technique and Hidden Markov Model for an Elderly Care Monitoring System. *Journal of Imaging*, *6*(6), 49. doi:10.3390/jimaging6060049 PMID:34460595

Kaur, A., Kaur, L., & Singh, A. (2021). State-of-the-art segmentation techniques and future directions for multiple sclerosis brain lesions. *Archives of Computational Methods in Engineering*, *28*(3), 951–977. doi:10.100711831-020-09403-7

Khairandish, M. O., Sharma, M., Jain, V., Chatterjee, J. M., & Jhanjhi, N. Z. (2021). A Hybrid CNN-SVM Threshold Segmentation Approach for Tumor Detection and Classification of MRI Brain Images. *IRBM*. Advance online publication. doi:10.1016/j.irbm.2021.06.003

Li, Y., Sun, J., Tang, C.-K., & Shum, H.-Y. (2004). Chi-Keung Tang, and Heung-Yeung Shum. Lazy snapping. *ACM Transactions on Graphics*, *23*(3), 303–308. doi:10.1145/1015706.1015719

Liu, J., & Guo, L. (2015, August). A new brain mri image segmentation strategy based on k-means clustering and svm. In *2015 7th International Conference on Intelligent Human-Machine Systems and Cybernetics* (Vol. 2, pp. 270-273). IEEE. 10.1109/IHMSC.2015.182

Maeno, K., Nagahara, H., Shimada, A., & Taniguchi, R. I. (2013). Light field distortion feature for transparent object recognition. *Proceedings of the IEEE Conference on Computer Vision and Pattern Recognition*, 2786-2793. 10.1109/CVPR.2013.359

Mihara, H., Funatomi, T., Tanaka, K., Kubo, H., Mukaigawa, Y., & Nagahara, H. (2016, May). 4D light field segmentation with spatial and angular consistencies. *2016 IEEE International Conference on Computational Photography (ICCP)*, 1-8. 10.1109/ICCPHOT.2016.7492872

Mirjalili, S. (2016). *Dragonfly algorithm: A new meta-heuristic optimization technique for solving single-objective*. Academic Press.

Mustaqeem, A., Javed, A., & Fatima, T. (2012). An efficient brain tumor detection algorithm using watershed & thresholding based segmentation. *International Journal of Image. Graphics and Signal Processing*, *4*(10), 34–39. doi:10.5815/ijigsp.2012.10.05

Orczyk, T., Doroz, R., & Porwik, P. (2021, June). Missing Value Imputation Method Using Separate Features Nearest Neighbors Algorithm. In *International Conference on Computational Science*. Springer. 10.1007/978-3-030-77967-2_12

Pascal, N. E., Pierre, E., & Emmanuel, T. (2014) Hybrid Method Segmentation for Medical Image Based on DWT, FCM and HMRF-EM. *International Journal of Computer and Information Technology*.

Pazhoohesh, M., Pourmirza, Z., & Walker, S. (2019, August). A comparison of methods for missing data treatment in building sensor data. In *2019 IEEE 7th International Conference on Smart Energy Grid Engineering (SEGE)* (pp. 255-259). IEEE. 10.1109/SEGE.2019.8859963

Rahman, S. A., Huang, Y., Claassen, J., Heintzman, N., & Kleinberg, S. (2015). Combining Fourier and lagged k-nearest neighbor imputation for biomedical time series data. *Journal of Biomedical Informatics*, *58*, 198–207. doi:10.1016/j.jbi.2015.10.004 PMID:26477633

Rother, C., Kolmogorov, V., & Blake, A. (2004). GrabCut" interactive foreground extraction using iterated graph cuts. *ACM Transactions on Graphics*, *23*(3), 309–314. doi:10.1145/1015706.1015720

Saeed, Abdullah, & Jhanjhi. (2021a). Performance analysis of machine learning algorithm for health care tools with High Dimension Segmentation. *Machine learning healthcare: Handling and managing data, 1*(1), 1-30.

Saeed, Abdullah, & Jhanjhi. (2021b). Comparison analysis of medical health care information of Graph Cutting using Multi Dimension Segmentation. *Machine learning healthcare: Handling and managing data, 1*(1), 1-23.

Saeed, Abdullah, & Jhanjhi. (2021c). Statistical Analysis the Pre and Post-Surgery of health care sector using High Dimension Segmentation. *Machine learning healthcare: Handling and managing data, 1*(1), 1-25.

Saeed, Abdullah, & Jhanjhi. (2021d). Combination of Brain Cancer with Hybrid K-NN Algorithm using statistical Analysis of Cerebrospinal Fluid (CSF) Surgery. *International Journal of Computer Science and Network Security, 21*(2), 120-130.

Saeed, Abdullah, Jhanjhi, & Naqvi. (2019). Implementation of Fourier transformation. *Indian Journal of Science & Technology, 12*(37), 1-16.

Saeed, S., Abdullah, A., & Jhanjhi, N. (2019). Investigation of a Brain Cancer with Interfacing of 3-Dimensional Image Processing. *Indian Journal of Science and Technology*, *12*(34), 1–12. doi:10.17485/ijst/2019/v12i34/146150

Saeed, S., & Naqvi, M. (2017). Implementation of Failure Enterprise Systems in Organizational Perspective Framework. *International Journal of Advanced Computer Science and Applications*, *8*(5), 54–63. doi:10.14569/IJACSA.2017.080508

Saeed, S., & Naqvi, S. M. (2017). Assessment of Brain Tumor Due to the Usage of MATLAB Performance. *Journal of Medical Imaging and Health Informatics*, *7*(6), 1454–1460. doi:10.1166/jmihi.2017.2187

Sedghi, A., O'Donnell, L. J., Kapur, T., Learned-Miller, E., Mousavi, P., & Wells, W. M. III. (2021). Image registration: Maximum likelihood, minimum entropy and deep learning. *Medical Image Analysis*, *69*, 101939. doi:10.1016/j.media.2020.101939 PMID:33388458

Singh, A. P., Pradhan, N. R., Luhach, A. K., Agnihotri, S., Jhanjhi, N. Z., Verma, S., Kavita, Ghosh, U., & Roy, D. S. (2020). A novel patient-centric architectural framework for blockchain-enabled healthcare applications. *IEEE Transactions on Industrial Informatics*, *17*(8), 5779–5789. doi:10.1109/TII.2020.3037889

Sokołowski, A., & Pardela, T. (2014). Application of Fourier transforms in classification of medical images. In *Human-computer systems interaction: backgrounds and applications* (Vol. 3, pp. 193–200). Springer.

Ullah, A., Azeem, M., Ashraf, H., Alaboudi, A. A., Humayun, M., & Jhanjhi, N. Z. (2021). Secure healthcare data aggregation and transmission in IoT—A survey. *IEEE Access: Practical Innovations, Open Solutions*, *9*, 16849–16865. doi:10.1109/ACCESS.2021.3052850

Ullah, A., Ishaq, N., Azeem, M., Ashraf, H., Jhanjhi, N. Z., Humayun, M., Tabbakh, T. A., & Almusaylim, Z. A. (2021). A Survey on Continuous Object Tracking and Boundary Detection Schemes in IoT Assisted Wireless Sensor Networks. *IEEE Access: Practical Innovations, Open Solutions*, *9*, 126324–126336. doi:10.1109/ACCESS.2021.3110203

Vijayalakshmi, B., Ramar, K., Jhanjhi, N. Z., Verma, S., Kaliappan, M., Vijayalakshmi, K., Vimal, S., Kavita, & Ghosh, U. (2021). An attention-based deep learning model for traffic flow prediction using spatiotemporal features towards sustainable smart city. *International Journal of Communication Systems*, *34*(3), e4609. doi:10.1002/dac.4609

Wang, L. (2019, December). Research and Implementation of Machine Learning Classifier Based on KNN. In *IOP Conference Series: Materials Science and Engineering*. IOP Publishing. 10.1088/1757-899X/677/5/052038

Wanner, S., & Goldluecke, B. (2012, June). Globally consistent depth labeling of 4D light fields. In *2012 IEEE Conference on Computer Vision and Pattern Recognition*. IEEE. 10.1109/CVPR.2012.6247656

Zhang, D. Q., & Chen, S. C. (2004). A novel kernelized fuzzy c-means algorithm with application in medical image segmentation. *Artificial Intelligence in Medicine*, *32*(1), 37–50. doi:10.1016/j.artmed.2004.01.012 PMID:15350623

Zhang, S., Cheng, D., Deng, Z., Zong, M., & Deng, X. (2018). A novel kNN algorithm with data-driven k parameter computation. *Pattern Recognition Letters*, *109*, 44–54. doi:10.1016/j.patrec.2017.09.036

Zhang, S., Li, X., Zong, M., Zhu, X., & Cheng, D. (2017). Learning k for knn classification. *ACM Transactions on Intelligent Systems and Technology*, *8*(3), 1–19.

Zhang, S., Zong, M., Sun, K., Liu, Y., & Cheng, D. (2014, December). Efficient kNN algorithm based on graph sparse reconstruction. In *International Conference on Advanced Data Mining and Applications* (pp. 356-369). Springer. 10.1007/978-3-319-14717-8_28

Zhang, Y., Brady, M., & Smith, S. (2001). Segmentation of brain MR images through a hidden Markov field model and the expectation-maximization algorithm. *IEEE Transactions on Medical Imaging*, *20*(1), 45–57. doi:10.1109/42.906424 PMID:11293691

Compilation of References

(2016). Deep Residual Learning for Image Recognition. In K. He, X. Zhang, S. Ren, & J. Sun (Eds.), Proceeding of the 2016 IEEE Conference on Computer Vision and Pattern Recognition (CVPR 2016) (pp. 770–778). IEEE. https://doi.org/10.1109/CVPR.2016.90.

(2017). Understanding of a Convolutional Neural Network. In S. Albawi, T. A. Mohammed, & S. Al-Zawi (Eds.), Proceeding of the 2017 International Conference on Engineering and Technology (ICET) (pp. 1–6). IEEE. https://doi.org/10.1109/ICEngTechnol.2017.8308186.

(2019). Overfitting and Underfitting Analysis for Deep Learning Based End-to-end Communication Systems. In H. Zhang, L. Zhang, & Y. Jiang (Eds.), Proceeding of the 11th International Conference on Wireless Communications and Signal Processing (WCSP) (pp. 1–6). IEEE. https://doi.org/10.1109/WCSP.2019.8927876.

Drukteinis, J. S., Mooney, B. P., Flowers, C. I., & Gatenby, R. A. (2013). Beyond mammography: New frontiers in breast cancer screening. *The American Journal of Medicine*, *126*(6), 472–479. doi:10.1016/j.amjmed.2012.11.025 PMID:23561631

Krafft, C., Shapoval, L., Sobottka, S. B., Geiger, K. D., Schackert, G., & Salzer, R. (2006). Identification of primary tumors of brain metastases by SIMCA classification of IR spectroscopic images. *Biochimica Biophysica Acta (BBA)-Biomembranes*, *1758*(7), 883–891. doi:10.1016/j.bbamem.2006.05.001 PMID:16787638

Krafft, C., Shapoval, L., Sobottka, S. B., Schackert, G., & Salzer, R. (2006). Identification of primary tumors of brain metastases by infrared spectroscopic imaging and linear discriminant analysis. *Technology in Cancer Research & Treatment*, *5*(3), 291–298. doi:10.1177/153303460600500311 PMID:16700626

Majeed, W., Aslam, B., Javed, I., Khaliq, T., Muhammad, F., Ali, A., & Raza, A. (2014). Breast cancer: Major risk factors and recent developments in treatment. *APJCP*, *15*(8), 3353–3358. doi:10.7314/APJCP.2014.15.8.3353 PMID:24870721

Nieder, C., Guckenberger, M., Gaspar, L. E., Rusthoven, C. G., Ruysscher, D. D., & ... . (2019). Management of patients with brain metastases from non-small cell lung cancer and adverse prognostic features: Multi-national radiation treatment recommendations are heterogeneous. *Radiation Oncology (London, England)*, *14*(1), 33. doi:10.118613014-019-1237-9 PMID:30770745

Sun, Y. S., Zhao, Z., Yang, Z. N., Xu, F., Lu, H. J., Zhu, Z. Y., & Zhu, H. P. (2014). Risk factors and preventions of breast cancer. *International Journal of Biological Sciences*, *13*(11), 1387–1397. doi:10.7150/ijbs.21635 PMID:29209143

Guillerey, C., Huntington, N. D., & Smyth, M. J. (2016). Targeting natural killer cells in cancer immunotherapy. *Nature Immunology*, *17*(9), 1025–1036. doi:10.1038/ni.3518 PMID:27540992

Maffini, M. V., Soto, A. M., Calabro, J. M., Ucci, A. A., & Sonnenschein, C. (2004). The stroma as a crucial target in rat mammary gland carcinogenesis. *Journal of Cell Science*, *117*(8), 1495–1502. doi:10.1242/jcs.01000 PMID:14996910

Hegan, D. C., Lu, Y., Stachelek, G. C., Crosby, M. E., Bindra, R. S., & Glazer, P. M. (2010). Inhibition of poly(ADP-ribose) polymerase down-regulates BRCA1 and RAD51 in a pathway mediated by E2F4 and p130. *Proceedings of the National Academy of Sciences of the United States of America*, *107*(5), 2201–2206. doi:10.1073/pnas.0904783107 PMID:20133863

Makarem, N., Chandran, U., Bandera, E. V., & Parekh, N. (2013). Dietary fat in breast cancer survival. *Annual Review of Nutrition*, *33*(1), 319–348. doi:10.1146/annurev-nutr-112912-095300 PMID:23701588

Nieder, Haukland, Mannsåker, Pawinski, & Yobuta. (2019). *Presence of Brain Metastases at Initial Diagnosis of Cancer: Patient Characteristics and Outcome.* Academic Press.

Catsburg, C., Miller, A. B., & Rohan, T. E. (2015). Active cigarette smoking and risk of breast cancer. *International Journal of Cancer*, *136*(9), 2204–2209. doi:10.1002/ijc.29266 PMID:25307527

Kaznowska, E., Depciuch, J., Szmuc, K., & Cebulski, J. (2017). Use of FTIR spectroscopy and PCA-LDC analysis to identify cancerous lesions within the human colon. *Journal of Pharmaceutical and Biomedical Analysis*, *134*(1), 259–268. doi:10.1016/j.jpba.2016.11.047 PMID:27930993

Hela, B., Hela, M., Kamel, H., Sana, B., & Najla, M. (2013). *Breast cancer detection: A review on mammograms analysis techniques. In 10th International Multi-Conferences on Systems.* Signals & Devices.

Kaznowska, E., Łach, K., Depciuch, J., Chaber, R., Koziorowska, A., Slobodian, S., Kiper, K., Chlebus, A., & Cebulski, J. (2018). Application of infrared spectroscopy for the identification of squamous cell carcinoma (lung cancer), Preliminary study. *Infrared Physics & Technology*, *89*(2), 282–290. doi:10.1016/j.infrared.2018.01.021

Belykh, E., Shaffer, K. V., Lin, C., Byvaltsev, V. A., Preul, M. C., & Chen, L. (2020). Blood-Brain Barrier, Blood-Brain Tumor Barrier, and Fluorescence-Guided Neurosurgical Oncology: Delivering Optical Labels to Brain Tumors. *Frontiers in Oncology*, *10*, 739. doi:10.3389/fonc.2020.00739 PMID:32582530

Blot, L., & Zwiggelaar, R. (2014). Background Texture Extraction for the Classification of Mammographic Parenchymal Patterns. *Medical Image Understanding and Analysis*, 1-5.

Bouyahia, S., Mbainaibeye, J., & Ellouze, N. (2009). Wavelet based microcalcifications detection in digitized mammograms. *Graphics. Vision and Image Processing Journal*, *8*, 1–12.

Putz, F., Mengling, V., Perrin, R., Masitho, S., Weissmann, T., Rösch, J., Bäuerle, T., Janka, R., Cavallaro, A., Uder, M., Amarteifio, P., Doussin, S., Schmidt, M. A., Dörfler, A., Semrau, S., Lettmaier, S., Fietkau, R., & Bert, C. (2020). Magnetic resonance imaging for brain stereotactic radiotherapy. *Strahlentherapie und Onkologie*, *196*(5), 1–13. doi:10.100700066-020-01604-0 PMID:32206842

Fakhro, A. E., Fateha, B. E., al-Asheeri, N., & al-Ekri, S. A. (1999). Breast cancer: Patient characteristics and survival analysis at Salmaniya Medical Complex, Bahrain. *Eastern Mediterranean Health Journal*, *5*(3), 430–439. doi:10.26719/1999.5.3.430 PMID:10793821

Hazra, A., Bera, N., & Mandal, A. (2017). Predicting lung cancer survivability using SVM and logistic regression algorithms. *International Journal of Computers and Applications*, *17*(2), 1–12.

Dheeba, J., & Jiji, G. C. (2010). Detection of Microcalcification Clusters in Mammograms using Neural Network. *International Journal of Advanced Science and Technology*, *130*, 31–45.

Großerueschkamp, F., Thieltges, A. K., Behrens, T., Brüning, T., Altmayer, M., & .... (2015). Marker-free automated histopathological annotation of lung tumour subtypes by FTIR imaging. *Analyst (London)*, *140*(7), 2114–2120. doi:10.1039/C4AN01978D PMID:25529256

Eddaoudi, F., Regragui, F., Mahmoudi, A., & Lamouri, N. (2011). Masses Detection Using SVM Classifier Based on Textures Analysis. *Applied Mathematical Sciences, 5*, 367–379.

Zhao, H., Li, G., Yu, C., & An, Z. (2016). The proceedings of brain metastases from lung cancer. *Open Life Sciences, 11*(1), 116–121. doi:10.1515/biol-2016-0016

Jasmine, J. S., Govardhan, A., & Baskaran, S. (2010). Classification of Microcalcification in Mammograms using NonsubsampledContourlet Transform and Neural Network. *European Journal of Scientific Research*, 531–539.

Klingemann, H. G. (2013). Cellular therapy of cancer with natural killer cells—Where do we stand? *Cytotherapy, 15*(10), 1185–1194. doi:10.1016/j.jcyt.2013.03.011 PMID:23768925

Aoyama, H., Tago, M., Kato, N., Toyoda, T., Kenjyo, M., Hirota, S., Shioura, H., Inomata, T., Kunieda, E., Hayakawa, K., Nakagawa, K., Kobashi, G., & Shirato, H. (2007). Neurocognitive function of patients with brain metastasis who received whole brain radiotherapy plus stereotactic radiosurgery or radiosurgery alone. *International Journal of Radiation Oncology, Biology, Physics, 68*(5), 1388–1395. doi:10.1016/j.ijrobp.2007.03.048 PMID:17674975

Beucher, S. S., & Lenteuejoul, C. (1979). Use of watersheds in contour detection. *Proceedings of the International Workshop on Image Processing: Real-Time Edge and Motion Detection/Estimation*, 1–12.

Davies, D. H., & Dance, D. R. (1990). Automatic computer detection of clustered calcifications in digital mammograms. *Physics in Medicine and Biology, 35*(8), 1111–1118. doi:10.1088/0031-9155/35/8/007 PMID:2217536

Yao, H., Shi, X., & Zhang, Y. (2014). The use of FTIR-ATR spectrometry for evaluation of surgical resection margin in colorectal cancer: A pilot study of 56 samples. *Journal of Spectroscopy, 2014*, 1–5. doi:10.1155/2014/213890

Bovis, K., & Singh, S. (2002). Classification of mammographic breast density using a combined classifier paradigm. *4th International Workshop on Digital Mammography*, 177–180.

Hands, J. R., Clemens, G., Stables, R., Ashton, K., Brodbelt, A., Davis, C., Dawson, T. P., Jenkinson, M. D., Lea, R. W., Walker, C., & Baker, M. J. (2016). Brain tumour differentiation: Rapid stratified serum diagnostics via attenuated total reflection Fourier-transform infrared spectroscopy. *Journal of Neuro-Oncology, 127*(3), 463–472. doi:10.100711060-016-2060-x PMID:26874961

Engh, J. A., Flickinger, J. C., Niranjan, A., Amin, D. V., Kondziolka, D. S., & Lunsford, L. D. (2007). Optimizing intracranial metastasis detection for stereotactic radiosurgery. *Stereotactic and Functional Neurosurgery, 85*(4), 162–168. doi:10.1159/000099075 PMID:17259753

Kestener, P. (2003). *Analysemultifractale 2D et 3D à l'aide de la transformation enondelettes: application enmammographie et en turbulence développée.* Université Bordeaux I, Ecoledoctorale de sciences physiques et de l'ingénieur, No d'ordre 2729.

Depciuch, J., Kaznowska, E., Koziorowska, A., & Cebulski, J. (2017). Verification of the effectiveness of the Fourier transform infrared spectroscopy computational model for colorectal cancer. *Journal of Pharmaceutical and Biomedical Analysis, 145*(1), 611–615. doi:10.1016/j.jpba.2017.07.026 PMID:28793272

Muhimmah, I., & Zwiggelaar, R. (2006). Mammographic Density Classification using Multiresolution Histogram Informatio. *Proceedings of the ITAB 2006*, 1-6.

Dong, K., Liu, L., Yu, Z., & Di Wu, Q. Z. (2019). Brain metastases from lung cancer with neuropsychiatric symptoms as the first symptoms. *Translational Lung Cancer Research, 8*(5), 682–691. doi:10.21037/tlcr.2019.10.02 PMID:31737504

Woods, K. S., & Bowyer, K. W. (1994). Computer detection of stellate lesions. *International Workshop on Digital Mammography*, 221–229.

Mandelblatt, J. S., Stout, N. K., Schechter, C. B., Broek, J. J. D., Miglioretti, D. L., Krapcho, M., Dietz, A. T., Munoz, D., Lee, S. J., Berry, D. A., Ravesteyn, N. T., Alagoz, O., Kerlikowske, K., Tosteson, A. N., Near, A. M., Hoeffken, A., Chang, Y., Heijnsdijk, E. A., Chisholm, G., ... Cronin, K. A. (2016). Collaborative modeling of the benefits and harms associated with different U.S. breast cancer screening strategies. *Annals of Internal Medicine*, 16(4), 164. doi:10.7326/M15-1536 PMID:26756606

Su, K. Y., & Lee, W. L. (2020). Fourier Transform Infrared Spectroscopy as a Cancer Screening and Diagnostic Tool: A Review and Prospects. *Cancers (Basel)*, 12(1), 115. doi:10.3390/cancers12010115 PMID:31906324

Bhowmik, A., Khan, R., & Ghosh, M. K. (2015). *Blood brain barrier: a challenge for effectual therapy of brain tumors.* BioMed.

Hamid, A., Tayeb, M. S., & Bawazir, A. A. (2001). Breast cancer in south-east Republic of Yemen. *Eastern Mediterranean Health Journal*, 7(06), 1012–1016. doi:10.26719/2001.7.6.1012 PMID:15332743

Oeffinger, K. C., Fontham, E. T. H., Etzioni, R., Herzig, A., Michaelson, J. S., Shih, Y.-C. T., Walter, L. C., Church, T. R., Flowers, C. R., LaMonte, S. J., Wolf, A. M. D., DeSantis, C., Lortet-Tieulent, J., Andrews, K., Manassaram-Baptiste, D., Saslow, D., Smith, R. A., Brawley, O. W., & Wender, R. (2015). Breast cancer screening for women at average risk: 2015 Guideline Update from the American Cancer Society. *Journal of the American Medical Association*, 314(15), 1599–1614. doi:10.1001/jama.2015.12783 PMID:26501536

Schouten, L. J., Rutten, J., Huveneers, H. A. M., & Twijnstra, A. (2002). Incidence of brain metastases in a cohort of patients with carcinoma of the breast, colon, kidney, and lung and melanoma. *Cancer*, 94(1), 2698–2705. doi:10.1002/cncr.10541 PMID:12173339

Monticciolo, D. L., Newell, M. S., Moy, L., Niell, B., Monsees, B., & Sickle, E. A. (2018). Breast cancer screening in women at higher-than-average risk: Recommendations from the ACR. *Journal of the American College of Radiology*, 15(3), 408–414. doi:10.1016/j.jacr.2017.11.034 PMID:29371086

Tahtamouni, L., Ahram, M., Koblinski, J., & Rolfo, C. (2019). Molecular regulation of cancer cell migration, invasion, and metastasis. *Analytical Cellular Pathology (Amsterdam)*, 2019, 1–2. doi:10.1155/2019/1356508 PMID:31218208

Kuhl, C. K., Schrading, S., Leutner, C. C., Morakkabati-Spitz, N., Wardelmann, E., Fimmers, R., Kuhn, W., & Schild, H. H. (2005). Mammography, breast ultrasound, and magnetic resonance imaging for surveillance of women at high familial risk for breast cancer. *Journal of Clinical Oncology*, 23(33), 8469–8476. doi:10.1200/JCO.2004.00.4960 PMID:16293877

Schad, L. R., Blüml, S., Hawighorst, H., Wenz, F., & Lorenz, W. J. (1994). Radiosurgical treatment planning of brain metastases based on a fast, three-dimensional MR imaging technique. *Magnetic Resonance Imaging*, 12(5), 811–819. doi:10.1016/0730-725X(94)92206-3 PMID:7934668

Campana, M., Rizzi, B., & Melani, C. (2008). A Framework for 4-D Biomedical Image Processing, Visualization and Analysis. GRAPP, 403-408.

Sung, J. S., Lee, C. H., Morris, E. A., Oeffinger, K. C., & Dershaw, D. D. (2011). Screening breast MRI imaging in women with a history of chest irradiation. *Radiology*, 259(1), 65–71. doi:10.1148/radiol.10100991 PMID:21325032

Leber, M. F., & Efferth, T. (2009). Molecular principles of cancer invasion and metastasis. *International Journal of Oncology*, 34(4), 881–895. PMID:19287945

Tieu, M. T., Cigsar, C., Ahmed, S., Ng, A., Diller, L., Millar, B. A., Crystal, P., & Hodgson, D. C. (2014). Crysta Pl, Hodgson DC. Breast cancer detection among young survivors of pediatric Hodgkin lymphoma with screening magnetic resonance imaging. *Cancer*, 120(16), 2507–2513. doi:10.1002/cncr.28747 PMID:24888639

Berg, W. A., Blume, J. D., & Cormack, J. B. (2008). Combined screening with ultrasound and mammography versus mammography alone in women at elevated risk of breast cancer. *Journal of the American Medical Association, 299*(18), 2151–2163. doi:10.1001/jama.299.18.2151 PMID:18477782

Niemiec, M., Głogowski, M., Tyc-Szczepaniak, D., Wierzchowski, M., & Kępka, L. (2011). Characteristics of long-term survivors of brain metastases from lung cancer. *Reports of Practical Oncology and Radiotherapy: Journal of Greatpoland Cancer Center in Poznan and Polish Society of Radiation Oncology, 16*(2), 49–53. doi:10.1016/j.rpor.2011.01.002 PMID:24376956

Brem, R. F., Tabar, L., & Duggy, S. W. (2015). Assessing improvement in detection of breast cancer with three-dimensional automated breast US in women with dense breast tissue: The SonoSight Study. *Radiology, 274*(3), 663–673. doi:10.1148/radiol.14132832 PMID:25329763

Brown, N. M. O., Pfau, S. J., & Gu, C. (2018). Bridging barriers: A comparative look at the blood–brain barrier across organisms. *Genes & Development, 32*(7-8), 466–478. doi:10.1101/gad.309823.117 PMID:29692355

Bergner, N., Romeike, B. F. M., Reichart, R., Kalff, R., Krafft, C., & Popp, J. (2013). Tumor margin identification and prediction of the primary tumor from brain metastases using FTIR imaging and support vector machines. *Analyst (London), 13*(14), 3983–3990. doi:10.1039/c3an00326d PMID:23563220

Ohuchi, N., Suzuki, A., Sobue, T., Kawai, M., Yamamoto, S., Zheng, Y.-F., Shiono, Y. N., Saito, H., Kuriyama, S., Tohno, E., Endo, T., Fukao, A., Tsuji, I., Yamaguchi, T., Ohashi, Y., Fukuda, M., & Ishida, T. (2016). Sensitivity and specificity of mammography and adjunctive ultrasonography to screen for breast cancer in the Japan Strategic Anti-Cancer Randomized Trial (JSTART): A randomized controlled trial. *Lancet, 387*(10016), 341–348. doi:10.1016/S0140-6736(15)00774-6 PMID:26547101

Anzalone, N., Essig, M., Lee, S. K., Dörfler, A., Ganslandt, O., Combs, S. E., & Picozzi, P. (2013). Optimizing contrast-enhanced magnetic resonance imaging characterization of brain metastases: Relevance to stereotactic radiosurgery. *Neurosurgery, 72*(5), 691–701. doi:10.1227/NEU.0b013e3182889ddf PMID:23381488

World Health Organization. (2006). Guidelines for the early detection and screening of breast cancer. *EMRO Technical Publications Series, 55*.

Lyon. (2002). IARC handbooks of cancer prevention. *International Agency for Research on Cancer, 7*, 9-12.

Taylor, O. G., Brzozowski, J. S., & Skelding, K. A. (2019). Glioblastoma multiforme: An overview of emerging therapeutic targets. *Frontiers in Oncology, 9*, 963. doi:10.3389/fonc.2019.00963 PMID:31616641

Bolourian, A., & Mojtahedi, Z. (2017). Possible damage to immune-privileged sites in natural killer cell therapy in cancer patients: Side effects of natural killer cell therapy. *Immunotherapy, 9*(3), 281–288. doi:10.2217/imt-2016-0137 PMID:28231718

Harirchi, I., Ebrahimi, M., Zamani, N., Jarvandi, S., & Montazeri, A. (2000). Breast cancer in Iran: A review of 903 case records. *Public Health. National Library of Medicine, 114*, 143–145. PMID:10800155

Baxter, N. (2001). Preventive health care. update: Should women be routinely taught breast self-examination to screen for breast cancer? *Canadian Medical Association Journal, 164*, 1837–1846. PMID:11450279

Martinive, P., & Houtte, P. V. (2018). The challenge of brain metastases from non-small cell lung cancer is not only an economical issue. *Annals of Palliative Medicine, 8*(2), 203–206. doi:10.21037/apm.2018.12.05 PMID:30691276

Lewis, P. D., Lewis, K. E., Ghosal, R., Bayliss, S., Lloyd, A. J., Wills, J., Godfrey, R., Kloer, P., & Mur, L. A. J. (2010). Evaluation of FTIR spectroscopy as a diagnostic tool for lung cancer using sputum. *BMC Cancer*, *10*(1), 640. doi:10.1186/1471-2407-10-640 PMID:21092279

Shitara, K., Özgüroğlu, M., Bang, Y. J., Bartolomeo, M. D., Mandalà, M., Ryu, M. H., Caglevic, C., Chung, H. C., Muro, K., Cutsem, E. V., Kobie, J., Cristescu, R., Garg, A. A., Lu, J., Shih, C. S., Adelberg, D., Cao, Z. A., & Fuchs, C. S. (2021). National breast screening programme: Organization and results. *Bulletin EpidemiologiqueHebdomadaire*, *32*(10), 39–40.

Barton, M., Harris, R., & Fletcher, S. W. (1999). Does this patient have breast cancer? The screening clinical breast examination: Should it be done? *Journal of the American Medical Association*, *282*(13), 1270–1280. doi:10.1001/jama.282.13.1270 PMID:10517431

Ostrom, Q. T., Cioffi, G., Gittleman, H., Patil, N., Waite, K., Kruchko, C., & Barnholtz-Sloan, J. S. (2019). Cbtrus statistical report: Primary brain and other central nervous system tumors diagnosed in the United States in 2012-2016. *Neuro-Oncology*, *21*(Supplement_5), 100. doi:10.1093/neuonc/noz150 PMID:31675094

Miller, T. T., Baines, C. J., & Wall, C. (2000). Canadian National Breast Screening Study-2: 13–year results of a randomized trial in women age 50–59 years. *Journal of the National Cancer Institute*, *92*(18), 1490–1499. doi:10.1093/jnci/92.18.1490 PMID:10995804

Saeed & Abdullah. (2021a). Performance analysis of machine learning algorithm for health care tools with High Dimension Segmentation. *Machine learning healthcare: Handling and managing data, 1*(1), 1-30.

Lyon. (2000). *International Agency for Research on Cancer.* Monographs on the evaluation of carcinogenic risks to humans, International Agency for Research on Cancer Press.

Saeed & Abdullah. (2021b). Comparison analysis of medical health care information of Graph Cutting using Multi Dimension Segmentation. *Machine learning healthcare: Handling and managing data, 1*(1), 1-23.

Zheng, Y., Keller, B. M., Ray, S., Wang, Y., Conant, E. F., Gee, J. C., & Kontos, D. (2015). Parenchymal texture analysis in digital mammography: A fully automated pipeline for breast cancer risk assessment. *Medical Physics*, *42*(7), 4149–4160. doi:10.1118/1.4921996 PMID:26133615

Li, H., Meng, X., Wang, T., Tang, Y., & Yin, Y. (2017). Breast masses in mammography classification with local contour features. *Biomedical Engineering Online*, *16*(1), 1–12. doi:10.118612938-017-0332-0 PMID:28410616

Cover, T., & Hart, P. (1967). Nearest neighbor pattern classification. IEEE Transactions on Information Theory, 1-12.

Saeed & Abdullah. (2021c). Statistical Analysis the Pre and Post-Surgery of health care sector using High Dimension Segmentation. *Machine learning healthcare: Handling and managing data, 1*(1), 1-25.

Kumar, S. M., & Balakrishnan, G. (2013). Classification of Microcalcification in Digital Mammogram using Stochastic Neighbor Embedding and KNN Classifier. International *Conference on Emerging Technology Trends on Advanced Engineering Research (ICETT'12)*, 1-9.

Saeed & Abdullah. (2021d). Combination of Brain Cancer with Hybrid K-NN Algorithm using statistical Analysis of Cerebrospinal Fluid (CSF) Surgery. *International Journal of Computer Science and Network Security, 21*(2), 120-130.

Harefa, J., Alexander, A., & Pratiwi, M. (2017). Comparison classifier: Support vector machine (SVM) and K-nearest neighbor (K-NN) in digital mammogram images. *Journal InformatikadanSistemInformasi*, *2*, 35–40.

Saeed & Afnizanfaizal. (2019). Implementation of Fourier transformation. *Indian Journal of Science & Technology, 12*(37), 1-16.

Barrow, A. D., & Colonna, M. (2017). Tailoring Natural Killer cell immunotherapy to the tumour microenvironment. Seminars in Immunology, 31, 30-36. doi:10.1016/j.smim.2017.09.001

Fattah, M. A., Zaki, A., Bassili, A., Shazly, M., & Tognoni, G. (2000). Breast self-examination practice and its impact on breast cancer diagnosis in Alexandria, Egypt. *Eastern Mediterranean Health Journal*, *6*(1), 34–40. doi:10.26719/2000.6.1.34 PMID:11370338

Jiang, W. G., Sanders, A. J., Katoh, M., Ungefroren, H., Gieseler, F., Prince, M., Thompson, S. K., Zollo, M., Spano, D., Dhawan, P., Sliva, D., Subbarayan, P. R., Sarkar, M., Honoki, K., Fujii, H., Georgakilas, A. G., Amedei, A., Niccolai, E., Amin, A., ... Santini, D. (2015). Tissue invasion and metastasis: Molecular, biological and clinical perspectives. *Seminars in Cancer Biology*, *35*, 244–275. doi:10.1016/j.semcancer.2015.03.008 PMID:25865774

Zhou, Y., Liu, C.-H., Pu, Y., Wu, B., Nguyen, T. A., Cheng, G., Zhou, L., Zhu, K., Chen, J., Li, Q., & Alfano, R. R. (2019). Combined spatial frequency spectroscopy analysis with visible resonance Raman for optical biopsy of human brain metastases of lung cancers. *Journal of Innovative Optical Health Sciences*, *12*(2), 1950010. doi:10.1142/S179354581950010X

Zhou, Y., Zhang, S., Wu, B., Yu, X., & Cheng, G. (2019). A portable visible resonance Raman analyzer with a handheld optical fiber probe for in vivo diagnosis of brain glioblastoma multiforme in an animal model. Proc. In Laser Science, 3-5. doi:10.1364/FIO.2019.JW3A.5

Zhou, Y., Zhang, S., Wu, B., Yu, X., & Cheng, G. (2020). Human glioma tumors detection by a portable visible resonance Raman analyzer with a hand-held optical fiber probe. *Biomedical Vibrational Spectroscopy, 11236*(1).

Ali, A., Goffin, J. R., Arnold, A., & Ellis, P. M. (2013). Survival of patients with non-small-cell lung cancer after a diagnosis of brain metastases. *Current Oncology (Toronto, Ont.)*, *20*(4), 300–306. doi:10.3747/co.20.1481 PMID:23904768

Dupont, W. D., & Page, D. L. (1985). Risk factors for breast cancer in women with proliferative disease. *The New England Journal of Medicine*, *312*(3), 146–151. doi:10.1056/NEJM198501173120303 PMID:3965932

Dohm, A., McTyre, E. R., Okoukoni, C., Henson, A., Cramer, C. K., LeCompte, M. C., Ruiz, J., Munley, M. T., Qasem, S., Lo, H.-W., Xing, F., Watabe, K., Laxton, A. W., Tatter, S. B., & Chan, M. D. (2018). Staged stereotactic radiosurgery for large brain metastases: Local control and clinical outcomes of a one-two punch technique. *Neurosurgery*, *83*(1), 114–121. doi:10.1093/neuros/nyx355 PMID:28973432

Key, T. J., Verkasalo, P. K., & Banks, E. (2001). Epidemiology of breast cancer. *The Lancet. Oncology*, *2*(3), 133–140. doi:10.1016/S1470-2045(00)00254-0 PMID:11902563

Salman, A., Sebbag, G., Argov, S., Mordechai, S., & Sahu, R. K. (2015). Early detection of colorectal cancer relapses by infrared spectroscopy in normal anastomosis tissue. *Journal of Biomedical Optics*, *20*(7), 75–107. doi:10.1117/1.JBO.20.7.075007 PMID:26178200

Stewart, B. W., & Wild, C. P. (2014). *World Cancer Report*. International Agency for Research on Cancer.

Siegel, R.L., Miller, K.D., & Jemal, A. (2017). Cancer Statistics. *A Cancer Journal for Clinicians*, *67*, 7-30.

Arvanitis, C. D., Ferraro, G. B., & Jain, R. K. (2020). The blood–brain barrier and blood–tumour barrier in brain tumours and metastases. *Nature Reviews. Cancer*, *20*(12), 26–41. doi:10.103841568-019-0205-x PMID:31601988

DeSantis, C.E., Fedewa, S.A., Sauer, A.G., Kramer, J.L., Smith, R.A., & Jemal, A. (2016). Breast cancer statistics, 2015: Convergence of incidence rates between black and white women. *A Cancer Journal for Clinicians*, *66*, 31-42.

Abbott, N. J., Pizzo, M. E., Preston, J. E., Janigro, D., & Thorne, R. G. (2018). The role of brain barriers in fluid movement in the CNS: Is there a 'glymphatic' system? *Acta Neuropathologica*, *135*(3), 387–407. doi:10.100700401-018-1812-4 PMID:29428972

Acharya, U. R., Vinitha Sree, S., Swapna, G., Martis, R. J., & Suri, J. S. (2013). Automated EEG analysis of epilepsy: A review. *Knowledge-Based Systems*, *45*, 147–165. doi:10.1016/j.knosys.2013.02.014

Adeli, H., Ghosh-Dastidar, S., & Dadmehr, N. (2007). A wavelet-chaos methodology for analysis of EEGs and EEG subbands to detect seizure and epilepsy. *IEEE Transactions on Biomedical Engineering*, *54*(2), 205–211. doi:10.1109/TBME.2006.886855 PMID:17278577

Adidja, M., & Robleh, H. A. (2020). Automated Blood Vessels Segmentation Method for Retinal Fundus Image Based on Mathematical Morphology Operations and Kirsch's Template. *International Journal of Computer Science and Network*, *9*(3), 114–122.

Agarwal, G., Gaur, L., & Bist, A. S. (2021). COVID-19 Real Time Impact Analysis India vs USA. In Futuristic Trends in Network and Communication Technologies. Springer. doi:10.1007/978-981-16-1480-4_29

Ahmed, M. M., & Mohamad, D. B. (2008). Segmentation of brain MR images for tumor extraction by combining kmeans clustering and perona-malik anisotropic diffusion model. *International Journal of Image Processing*, *2*(1), 27–34.

AlAfandy, K. A., Omara, H., Lazaar, M., & Al Achhab, M. (2020a). Investment of Classic Deep CNNs and SVM for Classifying Remote Sensing Images. *Advances in Science, Technology and Engineering Systems Journal*, *5*(5), 652-659. doi:10.25046/aj050580

AlAfandy, K. A., Omara, H., Lazaar, M., & Al Achhab, M. (2020b). Using Classic Networks for Classifying Remote Sensing Images: Comparative Study. *Advances in Science, Technology and Engineering Systems Journal*, *5*(5), 770-780. doi:10.25046/aj050594

AlAfandy, K. A., Omara, H., Lazaar, M., & Al Achhab, M. (Eds.). (2019). Artificial Neural Networks Optimization and Convolution Neural Networks to Classifying Images in Remote Sensing: A Review. *Proceeding of The 4th International Conference on Big Data and Internet of Things (BDIoT'19)*. 10.1145/3372938.3372945

Al-Amri, S. S., & Kalyankar, N. V. (2010). *Image segmentation by using threshold techniques.* arXiv preprint arXiv:1005.4020.

Andrzejak, R. G., Lehnertz, K., Rieke, C., Mormann, F., David, P., & Elger, C. E. (2001). Indications of nonlinear deterministic and finite dimensional structures in time series of brain electrical activity: Dependence on recording region and brain state. *Physical Review E: Statistical, Nonlinear, and Soft Matter Physics*, *64*(6), 061907. doi:10.1103/PhysRevE.64.061907 PMID:11736210

Angulakshmi, M., & Lakshmi Priya, G. G. (2017). Automated brain tumour segmentation techniques—A review. *International Journal of Imaging Systems and Technology*, *27*(1), 66–77. doi:10.1002/ima.22211

Asselborn, T., Chapatte, M., & Dillenbourg, P. (2020). Extending the Spectrum of Dysgraphia: A Data Driven Strategy to Estimate Handwriting Quality. *Scientific Reports*, *10*(1), 3140. Advance online publication. doi:10.103841598-020-60011-8 PMID:32081940

Avishka, I., Kumarawadu, K., Kudagama, A., Weerathunga, M., & Thelijjagoda, S. (2018). Mobile App to Support People with Dyslexia and Dysgraphia. *2018 IEEE International Conference on Information and Automation for Sustainability (ICIAfS)*. 10.1109/ICIAFS.2018.8913335

Banerjee, S., & Mitra, S. (2020). Novel volumetric sub-region segmentation in brain tumors. *Frontiers in Computational Neuroscience*, *14*, 3. doi:10.3389/fncom.2020.00003 PMID:32038216

Bauer, S., Wiest, R., Nolte, L. P., & Reyes, M. (2013). A survey of MRI-based medical image analysis for brain tumor studies. *Physics in Medicine and Biology*, *58*(13), R97–R129. doi:10.1088/0031-9155/58/13/R97 PMID:23743802

Baxter, D. M., & Warrington, E. K. (1994). Measuring Dysgraphia: A Graded-Difficulty Spelling Test. *Behavioural Neurology*, *7*(3–4), 107–116. doi:10.1155/1994/659593 PMID:24487323

Beevi, S. Z., Sathik, M. M., & Senthamaraikannan, K. (2010). *A robust fuzzy clustering technique with spatial neighborhood information for effective medical image segmentation.* arXiv preprint arXiv:1004.1679.

Bengio, Y., Goodfellow, I., & Courville, A. (2017). *Deep Learning.* MIT Press.

Berent, J., & Dragotti, P. L. (2007, September). Unsupervised Extraction of Coherent Regions for Image Based Rendering, In BMVC (pp. 1-10). doi:10.5244/C.21.28

Beretta, L., & Santaniello, A. (2016). Nearest neighbor imputation algorithms: A critical evaluation. *BMC Medical Informatics and Decision Making*, *16*(3), 197–208. doi:10.118612911-016-0318-z PMID:27454392

Bhide, A. S., Patil, P., & Dhande, S. (2012). Brain Segmentation using Fuzzy C means clustering to detect tumour Region. *International Journal of Advanced Research in Computer Science and Electronics Engineering*, *1*(2), 85–90.

Bishop, T. E., & Favaro, P. (2011). The light field camera: Extended depth of field, aliasing, and superresolution. *IEEE Transactions on Pattern Analysis and Machine Intelligence*, *34*(5), 972–986. doi:10.1109/TPAMI.2011.168 PMID:21844629

Blanchet, L., Krooshof, P. W. T., Postma, G. J., Idema, A. J., Goraj, B., Heerschap, A., & Buydens, L. M. C. (2011). Discrimination between metastasis and glioblastoma multiforme based on morphometric analysis of MR images. *AJNR. American Journal of Neuroradiology*, *32*(1), 67–73. doi:10.3174/ajnr.A2269 PMID:21051512

Blumenfeld, H. (2010). *Neuroanatomy through clinical cases.* Sinauer Associates.

Bohlen, M., Busch, C. J., Sehner, S., Forterre, F., Bier, J., Berliner, C., Bußmann, L., & Münscher, A. (2019). Tumor volume as a predictive parameter in the sequential therapy (induction chemotherapy) of head and neck squamous cell carcinomas. *European Archives of Oto-Rhino-Laryngology*, *276*(4), 1183–1189. doi:10.100700405-019-05323-w PMID:30725209

Bottou, L. (Ed.). (1991). Stochastic Gradient Learning in Neural Networks. In *Proceedings of the Neuro-Nîmes* (pp. 12-23). Academic Press.

Boykov, Y. Y., & Jolly, M. P. (2001, July). Interactive graph cuts for optimal boundary & region segmentation of objects in ND images. *Proceedings eighth IEEE international conference on computer vision. ICCV 2001*, 105-112. 10.1109/ICCV.2001.937505

Boykov, Y., & Kolmogorov, V. (2004). An experimental comparison of min-cut/max-flow algorithms for energy minimization in vision. *IEEE Transactions on Pattern Analysis and Machine Intelligence*, *26*(9), 1124–1137. doi:10.1109/TPAMI.2004.60 PMID:15742889

Boykov, Y., Veksler, O., & Zabih, R. (2001). Fast approximate energy minimization via graph cuts. *IEEE Transactions on Pattern Analysis and Machine Intelligence*, *23*(11), 1222–1239. doi:10.1109/34.969114

Boyle, J. R., & Joyce, R. L. (2019). Using Smartpens to Support Note-Taking Skills of Students with Learning Disabilities. *Intervention in School and Clinic*, *55*(2), 86–93. doi:10.1177/1053451219837642

Brinker, T., Stopa, E., Morrison, J., & Klinge, P. (2014). A new look at cerebrospinal fluid circulation. *Fluids and Barriers of the CNS*, *11*(1), 1–16. doi:10.1186/2045-8118-11-10 PMID:24817998

Bzdok, D., Krzywinski, M., & Altman, N. (2018). Machine learning: Supervised methods. *Nature Methods*, *15*(1), 5–6. doi:10.1038/nmeth.4551 PMID:30100821

Calabrese, C., Poppleton, H., Kocak, M., Hogg, T. L., Fuller, C., Hamner, B., Oh, E. Y., Gaber, M. W., Finklestein, D., Allen, M., Frank, A., Bayazitov, I. T., Zakharenko, S. S., Gajjar, A., Davidoff, A., & Gilbertson, R. J. (2007). A perivascular niche for brain tumor stem cells. *Cancer Cell, 11*(1), 69–82. doi:10.1016/j.ccr.2006.11.020 PMID:17222791

Cameron, Zimmet, Dunstan, Dalton, Shaw, Welborn, Owen, Salmon, & Jolly. (2003). *Overweight and obesity in Australia: the 1999–2000 Australian Diabetes, Obesity and Lifestyle Study (AusDiab)*. doi:10.5694/j.1326-5377.2003.tb05283.x

Centres for disease Control and Prevention. (2021). Sudden Unexpected Death in Epilepsy (SUDEP). *Epilepsy Features.* https://www.cdc.gov/epilepsy/communications/SUDEP

Cerri, S., Hoopes, A., Greve, D. N., Mühlau, M., & Van Leemput, K. (2020). A longitudinal method for simultaneous whole-brain and lesion segmentation in multiple sclerosis. In *Machine Learning in Clinical Neuroimaging and Radiogenomics in Neuro-oncology* (pp. 119–128). Springer. doi:10.1007/978-3-030-66843-3_12

Ceylan, M., & Yasar, H. (2016). A novel approach for automatic blood vessel extraction in retinal images: Complex ripplet-I transform and complex valued artificial neural network. *Turkish Journal of Electrical Engineering and Computer Sciences, 2016*(24), 3212–3227.

Chakraborty, T., Jha, D. K., Chowdhury, A. S., & Jiang, X. (2015). A Self-Adaptive matched filter for retinal blood vessel detection. *Machine Vision and Applications, 2015*(26), 55–68.

Chang, M. M., Sezan, M. I., Tekalp, A. M., & Berg, M. J. (1996). Bayesian segmentation of multislice brain magnetic resonance imaging using three-dimensional Gibbsian priors. *Optical Engineering (Redondo Beach, Calif.), 35*(11), 3206–3221. doi:10.1117/1.601059

Chatfield, C., & Xing, H. (2019). *The analysis of time series: an introduction with R.* Chapman and Hall/CRC. doi:10.1201/9781351259446

Chaturvedi, D. K., & Arya, M. (2013b). Correlation between Human Performance and Consciousness. *IEEE-International Conference on Human Computer Interaction.*

Chaturvedi, D. K., & Arya, M. (2013a). A Study of Correlation between Consciousness Level and Performance of Worker, *Industrial. Engineering Journal (New York), 6*(8), 40–43.

Chaturvedi, D. K., & Satsangi, R. (2013). The Correlation between Student Performance and Consciousness Level. *International Conference on Advanced Computing and Communication Technologies (ICACCT™-2013)*, 200-203.

Chen, D., Cohen, L. D., & Mirebeau, J. M. (2014). *Vessel Exraction using anisotropic minimal paths and path score.* https://projet.liris.cnrs.fr/imagine/pub/proceedings/ICIP-2014/Papers/1569899543.pdf

Cheng, L., De, J., Zhang, X., Lin, F., & Li, H. (2014). *Tracing Retinal blood vessels by Matrix-Forest theorem of Directed Graphs.* Doi:10.1007/978-3-319-10404-1_78

Choi, E., Schuetz, A., Stewart, W. F., & Sun, J. (2016). Using recurrent neural network models for early detection of heart failure onset. *Journal of the American Medical Informatics Association: JAMIA, 24*(2), 361–370. doi:10.1093/jamia/ocw112 PMID:27521897

Christ, M. J., & Parvathi, R. M. S. (2012). Segmentation of medical image using K-means clustering and marker controlled watershed algorithm. *European Journal of Scientific Research, 71*(2), 190–194.

Clarke, L. P., Velthuizen, R. P., Clark, M., Gaviria, J., Hall, L., Goldgof, D., Murtagh, R., Phuphanich, S., & Brem, S. (1998). MRI measurement of brain tumor response: Comparison of visual metric and automatic segmentation. *Magnetic Resonance Imaging, 16*(3), 271–279. doi:10.1016/S0730-725X(97)00302-0 PMID:9621968

Crouch, A. L., & Jakubecy, J. J. (2007). Dysgraphia: How It Affects A Student's Performance and What Can Be Done About It. *Teaching Exceptional Children-Plus, 3.*

Cura, A., Kucuk, H., Ergen, E., & Oksuzoglu, I. B. (2020). Driver profiling using long short term memory (LSTM) and convolutional neural network (CNN) methods. In *Preceding of the IEEE Transactions on Intelligent Transportation Systems (Early Access)* (pp. 1–11). IEEE. doi:10.1109/TITS.2020.2995722

Dai, P., Luo, H., Sheng, H., Zhao, Y., Li, L., & Wu, J. (2015). A New Approach to Segment Both Main and Peripheral Retinal Vessels Based on Gray Voting and Gaussian Mixture Model. *PLoS ONE, 10*(6). doi:10.1371/journal.pone.0127748

Dankovičová, Z., & Uchnár, M.Dankovičová. (2019). Extraction of parameters from dysgraphic handwriting for CDSS systems. *Acta Electrotechnica et Informatica, 19*(1), 48–54. doi:10.15546/aeei-2019-0007

Das, D., Nayak, M., & Pani, S. K. (2019). Missing Value Imputation-. *RE:view.*

Dash, J., Parida, P., & Bhoi, N. (2020). Retinal Blood Vessel Extraction from Fundus Images using Enhancement Filtering and Clustering. *ELCVIA. Electronic Letters on Computer Vision and Image Analysis, 19*(1), 38–52.

Das, S., & Majumder, S. (2021). A Review on Pattern Recognition based Retinal blood vessels extraction technique to detect Diabetic Retinopathy (DR). *2nd International Conference on Data Science and Applications (ICDSA 2021).*

Densely Connected Convolutional Networks. (2017). In G. Huang, Z. Liu, L. V. D. Maaten, & K. Q. Weinberger (Eds.), Proceeding of the 2017 IEEE Conference on Computer Vision and Pattern Recognition (CVPR 2017) (pp. 2261–2269). IEEE. https://doi.org/10.1109/CVPR.2017.243.

Dialameh, M., Hamzeh, A., & Rahmani, H. (2020). *DL-Reg: A Deep Learning Regularization Technique using Linear Regression.* https://arxiv.org/abs/2011.00368

Diaz, P., Rodriguez, A., Cuevas, E., Valdivia, A., Chavolla, E., Pérez-Cisneros, M., & Zaldívar, D. (2019). A hybrid method for blood vessel segmentation in images. *Biocybernetics and Biomedical Engineering, 39*(1-2). doi:10.1016/j.bbe.2019.06.009

Dong, L., Ogunbona, P., Li, W., Yu, G., Fan, L., & Zheng, G. (2006, August). A fast algorithm for color image segmentation. *First International Conference on Innovative Computing, Information and Control-Volume I (ICICIC'06)*, 685-688. 10.1109/ICICIC.2006.192

Dubey, S. R., Chakraborty, S., Roy, S. K., Mukherjee, S., Singh, S. K., & Chaudhuri, B. B. (2019). diffGrad: An Optimization Method for Convolutional Neural Networks. *IEEE Transactions on Neural Networks and Learning Systems, 31*(11), 4500–4511. https://doi.org/10.1109/TNNLS.2019.2955777

X. Du, Y. Cai, S. Wang, & L. Zhang (Eds.). (2016). Overview of Deep Learning. In *Proceeding of the 31st Youth Academic Annual Conference of Chinese Association of Automation (YAC)*. IEEE. 10.1109/YAC.2016.7804882

Ediger, M. (2002). Assessing handwriting achievement. *Reading Improvement, 39*, 103–110.

Ellis, K. R. (2016). *Students with disabilities' perceptions of assistive technology, the livescribe smartpen, audio recording, and note-taking service accommodations* (M.A. thesis). California State University, Sacramento, CA, United States. Retrieved from https://scholarworks.calstate.edu/concern/theses/th83kz62t

Fang, Z., Tian, R., Jia, Y. T., Xu, T. T., & Liu, Y. (2017). Treatment of cerebrospinal fluid leak after spine surgery. *Chinese Journal of Traumatology, 20*(2), 81–83. doi:10.1016/j.cjtee.2016.12.002 PMID:28336418

Feature Selection, L1 Vs. L2 Regularization, and Rotational Invariance. (2004). In A. Ng (Ed.), Proceedings of the 21st International Conference on Machine Learning (ICML '04) (pp. 78–85). ACM. https://doi.org/10.1145/1015330.1015435.

Gad, A. F. (2018). *Practical Computer Vision Applications Using Deep Learning with CNNs*. Apress. doi:10.1007/978-1-4842-4167-7

Galanopoulou, A. S., Buckmaster, P. S., Staley, K. J., Moshé, S. L., Perucca, E., Engel, J. Jr, Löscher, W., Noebels, J. L., Pitkänen, A., Stables, J., White, H. S., O'Brien, T. J., & Simonato for the American Epilepsy, M. (2012). Simonato for the American epilepsy, identification of new epilepsy treatments: Issues in preclinical methodology. *Epilepsia*, *53*(3), 571–582. doi:10.1111/j.1528-1167.2011.03391.x PMID:22292566

Gao, J., Chen, G., & Lin, W. (2020). *An Effective Retinal Blood Vessel Segmentation by Using Automatic Random Walks Based on Centerline Extraction*. Hindawi BioMed Research International.

Gaur, L., Singh, G., & Agarwal, V. (2021). Leveraging Artificial Intelligence Tools to Combat the COVID-19 Crisis. In *Futuristic Trends in Network and Communication Technologies*. Springer. doi:10.1007/978-981-16-1480-4_28

Gaur, L., Bhatia, U., & Jhanjhi, N. Z. (2021). Medical image-based detection of COVID-19 using Deep Convolution Neural Networks. *Multimedia Systems*. Advance online publication. doi:10.100700530-021-00794-6 PMID:33935377

Gaur, L., Solanki, A., Wamba, S. F., & Jhanjhi, N. Z. (2021). *Advanced AI Techniques and Applications in Bioinformatics*. CRC Press. doi:10.1201/9781003126164

Gharaibeh, N., Al-Hazaimeh, O. M., Al-Naami, B., & Nahar, K. M. O. (2018). An effective image processing method for detection of diabetic retinopathy diseases from retinal fundus images. *International Journal of Signal and Imaging Systems Engineering*, *11*(4), 206–216.

Gortler, S. J., Grzeszczuk, R., Szeliski, R., & Cohen, M. F. (1996, August). The lumigraph. *Proceedings of the 23rd annual conference on Computer graphics and interactive techniques*, 43-54.

Greig, D. M., Porteous, B. T., & Seheult, A. H. (1989). Exact maximum a posteriori estimation for binary images. *Journal of the Royal Statistical Society. Series B. Methodological*, *51*(2), 271–279. doi:10.1111/j.2517-6161.1989.tb01764.x

Gunavathi, C., & Premalatha, K. (2014). A Comparative Analysis of Swarm Intelligence Techniques for Feature Selection in Cancer Classification. *TheScientificWorldJournal*, *14*, 12. doi:10.1155/2014/693831 PMID:25157377

Guo, G., Wang, H., Bell, D., Bi, Y., & Greer, K. (2003, November). KNN model-based approach in classification. *OTM Confederated International Conferences On the Move to Meaningful Internet Systems*, 986-996. 10.1007/978-3-540-39964-3_62

Hamstra-Bletz, L., & Blöte, A. W. (1993). A Longitudinal Study on Dysgraphic Handwriting in Primary School. *Journal of Learning Disabilities*, *26*(10), 689–699. doi:10.1177/002221949302601007 PMID:8151209

Haney, S. M., Thompson, P. M., Cloughesy, T. F., Alger, J. R., & Toga, A. W. (2001). Tracking tumor growth rates in patients with malignant gliomas: A test of two algorithms. *AJNR. American Journal of Neuroradiology*, *22*(1), 73–82. PMID:11158891

Hanson, J., Yang, Y., Paliwal, K., & Zhou, Y. (2016). Improving protein disorder prediction by deep bidirectional long short-term memory recurrent neural networks. *Bioinformatics (Oxford, England)*, *33*, 685–692. doi:10.1093/bioinformatics/btw678 PMID:28011771

Hansson Mild, K., Lundström, R., & Wilén, J. (2019). Non-Ionizing radiation in Swedish health care—Exposure and safety aspects. *International Journal of Environmental Research and Public Health*, *16*(7), 1186. doi:10.3390/ijerph16071186 PMID:30987016

Hassan, G., Bendary, N. E., Hassanien, A. E., Fahmy, A., Shoeb, A. M., & Snasel, V. (2015). Retinal blood vessel segmentation approach based on mathematical morphology. *Procedia Computer Science*, *65*, 612–622.

Hawkins, D. M. (2004). The Problem of Overfitting. *Journal of Chemical Information and Computer Sciences, ACM, 44*(1), 1–12. https://doi.org/10.1021/ci0342472

Holmes, M. D. (2008). Dense array EEG: Methodology and new hypothesis on epilepsy syndromes. *Epilepsia, 49*(s3), 3–14. doi:10.1111/j.1528-1167.2008.01505.x PMID:18304251

Horn, D. R., & Chen, B. (2007, April). Lightshop: interactive light field manipulation and rendering. *Proceedings of the 2007 symposium on Interactive 3D graphics and games*, 121-128. 10.1145/1230100.1230121

Hrydziuszko, O., & Viant, M. R. (2012). Missing values in mass spectrometry based metabolomics: An undervalued step in the data processing pipeline. *Metabolomics, 8*(1), 161–174. doi:10.100711306-011-0366-4

Htun, S. N. N., Zin, T. T., & Tin, P. (2020). Image Processing Technique and Hidden Markov Model for an Elderly Care Monitoring System. *Journal of Imaging, 6*(6), 49. doi:10.3390/jimaging6060049 PMID:34460595

Hu, C., Song, L., Liu, M., Wang, J., & Zhang, L. (2018, October). A Novel Multi-Atlas and Multi-Channel (MAMC) Approach for Multiple Sclerosis Lesion Segmentation in Brain MRI. *Proceedings of the 2nd International Symposium on Image Computing and Digital Medicine*, 106-112. 10.1145/3285996.3286019

Ibrahim, W. A., & Morcos, M. M. (2002). Artificial intelligence and advanced mathematical tools for power quality applications: A survey. *IEEE Transactions on Power Delivery, 17*(2), 668–673. doi:10.1109/61.997958

Imani, E., Javidi, M., & Pourreza, H. R. (2015). Improvement of retinal blood vessel detection using morphological component analysis. *Computer Methods and Programs in Biomedicine, 118*(3), 263–279. PMID:25697986

Impedovo, D., & Pirlo, G. (2019). Dynamic Handwriting Analysis for the Assessment of Neurodegenerative Diseases: A Pattern Recognition Perspective. *IEEE Reviews in Biomedical Engineering, 12*, 209–220. doi:10.1109/RBME.2018.2840679 PMID:29993722

Jabbar, H. K., & Khan, R. Z. (2015). Methods to Avoid Over-fitting and Under-fitting in Supervised Machine Learning (Comparative Study). *Computer Science, Communication and Instrumentation Devices*, 163-172. doi:10.3850/978-981-09-5247-1_017

Jafri, M. Z. M., Abdulbaqi, H. S., Mutter, K. N., Mustapha, I. S., & Omar, A. F. (2017, June). Measuring the volume of brain tumour and determining its location in T2-weighted MRI images using hidden Markov random field: expectation maximization algorithm. In Digital Optical Technologies. International Society for Optics and Photonics.

Jain, G. (2017). *Hawan for Cleansing the Environment*. medium.com/@giftofforest192/hawan-for-cleansing-the-environment-a9e1746e38e0

Jain, R. (2019). Yoga & Epilepsy – What a Yoga Teacher Should Know. *Yoga and physical / mental health*. https://www.arhantayoga.org/blog/yoga-poses-epilepsy/

Jainish, G. R., Jiji, G. W., & Infant, P. A. (2020). A novel automatic retinal vessel extraction using maximum entropy based EM algorithm. Multimedia Tools and Applications, 79, 22337–22353. doi:10.100711042-020-08958-8

Jarabo, A., Masia, B., Bousseau, A., Pellacini, F., & Gutierrez, D. (2014). How do people edit light fields? *ACM Transactions on Graphics, 33*(4), 4. doi:10.1145/2601097.2601125

Jiang, K., Zhou, Z., Geng, X., Tang, L., Wu, H., & Dong, J. (2015). Isotropic Undecimated Wavelet Transform Fuzzy Algorithm for Retinal Blood Vessel Segmentation. *Journal of Medical Imaging and Health Informatics, 5*(7), 1524–1527. doi:10.1166/jmihi.2015.1561

Jiang, Y., Chung, F.-L., Wang, S., Deng, Z., Wang, J., & Qian, P. (2015). Collaborative fuzzy clustering from multiple weighted views. *IEEE Transactions on Cybernetics*, *45*(4), 688–701. doi:10.1109/TCYB.2014.2334595 PMID:25069132

Jiang, Y., Deng, Z., Chung, F.-L., Wang, G., Qian, P., Choi, K.-S., & Wang, S. (2017a). Recognition of Epileptic EEG signals using a novel multi-view TSK fuzzy system. *IEEE Transactions on Fuzzy Systems*, *25*(1), 3–20. doi:10.1109/TFUZZ.2016.2637405

Jiang, Y., Gu, X., Wu, D., Hang, W., Xue, J., & Qiu, S. (2020a). Novel negative-transfer-resistant fuzzy clustering model with a shared cross-domain transfer latent space and its application to brain CT image segmentation. In *Preceding of the IEEE/ACM Transactions on Computational Biology and Bioinformatics*. IEEE. doi:10.1109/TCBB.2019.2963873

Jiang, Y., Wu, D., Deng, Z., Qian, P., Wang, J., Wang, G., Chung, F.-L., Choi, K.-S., & Wang, S. (2017b). Seizure classification from EEG signals using transfer learning, semi-supervised learning and TSK fuzzy system. *IEEE Transactions on Neural Systems and Rehabilitation Engineering*, *25*(12), 2270–2284. doi:10.1109/TNSRE.2017.2748388 PMID:28880184

Kanai, S., Fujiwara, Y., Yamanaka, Y., & Adachi, S. (2018). *Sigsoftmax: Reanalysis of the softmax bottleneck.* arXiv preprint arXiv:1805.10829.

Kanungo, T., Mount, D. M., Netanyahu, N. S., Piatko, C. D., Silverman, R., & Wu, A. Y. (2002). An efficient k-means clustering algorithm: Analysis and implementation. *IEEE Transactions on Pattern Analysis and Machine Intelligence*, *24*(7), 881–892. doi:10.1109/TPAMI.2002.1017616

Kar, S. S., & Maity, S. P. (2016). Blood vessel extraction and optic disc removal using Curvelet Transform and Kernel Fuzzy C-means. Computers in Biology and Medicine, 1-16. doi:10.1016/j.compbiomed.2015.12.018

Karimi, M., Veni, G., & Yu, Y. Y. (2020). Illegible Text to Readable Text: An Image-to-Image Transformation using Conditional Sliced Wasserstein Adversarial Networks. *2020 IEEE/CVF Conference on Computer Vision and Pattern Recognition Workshops (CVPRW).* 10.1109/CVPRW50498.2020.00284

Karn, P. K., Biswal, B., & Samantaray, S. R. (2018). Robust retinal blood vessel segmentation using hybrid active contour model. *IET Image Processing*, 1–12. doi:10.1049/iet-ipr.2018.5413

Kaur, A., Kaur, L., & Singh, A. (2021). State-of-the-art segmentation techniques and future directions for multiple sclerosis brain lesions. *Archives of Computational Methods in Engineering*, *28*(3), 951–977. doi:10.100711831-020-09403-7

Ketkar, N. (2017). Introduction to Keras. In *Deep Learning with Python* (pp. 97-111). Apress. doi:10.1007/978-1-4842-2766-4_7

Khairandish, M. O., Sharma, M., Jain, V., Chatterjee, J. M., & Jhanjhi, N. Z. (2021). A Hybrid CNN-SVM Threshold Segmentation Approach for Tumor Detection and Classification of MRI Brain Images. *IRBM*. Advance online publication. doi:10.1016/j.irbm.2021.06.003

Khalil, H. A., Darwish, S., Ibrahim, Y. M., & Hassan, O. F. (2020). 3D-MRI brain tumor detection model using modified version of level set segmentation based on dragonfly algorithm. *Symmetry*, *12*(8), 1256. doi:10.3390ym12081256

Khan, B.K., Khaliq, A.A., & Shahid, M. (2016). A Morphological Hessian Based Approach for Retinal Blood Vessels Segmentation and Denoising Using Region Based Otsu Thresholding. *PLOS ONE, 11*(7), 1-19.

Khan, M. A., Lali, I. U., Rehman, A., Ishaq, M., Sharif, M., Saba, T., Zahoor, S., & Akram, T. (2019). Brain tumor detection and classification: A framework of marker-based watershed algorithm and multilevel priority features selection. *Microscopy Research and Technique*, *82*(6), 909–922. doi:10.1002/jemt.23238 PMID:30801840

Khan, M., Hussain, M., Ahsan, K., Saeed, M., Nadeem, A., Ali, S., Mahmood, N., & Rizwan, K. (2017). Augmented Reality Based Spelling Assistance to Dysgraphia Students. *Journal of Basic and Applied Sciences*, *13*, 500–507. doi:10.6000/1927-5129.2017.13.82

Kharrat, A., Benamrane, N., Messaoud, M. B., & Abid, M. (2009, November). Detection of brain tumor in medical images. In *2009 3rd International conference on signals, circuits and systems (SCS)*. IEEE. 10.1109/ICSCS.2009.5412577

Khojasteh, P., Aliahmad, B., & Kumar, D. K. (2018). Fundus images analysis using deep features for detection of exudates, hemorrhages and microaneurysms. *BMC Ophthalmology*, *18*, 288. doi:10.1186/s12886-018-0954-4

Kim, K.J., &Tagkopoulos, L. (2019). Application of Machine Learning Rheumatic Disease Research. *Korean J. Intern Med.*,*34*, 2.

Kingma, D. P., & Ba, J. L. (Eds.). (2015). Adam: A Method for Stochastic Optimization. *Proceeding of the 3rd International Conference on Learning Representations (ICLR 2015)*. https://arxiv.org/abs/1406.3269

Kolmogorov, V., & Zabih, R. (2002, May). Multi-camera scene reconstruction via graph cuts. In *European conference on computer vision*. Springer.

Kong, W., Dong, Z. Y., Jia, Y., Hill, D. J., Xu, Y., & Zhang, Y. (2019). Short-term residential load forecasting based on LSTM recurrent neural network. *IEEE Transactions on Smart Grid*, *10*(1), 841–851. doi:10.1109/TSG.2017.2753802

Kowdle, A., Sinha, S. N., & Szeliski, R. (2012, October). Multiple view object cosegmentation using appearance and stereo cues. In *European Conference on Computer Vision*. Springer. 10.1007/978-3-642-33715-4_57

KS, S. R., & Murugan, S. (2017). Memory based hybrid dragonfly algorithm for numerical optimization problems. *Expert Systems with Applications*, *83*, 63–78. doi:10.1016/j.eswa.2017.04.033

Kumar, S., Adarsh, A., Kumar, B., & Singh, A. K. (2020). An automated early diabetic retinopathy detection through improved blood vessel and optic disc segmentation. *Journal of Optics and Laser Technology*, *121*, 1-11.

Kumar, K., & Samal, D. (2019). Automated retinal vessel segmentation based on morphological preprocessing and 2D-Gabor wavelets. *Proceedings of ICACIE 2018*, 1. arXiv:1908.04123v1[eess.IV]

Kushol, R., Kabir, M. H., Abdullah-Al-Wadud, M., & Islam, M. S. (2020). Retinal blood vessel segmentation from fundus image using an efficient multiscale directional representation technique Bendlets. *Mathematical Biosciences and Engineering*, *17*(6), 7751–7771. PMID:33378918

Lahoty, P., & Rana, M. (2013). Agnihotra organic farming. *Popular Kheti*, *1*(4), 49-54.

Lavanyadevi, R., Machakowsalya, M., Nivethitha, J., & Kumar, A. N. (2017, April). Brain tumor classification and segmentation in MRI images using PNN. *2017 IEEE International Conference on Electrical, Instrumentation and Communication Engineering (ICEICE)*, 1-6. 10.1109/ICEICE.2017.8191888

LeCun, Y., Bengio, Y., & Hinton, G. (2015). Deep learning. *Nature*, *521*(7553), 436–444. doi:10.1038/nature14539 PMID:26017442

Lecun, Y., Bottou, L., Bengio, Y., & Haffner, P. (1998). Gradient-based Learning Applied to Document Recognition. *Proceedings of the IEEE*, *86*(11), 2278–2324. https://doi.org/10.1109/5.726791

Lee, C. H., Schmidt, M., Murtha, A., Bistritz, A., Sander, J., & Greiner, R. (2005, October). Segmenting brain tumors with conditional random fields and support vector machines. In *International Workshop on Computer Vision for Biomedical Image Applications*. Springer. 10.1007/11569541_47

Levoy, M., & Hanrahan, P. (1996, August). Light field rendering. *Proceedings of the 23rd annual conference on Computer graphics and interactive techniques*, 31-42.

Li, J., Cheng, J., Shi, J., & Huang, F. (2012). Brief Introduction of Back Propagation (BP) Neural Network Algorithm and Its Improvement. In D. Jin & S. Lin (Eds.), Advances in Computer Science and Information Engineering (pp. 553–558). Springer. https://doi.org/10.1007/978-3-642-30223-7_87.

Li, G., Citrin, D., Camphausen, K., Mueller, B., Burman, C., Mychalczak, B., Miller, R. W., & Song, Y. (2008). Advances in 4D medical imaging and 4D radiation therapy. *Technology in Cancer Research & Treatment, 7*(1), 67–81. doi:10.1177/153303460800700109 PMID:18198927

Liu, J., & Guo, L. (2015, August). A new brain mri image segmentation strategy based on k-means clustering and svm. In *2015 7th International Conference on Intelligent Human-Machine Systems and Cybernetics* (Vol. 2, pp. 270-273). IEEE. 10.1109/IHMSC.2015.182

Li, Y. H., Yeh, N. N., Chen, S. J., & Chung, Y. C. (2019). *Computer-Assisted Diagnosis for Diabetic Retinopathy Based on Fundus Images Using Deep Convolutional Neural Network.* doi:10.1155/2019/6142839

Li, Y., Sun, J., Tang, C.-K., & Shum, H.-Y. (2004). Chi-Keung Tang, and Heung-Yeung Shum. Lazy snapping. *ACM Transactions on Graphics, 23*(3), 303–308. doi:10.1145/1015706.1015719

Logeswari, T., & Karnan, M. (2010, February). An improved implementation of brain tumor detection using soft computing. *2010 Second International Conference on Communication Software and Networks*, 147-151. 10.1109/ICCSN.2010.10

Lu, C. Y., Xu, Z. S., & Ye, X. (2019). Evaluation of intraoperative MRI-assisted stereotactic brain tissue biopsy: A single-center experience in China. *Chinese Neurosurgical Journal, 5*(1), 1–8. doi:10.118641016-019-0152-0 PMID:32922904

Lumsdaine, A., & Georgiev, T. (2009, April). The focused plenoptic camera. *2009 IEEE International Conference on Computational Photography (ICCP*1-8.

Luo, M., Ma, Y. F., & Zhang, H. J. (2003, December). A spatial constrained k-means approach to image segmentation. *Fourth International Conference on Information, Communications and Signal Processing, 2003 and the Fourth Pacific Rim Conference on Multimedia. Proceedings of the 2003 Joint*, 738-742.

Luo, Z., Jia, Y., & He, J. (2019). An Optic Disc Segmentation Method Based on Active Contour Tracking. International Information and Engineering Technology Association. *Traitement du Signal., 36*(3), 265–271. doi:10.18280/ts.360310

Maeno, K., Nagahara, H., Shimada, A., & Taniguchi, R. I. (2013). Light field distortion feature for transparent object recognition. *Proceedings of the IEEE Conference on Computer Vision and Pattern Recognition*, 2786-2793. 10.1109/CVPR.2013.359

Maggiori, E., Tarabalka, Y., Charpiat, G., & Alliez, P. (2017). Convolutional Neural Networks for Large-Scale Remote-Sensing Image Classification. *IEEE Transactions on Geoscience and Remote Sensing, 55*(2), 645–657. https://doi.org/10.1109/TGRS.2016.2612821

Mahajan, P. (2016). Application of Pattern Recognition Algorithm in Health and Medicine: a review. *International Journal of Engineering and Computer Science, 5*(5), 16580-83.

Mallick, D., Kumar, K., & Agarwal, S. (2019). *Blood Vessel Detection using Modified Multiscale MF-FDOG Filters for Diabetic Retinopathy.* arXiv:1910.12028v1 [eess.IV]

Mao, W. L., Fathurrahman, H. I. K., Lee, Y., & Chang, T. W. (2020). EEG dataset classification using CNN method. *Journal of Physics: Conference Series, 1456*(1), 012017. doi:10.1088/1742-6596/1456/1/012017

Marjani, M., Nasaruddin, F., Gani, A., Karim, A., Hashem, I. A. T., Siddiqa, A., & Yakoob, I. (2017, March). Big IoT Data Analytics: Architecture, Opportunities, and Open Research Challenges. *IEEE Access: Practical Innovations, Open Solutions, 5*, 5247–5261. doi:10.1109/ACCESS.2017.2689040

Mateen, M., Wen, J., Nasrullah, N., Sun, S., & Hayat, S. (2020). *Exudate Detection for Diabetic Retinopathy Using Pretrained Convolutional Neural Networks.* doi:10.1155/2020/5801870

Mihara, H., Funatomi, T., Tanaka, K., Kubo, H., Mukaigawa, Y., & Nagahara, H. (2016, May). 4D light field segmentation with spatial and angular consistencies. *2016 IEEE International Conference on Computational Photography (ICCP)*, 1-8. 10.1109/ICCPHOT.2016.7492872

Mirjalili, S. (2016). *Dragonfly algorithm: A new meta-heuristic optimization technique for solving single-objective.* Academic Press.

Mirjalili, S. (2016). Dragonfly algorithm: A new meta-heuristic optimization technique for solving single-objective, discrete, and multi-objective problems. *Neural Computing & Applications, 27*(4), 1053–1073. doi:10.100700521-015-1920-1

Mishra, A., Chandra, P., Ghose, U., & Sodhi, S. S. (2017). Bi-modal Derivative Adaptive Activation Function Sigmoidal Feedforward Artificial Neural Networks. *Applied Soft Computing, Elsevier, 61*, 983–994. doi:10.1016/j.asoc.2017.09.002

Mistry, R., Tanwar, S., Tyagi, S., & Kumar, N. (2020). Blockchain for 5G-Enabled IoT for Industrial Automation: A Systematic Review, Solutions, and Challenges. *Mechanical Systems and Signal Processing, 135*, 1–19. doi:10.1016/j.ymssp.2019.106382

Mohd Ariffin, M., Zarith Nabilah Tengku Othman, T., Shakirah Aziz, N., Mehat, M., & Izza Arshad, N. (2018). Dysgraphi Coach: Mobile Application for Dysgraphia Children in Malaysia. *International Journal of Engineering & Technology, 7*(4.36), 440. doi:10.14419/ijet.v7i4.36.23912

Mucha, J., Mekyska, J., Faundez-Zanuy, M., Lopez-De-Ipina, K., Zvoncak, V., Galaz, Z., Kiska, T., Smekal, Z., Brabenec, L., & Rektorova, I. (2018). Advanced Parkinson's Disease Dysgraphia Analysis Based on Fractional Derivatives of Online Handwriting. *2018 10th International Congress on Ultra Modern Telecommunications and Control Systems and Workshops (ICUMT)*. 10.1109/ICUMT.2018.8631265

Mustaqeem, A., Javed, A., & Fatima, T. (2012). An efficient brain tumor detection algorithm using watershed & thresholding based segmentation. *International Journal of Image, Graphics and Signal Processing, 4*(10), 34–39. doi:10.5815/ijigsp.2012.10.05

Nagahashi, T., Fujiyoshi, H., & Kanade, T. (2009, September). Video segmentation using iterated graph cuts based on spatio-temporal volumes. In *Asian Conference on Computer Vision*. Springer.

Naqvi, S. S., Fatima, N., Khan, T. M., Rehman, Z. U., & Khan, M. A. (2019). Automatic optic disk detection and segmentation by variational active contour estimation in retinal fundus images. Springer. doi:10.100711760-019-01463-y

Natarajan, P., Krishnan, N., Kenkre, N. S., Nancy, S., & Singh, B. P. (2012, December). *Tumor detection using threshold operation in MRI brain images. In 2012 IEEE international conference on computational intelligence and computing research.* IEEE.

National Health Service. (2020). Epilepsy Treatment. *Conditions.* https://www.nhs.uk/conditions/epilepsy/treatment/

Ng, R., Levoy, M., Brédif, M., Duval, G., Horowitz, M., & Hanrahan, P. (2005). *Light field photography with a hand-held plenoptic camera* (Doctoral dissertation). Stanford University.

Nivetha, C., Sumathi, S., & Chandrasekaran, M. (2017). Retinal Blood Vessels Extraction and Detection of Exudates Using Wavelet Transform and PNN Approach for the Assessment of Diabetic Retinopathy. *IEEE International Conference on Communication and Signal Processing*, 1962-1966.

Oliveira, W.S., Teixeira, J.V., Ren, T.I., & Cavalcanti, G.D.C. (2016). Unsupervised Retinal Vessel Segmentation Using Combined Filters. *PLoS ONE, 11*(2). doi:10.1371/journal.pone.0149943

Ooyen, A. V., & Nienhuis, B. (1992). Improving the Convergence of the Back-propagation Algorithm. *Neural Networks, 5*(3), 465-471. doi:10.1016/0893-6080(92)90008-7

Orczyk, T., Doroz, R., & Porwik, P. (2021, June). Missing Value Imputation Method Using Separate Features Nearest Neighbors Algorithm. *International Conference on Computational Science*, 128-141. 10.1007/978-3-030-77967-2_12

Osher, S., & Sethian, J. A. (1988). Fronts propagating with curvature-dependent speed: Algorithms based on Hamilton-Jacobi formulations. *Journal of Computational Physics, 79*(1), 12–49. doi:10.1016/0021-9991(88)90002-2

Panchal, P., Bhojani, R., & Panchal, T. (2016). An Algorithm for Retinal Feature Extraction using Hybrid Approach. *Procedia Computer Science, 79*, 61–68. doi:10.1016/j.procs.2016.03.009

Panebianco, Sridharan, Ramaratnam, & Cochrane Epilepsy Group. (2017). *Yoga for Epilepsy. In The Cochrane Collaboration*. John Wiley & Sons, Ltd. doi:10.1002/14651858.CD001524.pub3

Pan, S. J., & Yang, Q. (2010). A Survey on Transfer Learning. *IEEE Transactions on Knowledge and Data Engineering, 22*(10), 1345–1359. https://doi.org/10.1109/TKDE.2009.191

Pan, W., Gu, W., Nagpal, S., Gephart, M. H., & Quake, S. R. (2015). Brain tumor mutations detected in cerebral spinal fluid. *Clinical Chemistry, 61*(3), 514–522. doi:10.1373/clinchem.2014.235457 PMID:25605683

Paola, J. D., & Schowengerdt, R. A. (1995). A Review and Analysis of Backpropagation Neural Networks for Classification of Remotely-sensed Multi-spectral Imagery. *International Journal of Remote Sensing, 16*(16), 3033-3058. doi:10.1080/01431169508954607

Pascal, N. E., Pierre, E., & Emmanuel, T. (2014) Hybrid Method Segmentation for Medical Image Based on DWT, FCM and HMRF-EM. *International Journal of Computer and Information Technology*.

Pascal, N. E., Pierre, E., & Emmanuel, T. (2014). Hybrid Method Segmentation for Medical Image Based on DWT, FCM and HMRF-EM. *International Journal of Computer and Information Technology*.

Patro, S. G. K., & Sahu, K. K. (2015). *Normalization: A Preprocessing Stage*. arXiv e-prints arXiv:1503.06462.

Pazhoohesh, M., Pourmirza, Z., & Walker, S. (2019, August). A comparison of methods for missing data treatment in building sensor data. In *2019 IEEE 7th International Conference on Smart Energy Grid Engineering (SEGE)* (pp. 255-259). IEEE. 10.1109/SEGE.2019.8859963

Pedregosa, F., Varoquaux, G., Gramfort, A., Michel, V., Thirion, B., Grisel, O., Blondel, M., Prettenhofer, P., Weiss, R., Dubourg, V., Vanderplas, J., Passos, A., Cournapeau, D., Brucher, M., Perrot, M., & Duchesnay, É. (2011). Scikit-learn: Machine Learning in Python. *Journal of Machine Learning Research, 12*, 2825–2830.

Popoola, J. J., Godson, T. E., Olasoji, Y. O., & Adu, M. R. (2019). Study on capabilities of different segmentation algorithms in detecting and reducing brain tumor size in magnetic resonance imaging for effective telemedicine services. *European Journal of Engineering and Technology Research, 4*(2), 23–29. doi:10.24018/ejers.2019.4.2.1142

Pradhan, S. (2010). *Development of Unsupervised Image Segmentation Schemes for Brain MRI using HMRF model* (Doctoral dissertation).

Prastawa, M., Bullitt, E., Moon, N., Van Leemput, K., & Gerig, G. (2003). Automatic brain tumor segmentation by subject specific modification of atlas priors1. *Academic Radiology*, *10*(12), 1341–1348. doi:10.1016/S1076-6332(03)00506-3 PMID:14697002

Qian, N. (1999). On the Momentum Term in Gradient Descent Learning Algorithms. *Neural Networks, 12*(1), 145-151. doi:10.1016/S0893-6080(98)00116-6

Quenneville, J. (2001). Tech Tools for Students with Learning Disabilities: Infusion into Inclusive Classrooms. *Preventing School Failure*, *45*(4), 167–170. doi:10.1080/10459880109603332

Rad, A. E. R., Safry, M., Rahim, M., Kolivand, H., & Amin, I. B. M. (2016). Morphological Region-Based Initial Contour Algorithm for Level Set Methods in Image Segmentation. *Multimedia Tools and Applications*, 1–16.

Radenovic, F., Tolias, G., & Chum, O. (2019). Fine-tuning CNN image retrieval with no human annotation. *IEEE Transactions on Pattern Analysis and Machine Intelligence*, *41*(7), 1655–1668. doi:10.1109/TPAMI.2018.2846566 PMID:29994246

Rahman, C. M., & Rashid, T. A. (2019). Dragonfly algorithm and its applications in applied science survey. *Computational Intelligence and Neuroscience*, *2019*, 1–21. doi:10.1155/2019/9293617 PMID:31885533

Rahman, S. A., Huang, Y., Claassen, J., Heintzman, N., & Kleinberg, S. (2015). Combining Fourier and lagged k-nearest neighbor imputation for biomedical time series data. *Journal of Biomedical Informatics*, *58*, 198–207. doi:10.1016/j.jbi.2015.10.004 PMID:26477633

Rajalakshmi, N., & Prabha, V. L. (2012). Brain tumor detection of mr images based on color-converted hybrid pso+ k-means clustering segmentation. *European Journal of Scientific Research*, 5-14.

Raja, P. S., & Thangavel, K. (2020). Missing value imputation using unsupervised machine learning techniques. *Soft Computing*, *24*(6), 4361–4392. doi:10.100700500-019-04199-6

Rajasekaran, K. A., & Gounder, C. C. (2018). Advanced Brain Tumour Segmentation from MRI Images. *Basic Physical Principles and Clinical Applications, High-Resolution Neuroimaging*, 83-108.

A. D. Rasamoelina, F. Adjailia, & P. Sinčák (Eds.). (2020). A Review of Activation Function for Artificial Neural Network. In *Proceeding of the 2020 IEEE 18th World Symposium on Applied Machine Intelligence and Informatics (SAMI)*. IEEE. 10.1109/SAMI48414.2020.9108717

Rastogi, R., Chaturvedi, D. K., Satya, S., Arora, N., Gupta, M., Verma, H., & Saini, H. (2020c). An Optimized Biofeedback EMG and GSR Biofeedback Therapy for Chronic TTH on SF-36 Scores of Different MMBD Modes on Various Medical Symptoms. Studies Comp. Intelligence, 841. doi:10.1007/978-981-13-8930-6_8

Rastogi, R., Chaturvedi, D. K., Satya, S., Arora, N., Saini, H., & Verma, H. (2018c). Comparative Efficacy Analysis of Electromyography and Galvanic Skin Resistance Biofeedback on Audio Mode for Chronic TTH on Various Indicators. *Proceedings of International Conference on Computational Intelligence &IoT (ICCIIoT) 2018*.

Rastogi, R., Chaturvedi, D. K., Satya, S., Arora, N., Sirohi, H., Singh, M., Verma, P., & Singh, V. (2018b). Which One is Best: Electromyography Biofeedback Efficacy Analysis on Audio, Visual and Audio-Visual Modes for Chronic TTH on Different Characteristics. *Proceedings of International Conference on Computational Intelligence &IoT (ICCIIoT) 2018*.

Rastogi, R., Chaturvedi, D. K., Sharma, S., Bansal, A., & Agrawal, A. (2018a). Audio Visual EMG & GSR Biofeedback Analysis for Effect of Spiritual Techniques on Human Behaviour and Psychic Challenges. *Proceedings of the 12th INDIACom*, 252-258.

Rastogi, R., Chaturvedi, D. K., Verma, H., Mishra, Y., & Gupta, M. (2020a). Identifying Better? Analytical Trends to Check Subjects' Medications Using Biofeedback Therapies. *International Journal of Applied Research on Public Health Management, 5*(1). https://www.igi-global.com/article/identifying-better/240753 doi:10.4018/IJARPHM.2020010102

Rastogi, R., Gupta, M., & Chaturvedi, D.K. (2020b). Efficacy of Study for Correlation of TTH vs Age and Gender Factors using EMG Biofeedback Technique. *International Journal of Applied Research on Public Health Management, 5*(1), 49-66. doi:10.4018/IJARPHM.2020010104

Rastogi, R., Saxena, M., Gupta, U. S., Sharma, S., Chaturvedi, D. K., Singhal, P., Gupta, M., Garg, P., Gupta, M., & Maheshwari, M. (2019b). Yajna and Mantra Therapy Applications on Diabetic Subjects: Computational Intelligence Based Experimental Approach. *Proceedings of The 2nd edition of International Conference on Industry Interactive Innovations in Science, Engineering and Technology (I3SET2K19).* https://papers.ssrn.com/sol3/papers.cfm?abstract_id=3515800

Rastogi, R., Saxena, M., Sharma, S. K., Muralidharan, S., Beriwal, V. K., Singhal, P., Rastogi, M., & Shrivastava, R. (2019a). Evaluation of efficacy of Yagya therapy on t2- diabetes mellitus patients. *Proceedings of the 2nd edition of International Conference on Industry Interactive Innovations in Science, Engineering and Technology (I3SET2K19).* https://papers.ssrn.com/sol3/papers.cfm?abstract_id=3514326

Rastogi, R., Saxena, M., Sharma, S. K., Murlidharan, S., Berival, V. K., Jaiswal, D., Sharma, A., & Mishra, A. (2019c). Statistical Analysis on Efficacy of Yagya Therapy for Type-2 Diabetic Mellitus Patients through Various Parameters. In On Computational Intelligence in Pattern Recognition (CIPR). doi:10.1007/978-981-15-2449-3_15

Rastogi, R. (2012). Current Approaches for Researches in Naturopathy: How far is its Evidence Base? *J of Homeopathy & Ayurvedic Medicine, 1*(2), 1–107. doi:10.4172/2167-1206.1000107

Ravichandran, C., & Raja, J. B. (2014). A Fast Enhancement/Thresholding Based Blood Vessel Segmentation for Retinal Image Using Contrast Limited Adaptive Histogram Equalization. *Journal of Medical Imaging and Health Informatics, 4*(4), 567–575.

Ray, S., & Turi, R. H. (1999, December). Determination of number of clusters in k-means clustering and application in colour image segmentation. *Proceedings of the 4th international conference on advances in pattern recognition and digital techniques*, 137-143.

Rosenblum, S., Dvorkin, A. Y., & Weiss, P. L. (2006). Automatic segmentation as a tool for examining the handwriting process of children with dysgraphic and proficient handwriting. *Human Movement Science, 25*(4–5), 608–621. doi:10.1016/j.humov.2006.07.005 PMID:17011656

Rosenblum, S., Weiss, P. L., & Parush, S. (2004). Handwriting evaluation for developmental dysgraphia: Process versus product. *Reading and Writing, 17*(5), 433–458. doi:10.1023/B:READ.0000044596.91833.55

Rother, C., Kolmogorov, V., & Blake, A. (2004). GrabCut" interactive foreground extraction using iterated graph cuts. *ACM Transactions on Graphics, 23*(3), 309–314. doi:10.1145/1015706.1015720

Roy, S., Nag, S., Maitra, I. K., & Bandyopadhyay, S. K. (2013). *A review on automated brain tumor detection and segmentation from MRI of brain.* arXiv preprint arXiv:1312.6150.

Ruan, S., Lebonvallet, S., Merabet, A., & Constans, J. M. (2007, April). Tumor segmentation from a multispectral MRI images by using support vector machine classification. *2007 4th IEEE International Symposium on Biomedical Imaging: From Nano to Macro*, 1236-1239. 10.1109/ISBI.2007.357082

Ruder, S. (2016). *An Overview of Gradient Descent Optimization Algorithms.* arXiv preprint arXiv:1609.04747.

Rustin, G. J., Quinn, M., Thigpen, T., Du Bois, A., Pujade-Lauraine, E., Jakobsen, A., Eisenhauer, E., Sagae, S., Greven, K., Vergote, I., Cervantes, A., & Vermorken, J. (2004). Re: New guidelines to evaluate the response to treatment in solid tumors (ovarian cancer). *Journal of the National Cancer Institute, 96*(6), 487–488. doi:10.1093/jnci/djh081 PMID:15026475

Saeed & Abdullah. (2021). Combination of Brain Cancer with Hybrid K-NN Algorithm using statistical Analysis of Cerebrospinal Fluid (CSF) Surgery. *International Journal of Computer Science and Network Security, 21*(2), 120-130.

Saeed & Abdullah. (2021). Performance analysis of machine learning algorithm for health care tools with High Dimension Segmentation. *Machine learning healthcare: Handling and managing data, 1*(1), 1-30.

Saeed & Abdullah. (2021). Statistical Analysis the Pre and Post-Surgery of health care sector using High Dimension Segmentation. *Machine learning healthcare: Handling and managing data, 1*(1), 1-25.

Saeed & Naqvi. (2019). Implementation of Fourier transformation. *Indian Journal of Science & Technology, 12*(37), 1-16.

Saeed & Naqvi. (n.d.). Assessment of Brain Tumor Due to the Usage of MATLAB Performance. *Journal of Medical Imaging and Health Informatics, 7*(6), 1454–1460. doi:10.1166/jmihi.2017.2187

Saeed, Abdullah, & Jhanjhi. (2021a). Performance analysis of machine learning algorithm for health care tools with High Dimension Segmentation. *Machine learning healthcare: Handling and managing data, 1*(1), 1-30.

Saeed, Abdullah, & Jhanjhi. (2021b). Comparison analysis of medical health care information of Graph Cutting using Multi Dimension Segmentation. *Machine learning healthcare: Handling and managing data, 1*(1), 1-23.

Saeed, Abdullah, & Jhanjhi. (2021c). Statistical Analysis the Pre and Post-Surgery of health care sector using High Dimension Segmentation. *Machine learning healthcare: Handling and managing data, 1*(1), 1-25.

Saeed, Abdullah, & Jhanjhi. (2021d). Combination of Brain Cancer with Hybrid K-NN Algorithm using statistical Analysis of Cerebrospinal Fluid (CSF) Surgery. *International Journal of Computer Science and Network Security, 21*(2), 120-130.

Saeed, Abdullah, Jhanjhi, & Naqvi. (2019). Implementation of Fourier transformation. *Indian Journal of Science & Technology, 12*(37), 1-16.

Saeed, S., & Abdullah, A. (20121). Statistical Analysis the Pre and Post-Surgery of health care sector using High Dimension Segmentation. *Machine Learning Healthcare: Handling and Managing Data, 1*(1), 1-25.

Saeed, S., & Naqvi, S. M. (2018). Impact of Data Mining Techniques to Analyze Health Care Data. *Journal of Medical Sciences and Health.*

Saeed, S., Abdullah, A., & Jhanjhi, N. (2019). Investigation of a Brain Cancer with Interfacing of 3-Dimensional Image Processing. *Indian Journal of Science and Technology, 12*(34), 1–12. doi:10.17485/ijst/2019/v12i34/146150

Saeed, S., & Naqvi, M. (2017). Implementation of Failure Enterprise Systems in Organizational Perspective Framework. *International Journal of Advanced Computer Science and Applications, 8*(5), 54–63. doi:10.14569/IJACSA.2017.080508

Sainath, T. N., Vinyals, O., Senior, A., & Sak, H. (2015). Convolutional, long short-term memory, fully connected deep neural networks, ICASSP. *Preceding of the IEEE International Conference on Acoustics, Speech and Signal Processing (ICASSP)*, 4580–4584.

Sajid, S., Hussain, S., & Sarwar, A. (2019). Brain tumor detection and segmentation in MR images using deep learning. *Arabian Journal for Science and Engineering, 44*(11), 9249–9261. doi:10.100713369-019-03967-8

Sakka, L., Coll, G., & Chazal, J. (2011). Anatomy and physiology of cerebrospinal fluid. *European Annals of Otorhinolaryngology, Head and Neck Diseases, 128*(6), 309–316. doi:10.1016/j.anorl.2011.03.002 PMID:22100360

San-Segundo, R., Gil-Martín, M., D'Haro-Enríquez, L. F., & Pardo, J. M. (2019). Classification of epileptic EEG recordings using signal transforms and convolutional neural networks. *Computers in Biology and Medicine, 109*, 148–158. doi:10.1016/j.compbiomed.2019.04.031 PMID:31055181

Sattar, S., Alibhai, S. M., Spoelstra, S. L., & Puts, M. T. (2019). The assessment, management, and reporting of falls, and the impact of falls on cancer treatment in community-dwelling older patients receiving cancer treatment: Results from a mixed-methods study. *Journal of Geriatric Oncology, 10*(1), 98–104. doi:10.1016/j.jgo.2018.08.006 PMID:30174258

Saxena, M., Kumar, B., & Matharu, S. (2018). Impact of Yagya on Particulate Matters. *Interdisciplinary Journal of Yagya Research, 1*(1), 1-8.

Saxena, M., Sharma, S. K., Muralidharan, S., Beriwal, V., Rastogi, R., Singhal, P., Sharma, V., & Sangam, U. (2020). Statistical Analysis Of Efficacy Of Yagya Therapy On Type-2 Diabetic Mellitus Patients on Various Parameters. *Proceedings Of 2nd International Conference on Computational Intelligence In Pattern Recognition (CIPR – 2020)*.

Saxena, M., Sengupta, B., & Pandya, P. (2008, September). Controlling the Microflora in Outdoor Environment: Effect of Yagya. *Indian Journal of Air Pollution Control, 8*(2), 30–36.

Schachter & Shafer. (2017). Challenges with Epilepsy. *Social Concerns of Seizures*. https://www.epilepsy.com/learn/challenges-epilepsy/social-concerns

Scheidl, H. (2011). *Handwritten Text Recognition in Historical Documents* [Unpublished diploma thesis]. Technische Universität Wien, Austria.

Scheidl, H., Fiel, S., & Sablatnig, R. (2018). Word Beam Search: A Connectionist Temporal Classification Decoding Algorithm. *2018 16th International Conference on Frontiers in Handwriting Recognition (ICFHR)*. 10.1109/ICFHR-2018.2018.00052

Schmidhuber, J. (2015). Deep Learning in neural networks: An overview. *Neural Networks, 61*, 5–117. doi:10.1016/j.neunet.2014.09.003 PMID:25462637

Sedghi, A., O'Donnell, L. J., Kapur, T., Learned-Miller, E., Mousavi, P., & Wells, W. M. III. (2021). Image registration: Maximum likelihood, minimum entropy and deep learning. *Medical Image Analysis, 69*, 101939. doi:10.1016/j.media.2020.101939 PMID:33388458

Selvy, P. T., Palanisamy, V., & Purusothaman, T. (2011). Performance analysis of clustering algorithms in brain tumor detection of MR images. *European Journal of Scientific Research, 62*(3), 321–330.

Setiawan, W., Utoyo, M. I., & Rulaningtyas, R. (2018). Retinal Vessel Segmentation using a Modified Morphology Process and Global Thresholding. *The 8th Annual Basic Science International Conference. AIP Conference Proceedings 2021*. 10.1063/1.5062795

Shanmuganathan, S. (2016). Artificial Neural Network Modelling: An Introduction. In S. Shanmuganathan & S. Samarasinghe (Eds.), *Artificial Neural Network Modelling* (pp. 1–14). Springer. doi:10.1007/978-3-319-28495-8_1

U. S. Shanthamallu, A. Spanias, C. Tepedelenlioglu, & M. Stanley (Eds.). (2017). A Brief Survey of Machine Learning Methods and Their Sensor and IoT Applications. In *Proceeding of the 8th International Conference on Information, Intelligence, Systems & Applications (IISA)*. IEEE. 10.1109/IISA.2017.8316459

Sharma, S.R. (2013). Shabd Brahma—Naad Brahm. *BrahmVarchas, Shantikunj,* 55.

Sharma, S.R. (2015a). Shabd Brahma—Naad Brahm. *BrahmVarchas, Shantikunj,* 98.

Sharma, S.R. (2015b). Gayatri MahaVigyan. *BrahmVarchas, Shantikunj,* 235.

Sharma, S.R. (2015c). Shabd Brahma—Naad Brahm. *BrahmVarchas, Shantikunj,* 34

Sharma, S.R. (2015d). Shabd Brahma—Naad Brahm. *BrahmVarchas, Shantikunj,* 61

Shen, S., Sandham, W. A., & Granat, M. H. (2003, April). Preprocessing and segmentation of brain magnetic resonance images. *4th International IEEE EMBS Special Topic Conference on Information Technology Applications in Biomedicine,* 149-152. 10.1109/ITAB.2003.1222495

Shenwai & Tare. (2017). Integrated Approach towards Holistic Health: Current Trends and Future Scope. *Int. J. of Cur. Rec. Rev., 9*(7), 11-14.

Shirly, S., & Ramesh, K. (2019). Review on 2D and 3D MRI image segmentation techniques. *Current Medical Imaging, 15*(2), 150–160. doi:10.2174/1573405613666171123160609 PMID:31975661

Shokouhifar, M., & Abkenar, G. S. (2011). An artificial bee colony optimization for mri fuzzy segmentation of brain tissue. *2011 International Conference on Management and Artificial Intelligence IPEDR.*

Shorten, C., & Khoshgoftaar, T. M. (2019). A Survey on Image Data Augmentation for Deep Learning. *Journal of Big Data, 6*(1), 1–48. https://doi.org/10.1186/s40537-019-0197-0

Shrivastava, V., Batham, L., Mishra, A. (2019). Yagyopathy (Yagya Therapy) for Various Diseases - An Overview. *Ayurveda Evam Samagra Swasthya Shodhamala, 1*(1), 1-11.

Siddiqui, A. T., & Muntjir, M. (2017). An Approach to Smart Study using Pen and Paper Learning. *International Journal of Emerging Technologies in Learning, 12*(05), 117. doi:10.3991/ijet.v12i05.6798

Simonyan, K., & Zisserman, A. (Eds.). (2015). Very deep convolutional networks for large-scale image recognition. *Proceeding of the 3rd International Conference on Learning Representations (ICLR 2015).* https://arxiv.org/abs/1409.1556

Singh, A., Pokharel, R., & Principe, J. (2014). The C-loss Function for Pattern Classification. *Pattern Recognition, 47*(1), 441-453. doi:10.1016/j.patcog.2013.07.017

Singh, A. P., Pradhan, N. R., Luhach, A. K., Agnihotri, S., Jhanjhi, N. Z., Verma, S., Kavita, Ghosh, U., & Roy, D. S. (2020). A novel patient-centric architectural framework for blockchain-enabled healthcare applications. *IEEE Transactions on Industrial Informatics, 17*(8), 5779–5789. doi:10.1109/TII.2020.3037889

Singh, N. P., & Srivastava, R. (2016). Retinal blood vessels segmentation by using Gumbel Probability Distribution Function based matched filter. *Computer Methods and Programs in Biomedicine,* 1–15. doi:10.1016/j.cmpb.2016.03.001 PMID:27084319

Sirven & Shafer. (2014). What is Epilepsy. *Epilepsy. Foundation.*https://www.epilepsy.com/learn/about-epilepsy-basics/what-epilepsy

Smith, S. J. M. (2005). EEG in the diagnosis, classification, and management of patients with epilepsy. *Journal of Neurology, Neurosurgery, and Psychiatry, 76*(suppl_2), ii2–ii7. doi:10.1136/jnnp.2005.069245 PMID:15961864

Sokołowski, A., & Pardela, T. (2014). Application of Fourier transforms in classification of medical images. In *Human-computer systems interaction: backgrounds and applications* (Vol. 3, pp. 193–200). Springer.

Spector, R., Snodgrass, S. R., & Johanson, C. E. (2015). A balanced view of the cerebrospinal fluid composition and functions: Focus on adult humans. *Experimental Neurology, 273,* 57–68. doi:10.1016/j.expneurol.2015.07.027 PMID:26247808

Srikanth. (2019). *15 Benefits of Machine Learning in Health Care.* https://techiexpert.com/benefits-of-machine-learning-in-health-care/

Srivastava, N., Hinton, G., Krizhevsky, A., Sutskever, I., & Salakhutdinov, R. (2014). Dropout: A Simple Way to Prevent Neural Networks from Overfitting. *Journal of Machine Learning Research, 15,* 1929–1958.

Srivedmata Gayatri Trust. Gayatri Parivar, UK. (2011). *Yagya's Effect On The Environment.* https://home.awgpuk.org/index.php/yagya/42-yagya-s-effect-on-the-environment

Strate School of Design. Paris and Singapore. (2016). *IoT applications in healthcare, Supporting Robust Health and Medical Practices.* https://www.strate.education/gallery/news/healthcare-iot

Sultan, H. H., Salem, N. M., & Al-Atabany, W. (2019). Multi-classification of brain tumor images using deep neural network. *IEEE Access: Practical Innovations, Open Solutions, 7,* 69215–69225. doi:10.1109/ACCESS.2019.2919122

Sundaram, R. (2019). Extraction of Blood Vessels in Fundus Images of Retina through Hybrid Segmentation Approach. *Mathematics, 7*(169), 1–17. doi:10.3390/math7020169

Sun, Y., Lo, F. P.-W., & Lo, B. (2019). EEG-based user identification system using 1D-convolutional long short-term memory neural networks. *Expert Systems with Applications, 125,* 259–267. doi:10.1016/j.eswa.2019.01.080

Taheri, S., Ong, S. H., & Chong, V. F. H. (2010). Level-set segmentation of brain tumors using a threshold-based speed function. *Image and Vision Computing, 28*(1), 26–37. doi:10.1016/j.imavis.2009.04.005

Tamim, N., Elshrkawey, M., Azim, G.A., & Nassar, H. (2020). Retinal Blood Vessel Segmentation Using Hybrid Features and Multi-Layer Perceptron Neural Networks. *Symmetry 2020, 12,* 894. doi:10.3390/sym12060894

Tatiraju, S., & Mehta, A. (2008). Image Segmentation using k-means clustering, EM and Normalized Cuts. *Department of EECS, 1,* 1–7.

Telano, L. N., & Baker, S. (2020). *Physiology, Cerebral Spinal Fluid (CSF).* StatPearls.

Tsubouchi, Y., Tanabe, A., Saito, Y., Noma, H., & Maegaki, Y. (2019). Long−term prognosis of epilepsy in patients with cerebral palsy. *Developmental Medicine and Child Neurology, 61*(9), 1067–1073. doi:10.1111/dmcn.14188 PMID:30854645

Tzika, A. A., Astrakas, L., & Zarifi, M. (2011). Pediatric Brain Tumors: Magnetic Resonance Spectroscopic Imaging. *Diagnostic Techniques and Surgical Management of Brain Tumors, 205.*

Ullah, A., Azeem, M., Ashraf, H., Alaboudi, A. A., Humayun, M., & Jhanjhi, N. Z. (2021). Secure healthcare data aggregation and transmission in IoT—A survey. *IEEE Access: Practical Innovations, Open Solutions, 9,* 16849–16865. doi:10.1109/ACCESS.2021.3052850

Ullah, A., Ishaq, N., Azeem, M., Ashraf, H., Jhanjhi, N. Z., Humayun, M., Tabbakh, T. A., & Almusaylim, Z. A. (2021). A Survey on Continuous Object Tracking and Boundary Detection Schemes in IoT Assisted Wireless Sensor Networks. *IEEE Access: Practical Innovations, Open Solutions, 9,* 126324–126336. doi:10.1109/ACCESS.2021.3110203

Van Leemput, K., Maes, F., Vandermeulen, D., & Suetens, P. (1998, October). Automatic segmentation of brain tissues and MR bias field correction using a digital brain atlas. In *International Conference on Medical Image Computing and Computer-Assisted. Intervention.* Springer. 10.1007/BFb0056312

Vasuda, P., & Satheesh, S. (2010). Improved fuzzy C-means algorithm for MR brain image segmentation. *International Journal on Computer Science and Engineering, 2*(5).

Verma, S., Mishra, A., & Shrivastava, V. (2018). Yagya Therapy in Vedic and Ayurvedic Literature: A Preliminary exploration. *Interdisciplinary Journal of Yagya Research, 1*(1), 15-20. http://ijyr.dsvv.ac.in/index.php/ijyr/article/view/7/13

Vijayalakshmi, B., Ramar, K., Jhanjhi, N. Z., Verma, S., Kaliappan, M., Vijayalakshmi, K., Vimal, S., Kavita, & Ghosh, U. (2021). An attention-based deep learning model for traffic flow prediction using spatiotemporal features towards sustainable smart city. *International Journal of Communication Systems*, *34*(3), e4609. doi:10.1002/dac.4609

Wang, D. (2019). Efficient level-set segmentation model driven by the local GMM and split Bregman method. *IET Image Processing*, *13*(5), 761–770. doi:10.1049/iet-ipr.2018.6216

Wang, L. (2019, December). Research and Implementation of Machine Learning Classifier Based on KNN. In *IOP Conference Series: Materials Science and Engineering*. IOP Publishing. 10.1088/1757-899X/677/5/052038

Wanner, S., & Goldluecke, B. (2012, June). Globally consistent depth labeling of 4D light fields. In *2012 IEEE Conference on Computer Vision and Pattern Recognition*. IEEE. 10.1109/CVPR.2012.6247656

Wanner, S., Straehle, C., & Goldluecke, B. (2013). Globally consistent multi-label assignment on the ray space of 4d light fields. *Proceedings of the IEEE Conference on Computer Vision and Pattern Recognition*, 1011-1018. 10.1109/CVPR.2013.135

Wei, B., Sun, X., Ren, X., & Xu, J. (2017). *Minimal Effort Back Propagation for Convolutional Neural Networks*. arXiv preprint arXiv:1709.05804.

Xu, Y., Nagahara, H., Shimada, A., & Taniguchi, R. I. (2019). TransCut2: Transparent Object Segmentation From a Light-Field Image. *IEEE Transactions on Computational Imaging*, *5*(3), 465–477. doi:10.1109/TCI.2019.2893820

Yamashita, R., Nishio, M., Do, R. K. G., & Togashi, K. (2018). Convolutional Neural Networks: An Overview and Application in Radiology. *Insights into Imaging*, *9*, 611-629. doi:10.1007/s13244-018-0639-9

Yu, H., Barriga, S., Agurto, S., Zamora, G., Bauman, W., & Soliz, P. (2012). Fast Vessel Segmentation in Retinal Images Using Multiscale Enhancement and Second-order Local Entropy. *Medical Imaging 2012: Computer-Aided Diagnosis, Proc. of SPIE*, 8315, 1-12.

Yuan, X., Li, L., & Wang, Y. (2020). Nonlinear dynamic soft sensor modeling with supervised long short-term memory network. In *Preceding of the IEEE Transactions on Industrial Informatics* (pp. 3168–3176). IEEE. doi:10.1109/TII.2019.2902129

Zhang, J., Bekkers, E., Abbasi, S., & Dashtbozorg, R. B. H. (2015). *Robust and Fast Vessel Segmentation via Gaussian Derivatives in Orientation Scores*. Springer International Publishing.

Zhang, D. Q., & Chen, S. C. (2004). A novel kernelized fuzzy c-means algorithm with application in medical image segmentation. *Artificial Intelligence in Medicine*, *32*(1), 37–50. doi:10.1016/j.artmed.2004.01.012 PMID:15350623

Zhang, J., Ma, K. K., Er, M. H., & Chong, V. (2004, January). Tumor segmentation from magnetic resonance imaging by learning via one-class support vector machine. *International Workshop on Advanced Image Technology (IWAIT'04)*, 207-211.

Zhang, S., Cheng, D., Deng, Z., Zong, M., & Deng, X. (2018). A novel kNN algorithm with data-driven k parameter computation. *Pattern Recognition Letters*, *109*, 44–54. doi:10.1016/j.patrec.2017.09.036

Zhang, S., Li, X., Zong, M., Zhu, X., & Cheng, D. (2017). Learning k for knn classification. *ACM Transactions on Intelligent Systems and Technology*, *8*(3), 1–19.

Zhang, S., Zong, M., Sun, K., Liu, Y., & Cheng, D. (2014, December). Efficient kNN algorithm based on graph sparse reconstruction. In *International Conference on Advanced Data Mining and Applications* (pp. 356-369). Springer. 10.1007/978-3-319-14717-8_28

Zhang, Y., Brady, M., & Smith, S. (2001). Segmentation of brain MR images through a hidden Markov field model and the expectation-maximization algorithm. *IEEE Transactions on Medical Imaging*, *20*(1), 45–57. doi:10.1109/42.906424 PMID:11293691

Zhang, Z. (2016). *Derivation of Backpropagation in Convolutional Neural Network (CNN)*. University of Tennessee.

Zhao, Y., Rada, L., Chen, K., Harding, S. P., & Zheng, Y. (2015). Automated Vessel Segmentation Using Infinite Perimeter Active Contour Model with Hybrid Region Information with Application to Retinal Images. *IEEE Transactions on Medical Imaging*, 1–11. doi:10.1109/TMI.2015.2409024 PMID:25769147

Zhou, J., Chan, K. L., Chong, V. F. H., & Krishnan, S. M. (2006, January). Extraction of brain tumor from MR images using one-class support vector machine. *2005 IEEE Engineering in Medicine and Biology 27th Annual Conference*, 6411-6414.

Zhuge, Y., Krauze, A. V., Ning, H., Cheng, J. Y., Arora, B. C., Camphausen, K., & Miller, R. W. (2017). Brain tumor segmentation using holistically nested neural networks in MRI images. *Medical Physics*, *44*(10), 5234–5243. doi:10.1002/mp.12481 PMID:28736864

Zoph, B., & Le, Q. V. (Eds.). (2017). Neural Architecture Search with Reinforcement Learning. *Proceeding of the 5ᵗʰ International Conference on Learning Representations (ICLR 2017)*. https://openreview.net/forum?id=r1Ue8Hcxg

About the Contributors

Noor Zaman received the Ph.D. degree in IT from UTP, Malaysia. He has great international exposure in academia, research, administration, and academic quality accreditation. He was with ILMA University, KFU for a decade, and currently with Taylor's University, Malaysia. He has 19 years of teaching & administrative experience. He has an intensive background of academic quality accreditation in higher education besides scientific research activities, he had worked a decade for academic accreditation and earned ABET accreditation twice for three programs at CCSIT, King Faisal University, Saudi Arabia. Dr. Noor Zaman has awarded as top reviewer 1% globally by WoS/ISI (Publons) recently. He has edited/authored more than 11 research books with international reputed publishers, earned several research grants, and a great number of indexed research articles on his credit. He has supervised several postgraduate students including masters and Ph.D. Dr. Jhanjhi is an Associate Editor of IEEE ACCESS, Guest editor of several reputed journals, member of the editorial board of several research journals, and active TPC member of reputed conferences around the globe.

Loveleen Gaur is currently working as Professor, Program Director Artificial Intelligence and Data Analytics at Amity International Business School, Amity University, India. She has more than 20 years of teaching, research, and administrative experience internationally. She is the founding director of MBA in Artificial Intelligence and Data Analytics in Amity International Business School. She is supervising number of Ph.D. scholars, Post Graduate students, mainly in Artificial Intelligence and Data Analytics for business and management. Under her guidance, the AI/Data Analytics research cluster has published extensively in high-impact factor journals and has established extensive research collaboration globally with several renowned professionals. She is a senior IEEE member and Series Editor with CRC and Wiley. She has high indexed publications in SCI/ABDC/WoS/Scopus and has several Patents/copyrights on her account, edited/authored more than 20 research books published by world-class publishers. She has excellent experience in supervising and co-supervising postgraduate students internationally. An ample number of Ph.D. and Master's students graduated under her supervision. She is an external Ph.D./ Master thesis examiner/evaluator for several universities globally. She has completed internationally funded research grants successfully. She has also served as Keynote speaker for several international conferences, presented several Webinars worldwide, chaired international conference sessions. Prof. Gaur has significantly contributed to enhancing scientific understanding by participating in over three hundred scientific conferences, symposia, and seminars, by chairing technical sessions and delivering plenary and invited talks.

* * *

Afnizanfaizal Abdullah is a senior lecturer at the School of Computing, with a PhD. in Computer Science, specializing in artificial intelligence techniques for analyzing biological data. My research interests are in the designing of machine learning algorithms for healthcare applications in the cloud environments. In 2015, I have co-founded Synthetic Biology Research Group to drive innovation in research and development of healthcare, biotechnology, and environment areas through computing and engineering. I am also active in engaging with industrial partners and professional communities to contribute the knowledge and skills for the public.

Mohammed Al Achhab received his PhD in December 2006 from the University of Franche-Comté, Besançon, France, in the field of formal verification of reactive systems. He received a Master degree in July 2003 from University of Franche-Comté, in the field of software engineering and artificial intelligence. He was Temporary Lecturer and Research Assistant, at the University of Franche-Comté. He was an assistant professor at Faculty of Sciences Dhar El mehraz, Fez from 2007 to 2012. Currently, he is a professor at the National School of Applied Sciences of Tetuan. He is a member of the steering committee of the department of computer sciences and member of the National School board. His research focuses on analysis and validation of business process, natural language processing, case of study Arabic and adaptive e-learning. He is the co-author of more than 20 peer-reviewed publications. To his credit also, is being Member in many scientific associations notably IEEE, innove, and mocit. He has been participating in many national and international scientific and organizing committees. He is the mentor of the IEEE UAE Student Branch since 2015. He is the conference chair of the 2014 and 2016 IEEE CiSt editions.

Khalid A. AlAfandy was born in Sharkia, Egypt, in 1975. He received the B.Sc. degree in Electronic Engineering - Department of Computer Science and Engineering from Menoufia University, Menouf, Egypt, in 1997, the M.Sc. degree in Engineering Science - Department of Computer Science and Engineering was received from Menoufia University, Menouf, Egypt, in 2017, and now he is PhD student in National School for applied Science (ENSA) in Tetouan, Abdelmalek Essaadi University, Tetouan, Morocco. Through his Master research, he had Authored 3 conference Papers and 3 journal papers, and after finishing his Master research he had authored another 1 journal paper. Through his PhD research, he had Authored 2 conference papers, 3 journal papers, and 2 book chapters, there is 1 journal paper is under review. So, the total publications are 5 conference papers, 7 journal papers, and 2 book chapters.

Devershi Pallavi Bhatt, Ph.D. (Computer Science), M. Tech Computer Science and Engineering with Gold Medal, MCA, is a Professor & HoD, Department of Computer Applications, Manipal University Jaipur with 15 years of experience Senior member of IEEE Professional Member of ACM Certified Ethical Hacker (C|EH) Certified EC-Council Security Specialist (ECSS) Certified EC-Council Instructor (C|EI) Previously worked for reputed institutes like Banasthali Vidyapith, Niwai, Tonk; Pune University, Pune; and Punjab Technical University One Ph.D. has been successfully awarded under her guidance, currently supervising Four Ph.D. scholars in Manipal University Jaipur in Information and Network Security, Image and Video Forensics, behavioral biometric and IoT. More than 35 research publications i.e. in reputed Journals and presented in International Conferences of repute in India and Abroad. She has 1 patent 4 Copyrights in her account. Dr. Bhatt has successfully completed 2 research projects of 2 years each as a principal investigator funded by Manipal University Jaipur and Pune University. Delivered Keynotes and invited lectures in India and Abroad including MeitY, BIS, NITs, IITs to name a few.

Awarded Pratibha Samman and Shodh Shashtri Samman for doing Ph.D. in Wireless Sensor Networks, best researcher award by Manipal University Jaipur in 2020 November and best researcher by Institute of Technical and Scientific Research for doing good quality research publications.

Smita Das is presently working as an Assistant Professor in the Department of IT at MBB College, Agartala, Tripura, India.

Vipul Goyal is a final year student at Amity University, Uttar Pradesh. He currently lives in Surat, Gujarat but was born and raised in Ghaziabad, Uttar Pradesh.

Habibollah Haron is a Professor in Soft Computing, Universiti Teknologi Malaysia (UTM). He has held various administrative positions including being the Head of Department of Department of Modeling and Industrial Computing and Department of Computer Science before assuming the post of Deputy Dean (Academic), Faculty of Computing. During his tenure, he was in charge of proposing new curriculum and revising existing curriculum for bachelor and master program, managing and facilitate his academic staff for pursuing studies and preparing research proposal, and advising students on academic matters. He has taught various courses at the faculty including industrial computing related courses example robotic, automation, programming languages and computational mathematic related subject at both undergraduate and postgraduate levels. He also supervises both Master and PhD students in related fields. She has been written few books and Editor for few conference proceeding, Editorial Board and Reviewer of various journals related to the computer science, and has been appointed as keynote speaker for various conferences. His research interests include optimization in various domain such as medical problems, manufacturing, robotic and image processing. He has also project leader for various research projects at university, national and international level.

Noor Zaman Jhanjhi (NZ Jhanjhi) is currently working as Associate Professor, Director Center for Smart society 5.0 [CSS5], and Cluster Head for Cybersecurity cluster, at School of Computer Science and Engineering, Faculty of Innovation and Technology, Taylor's University, Malaysia. He is supervising a great number of Postgraduate students, mainly in cybersecurity for Data Science. The cybersecurity research cluster has extensive research collaboration globally with several institutions and professionals. Dr Jhanjhi is Associate Editor and Editorial Assistant Board for several reputable journals, including IEEE Access Journal, PeerJ Computer Science, PC member for several IEEE conferences worldwide, and guest editor for the reputed indexed journals. Active reviewer for a series of top tier journals has been awarded globally as a top 1% reviewer by Publons (Web of Science). He has been awarded as outstanding Associate Editor by IEEE Access for the year 2020. He has high indexed publications in WoS/ISI/SCI/Scopus, and his collective research Impact factor is more than 350 points as of the first half of 2021. He has international Patents on his account, edited/authored more than 30 plus research books published by world-class publishers. He has great experience supervising and co-supervising postgraduate students. An ample number of PhD and Master students graduated under his supervision. He is an external PhD/Master thesis examiner/evaluator for several universities globally. He has completed more than 22 international funded research grants successfully. He has served as Keynote speaker for several international conferences, presented several Webinars worldwide, chaired international conference sessions. His research areas include Cybersecurity, IoT security, Wireless security, Data Science, Software Engineering, UAVs.

Navirah Kamal is a Computer Science Engineering graduate from Amity Univerisity Uttar Pradesh, India. Her primary interest includes working in the field of machine learning and data science.

Mohamed Lazaar received his PhD in March 2013 from the Faculty of Sciences and Technics, Sidi Mohammed Ben Abdellah university of Fez. He is a Professor of Computer Science and Artificial Intelligence at National School of Computer Sciences and Systems Analysis, Mohammed V University in Rabat. Dr. Mohamed Lazaar is a member in Smart Systems Laboratory and in Rabat IT Center at ENSIAS. His research interests include the performance of Machine Learning Methods and their applications in NLP, Recommender Systems, Multimedia Processing, etc.

Swanirbhar Majumder is presently working as Professor in the Dept of IT in Tripura University. Previously he had worked as Assistant Prof. in Dept of ECE, NERIST, a Deemed to be University of Arunachal Pradesh since 2006. He did his PhD, PG and UG from Jadvpur University, University of Calcutta and North Eastern Hill University, respectively. His areas of research work comprises of Biomedical Signal Processing, Image Processing, Embedded Systems and Soft Computing.

Syed Mehmood Naqvi is a Professor in the School of Applied Computing at Sheridan College, Canada. Formerly, he was Dean of Faculty of Computer Science and Information Technology at Institute of Business and Technology, Pakistan. He received Ph.D. in Computer Application Technology from Beihang University (formerly Beijing University of Aeronautics and Astronautics), Beijing, China in 1999. He did his postdoctoral research in the area of signal processing at the University of Northern British Columbia, Canada. Syed Naqvi has more than twenty years of teaching, research, and administrative experience at various universities, colleges, and institutes in Canada, Pakistan, and the UAE. He has served as an active member of many curricula development and revision committees for undergraduate and graduates computer science and information technology programs. His current areas of research include educational technology, medical image processing, and software development methodologies and models.

Hicham Omara is currently Professor in the Department of Computer Science in the Faculty of Science, Abdelmalek Essaadi University. His current research interests include recommender systems and machine learning.

T. Rajeshwari, a psychotherapist specializing in nutrition and mental health, practises freelance and has been working with children of all ages for around 35 years including as a therapist in Montessori schools. Lives in Kolkata and runs a center called Sneh Sri, which is centered on empowering women from low income backgrounds by training them to make utility products and handicrafts. Also a motivational speaker conducts workshops on effective parenting and healing meditation around the country. Also conducted nutrition and lifestyle management workshop and mind training workshop to engineers, different professionals, students and home makers. Now in a research program of " the sounds of vedic mantras and its impact on human behaviour" with a project on yagyopathy. Treatment through ancient yagya(smokelessyagya in 10 minutes) . I'm also a karmakandi attached to AWGP. Akhilawishwa Gayatri pariwar. Also with GPYG Kolkata (Gayatripariwar youth group). She is MS in psychotherapy and dip. in Nutrition.

Rohit Rastogi received his B.E. degree in Computer Science and Engineering from C.C.S.Univ. Meerut in 2003, the M.E. degree in Computer Science from NITTTR-Chandigarh (National Institute of Technical Teachers Training and Research-affiliated to MHRD, Govt. of India), Punjab Univ. Chandigarh in 2010. Currently he is pursuing his Ph.D. In computer science from Dayalbagh Educational Institute, Agra under renowned professor of Electrical Engineering Dr. D.K. Chaturvedi in area of spiritual consciousness. Dr. Santosh Satya of IIT-Delhi and dr. Navneet Arora of IIT-Roorkee have happily consented him to co supervise. He is also working presently with Dr. Piyush Trivedi of DSVV Hardwar, India in center of Scientific spirituality. He is a Associate Professor of CSE Dept. in ABES Engineering. College, Ghaziabad (U.P.-India), affiliated to Dr. A.P. J. Abdul Kalam Technical Univ. Lucknow (earlier Uttar Pradesh Tech. University). Also, he is preparing some interesting algorithms on Swarm Intelligence approaches like PSO, ACO and BCO, etc. Rohit Rastogi is involved actively with Vichaar Krnati Abhiyaan and strongly believe that transformation starts within self.

Soobia Saeed is working as an Assistant Professor, Head of publication Department, and Coordinator of Seminars and Training at Institute of Business & Technology-IBT, Karachi, Pakistan. Currently, she is a Ph.D. Scholar in software engineering, from University Teknologi Malaysia-UTM, Malaysia She did MS in Software Engineering from Institute of Business & Technology- IBT, Karachi, Pakistan, and Masters in Computer Science fromInstitute of Business & Technology-IBT, Karachi, Pakistan and Bachelors in Mathematical Science from Federal Urdu University of Art, Science & Technology (FUUAST), and Karachi, Pakistan. She is a farmer research Analytic from University Teknologi Malaysia and supervises ICT & R and D funded Final Year Project (FYP).

Sheelu Sagaris a research scholar pursuing her PhD in Management from Amity University (AUUP). She graduated with a Bachelor Degree of Science from Delhi University. She received her Post Graduate Degree in Master of Business Administration with distinction from Amity University Uttar Pradesh India in 2019. She is working at a post of Asst. Controller of Examinations, Amity University, Uttar Pradesh. She is associated with various NGOs - in India. She is an Active Member of Gayatri Teerth, ShantiKunj, Haridwar, Trustee - ChaturdhamVedBhawanNyas (having various centers all over India), Member Executive Body -Shree JeeGauSadan, Noida. She is a social worker and has been performing Yagya since last 35 years and working for revival of Indian Cultural Heritage through yagna (Hawan), meditation through Gayatri Mantra and pranayama. She is doing her research on Gayatri Mantra.

Gauri Sharma is a student at Manipal University Jaipur pursuing B-Tech in Computer Science and Engineering (2nd Year).

Preeti Sharma is a research scholar at Manipal University Jaipur. She is currently working on medical image processing.

Bhavna Singh is Ayurvedic Practitioner and currently acting as Principal in Ayurvedic College, Hapur, U.P., India. She has keen interest to stud the herbal and their effects on human body. She has done scientific experiments of different herbals and their vaporized state through Yajna on patient diseases. She is also fond of scientific writings and establishing Indian Vedic wisdom through logical explanations. She has been actively working in Thought Transformation movement and strongly feels that science and spirituality can move together to enrich each other. Her many papers are imprinted on various scientific journals.

Neeti Tandon is research scholar in Fundamental Physics at Vikram University Ujjain. She is keen researcher in Yagyopathy. She is scientist by thought and working on the study of effect of Yajna, Mantra and Yoga on mental patients, patients suffering with various diseases like diabetes, stress, arthritis, lever infection and hypertension. She is also Active Volunteer of Gayatri Parivaar and Thought Transformation Movement. She keeps herself engaged in many philanthropic activities like plantation, slum area kid education and anti-addiction movement. She is gold medalist and honors throughout her education and obtained graduation and post-graduation in Physics Science.

Index

A

ANNs 127-132, 135-137, 139, 146, 150, 154-156, 167
Anti-Epileptic drugs 81, 83, 85, 93, 95
anxiety 45, 85-87, 99, 116

B

brain 1-6, 10-12, 14-23, 25, 28, 63, 80, 82-84, 88, 92-94, 96-97, 106, 128, 161, 168-173, 178-188, 193-211, 213, 215-221, 236, 239-240, 243-244, 247, 249, 252, 255-259
breast cancer 24-28, 30-37, 39, 41-42, 45-51, 206-207

C

CNN 12, 15-19, 63-65, 81, 87, 89, 91-92, 96-97, 127, 147, 159, 166, 225, 227
CSF low-grade tumor 168, 202, 236

D

death 24, 27-28, 36, 92-94, 96
deep learning 1-3, 10-12, 15-16, 18-23, 81, 84, 87, 92, 97, 127-128, 132, 134-135, 141-142, 144, 161-166, 199, 210, 258
deep neural network 1, 10-11, 16-17, 92, 200
DenseNet 127, 156, 159-160, 167
depression 84, 99, 116
DFT LELPP-TC 236
Diabetic Retinopathy 52-53, 77-79
Digital image processing 2-3, 7-10, 13, 22-23
dysgraphia 222-235
dysgraphic handwriting 222-223, 226-228, 232-234

E

EEG 4, 81, 83-84, 87-92, 94, 96-98
extraction 16, 19, 21, 47, 52-63, 65-66, 68, 70-71, 73-

80, 87, 174, 179, 193, 199, 201, 215, 224, 234, 244, 250, 252, 255, 257

F

females 24, 27-28, 30-36, 38-39, 42, 47, 100-101
Fourier transformation 168, 178, 191-193, 199, 202, 204, 207, 213, 220, 236, 238, 240, 242, 245, 257
Fourier transformation Laplace 168, 202
fundus images 52-53, 57, 61, 63, 71, 73, 76-80

G

GCHMkC CM 236

H

Handwriting Analysis 222, 224, 227, 234
handwritten text recognition 225-226, 233, 235
hybrid approaches 52-53, 70-71, 76, 80

I

Illegible Text 222, 226, 234
image processing 1-3, 7-10, 13, 15-16, 19, 22-23, 47, 70, 77-78, 191, 193, 199, 201, 203-204, 218, 220, 247, 255-257
image segmentation 1-3, 8, 13-14, 16, 18-19, 21, 23, 34, 44, 79, 97, 168, 170-172, 174, 178, 182-183, 190-193, 195, 197-201, 204, 236, 244, 256, 258

L

Lack of Correct and Timely Treatment 81
Laplace Transformation 168, 177-178, 192-193, 202, 238, 240, 242, 246, 249
Learning Disabilities 222, 229-230, 232, 234
LSTM 81, 87, 89-91, 96-97, 227

M

machine learning 1-2, 10, 15-16, 18, 22-24, 45, 54, 63, 65, 71, 87, 113-115, 127-128, 133, 139, 161-162, 164-166, 168, 178, 187, 192, 194-195, 198-199, 201, 215, 220, 225, 257-258

mammography 24, 26-28, 30, 32-34, 36-37, 39-42, 45, 47-51, 181

Mantra 99-101, 105, 107, 109-111, 114, 116-119

Matched Filtering Method 60, 80

Mathematical Morphology-Based Method 80

Medical Imaging 1-3, 11, 14, 18, 20, 22-23, 78-79, 178, 181, 183-184, 197, 199-201, 220, 258-259

mental fitness 99, 110-111

Model-Based Method 80

MRI 1-7, 9, 15-21, 24, 26, 28, 31-34, 46-47, 50, 68, 81, 168-172, 176, 178, 180-186, 191-193, 195-201, 204, 208-211, 215, 217, 237-238, 240-245, 247, 249-250, 252-253, 255-256

Multiscale 19, 55, 57-58, 61, 78-79

Multiscale-Based Method 80

N

NASNet 127, 156, 160, 167

Neural Network-Based Method 80

Neural Networks 10-12, 15, 18-22, 63, 77-79, 87, 96-98, 163-167, 172, 201, 230

Neuroscience 1, 23, 193, 198, 247, 256

P

Pattern Recognition 22, 52-54, 77, 113-114, 163, 166-167, 172, 197, 199, 201, 224, 234, 256, 258

R

Radiology 1-2, 5, 48, 50, 166, 198

ResNets 127, 159

S

screening 24, 26-28, 30-37, 39-41, 45, 47-48, 50-51, 53, 207, 215, 221

segmentation 1-3, 8, 12-24, 34, 44, 52-62, 66-73, 76-80, 97, 114, 168-175, 178-186, 188, 190-204, 209, 220, 226, 228, 234, 236-238, 240, 244, 247, 249-252, 255-259

SLR CSF low-grade tumor 168, 236

stress 85-86, 93, 99-100, 109-110, 116-117, 185

SUDEP 81, 92-94, 96

supervised 15, 22, 52, 54-55, 63, 92, 98, 128, 139, 162, 164, 168, 172, 174, 178, 186, 190, 194, 208

T

transformation segmentation 168, 202

tumor 1-3, 5, 12, 15-23, 25, 27-28, 30, 37, 42, 44, 168-173, 178-189, 193-203, 205, 208, 213, 217-218, 220, 236, 239-241, 247, 249-253, 255-258

types of seizures 81-82

U

unsupervised 15, 22, 54-55, 63, 79, 162, 174, 187, 190, 193, 198, 208

V

Vessel Tracking Method 66, 80

VGG 127, 156-157, 167

W

Writing Aids 222, 229

Y

Yajna 99, 101, 103-112, 114

Yoga 81, 85-87, 96-97, 101, 107, 117

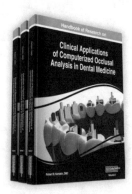
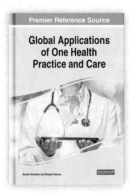
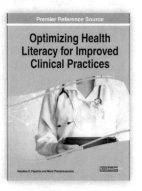
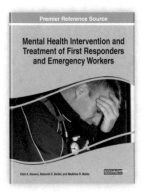
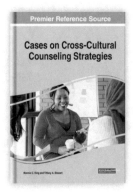
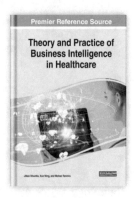
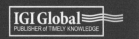

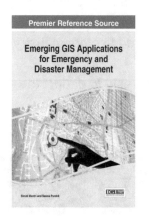
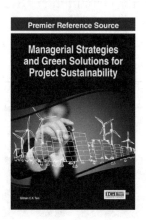
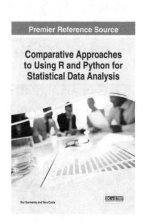
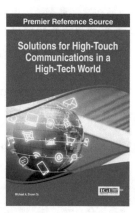

IGI Global Author Services

Providing a high-quality, affordable, and expeditious service, IGI Global's Author Services enable authors to streamline their publishing process, increase chance of acceptance, and adhere to IGI Global's publication standards.

Benefits of Author Services:

- **Professional Service:** All our editors, designers, and translators are experts in their field with years of experience and professional certifications.

- **Quality Guarantee & Certificate:** Each order is returned with a quality guarantee and certificate of professional completion.

- **Timeliness:** All editorial orders have a guaranteed return timeframe of 3-5 business days and translation orders are guaranteed in 7-10 business days.

- **Affordable Pricing:** IGI Global Author Services are competitively priced compared to other industry service providers.

- **APC Reimbursement:** IGI Global authors publishing Open Access (OA) will be able to deduct the cost of editing and other IGI Global author services from their OA APC publishing fee.

Author Services Offered:

English Language Copy Editing
Professional, native English language copy editors improve your manuscript's grammar, spelling, punctuation, terminology, semantics, consistency, flow, formatting, and more.

Scientific & Scholarly Editing
A Ph.D. level review for qualities such as originality and significance, interest to researchers, level of methodology and analysis, coverage of literature, organization, quality of writing, and strengths and weaknesses.

Figure, Table, Chart & Equation Conversions
Work with IGI Global's graphic designers before submission to enhance and design all figures and charts to IGI Global's specific standards for clarity.

Translation
Providing 70 language options, including Simplified and Traditional Chinese, Spanish, Arabic, German, French, and more.

Hear What the Experts Are Saying About IGI Global's Author Services

"Publishing with IGI Global has been **an amazing experience** for me for sharing my research. The **strong academic production** support ensures quality and timely completion." – **Prof. Margaret Niess, Oregon State University, USA**

"The service was **very fast, very thorough, and very helpful** in ensuring our chapter meets the criteria and requirements of the book's editors. I was **quite impressed and happy** with your service." – **Prof. Tom Brinthaupt, Middle Tennessee State University, USA**

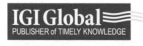

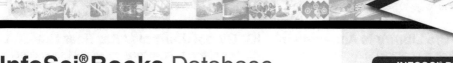

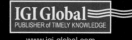

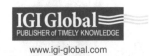

www.igi-global.com

Publisher of Peer-Reviewed, Timely, and
Innovative Academic Research Since 1988

IGI Global's Transformative Open Access (OA) Model:
How to Turn Your University Library's Database Acquisitions Into a Source of OA Funding

Well in advance of Plan S, IGI Global unveiled their OA Fee Waiver (Read & Publish) Initiative. Under this initiative, librarians who invest in IGI Global's InfoSci-Books and/or InfoSci-Journals databases will be able to subsidize their patrons' OA article processing charges (APCs) when their work is submitted and accepted (after the peer review process) into an IGI Global journal.

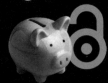

How Does it Work?

Step 1: **Library Invests in the InfoSci-Databases:** A library perpetually purchases or subscribes to the InfoSci-Books, InfoSci-Journals, or discipline/subject databases.

Step 2: **IGI Global Matches the Library Investment with OA Subsidies Fund:** IGI Global provides a fund to go towards subsidizing the OA APCs for the library's patrons.

Step 3: **Patron of the Library is Accepted into IGI Global Journal (After Peer Review):** When a patron's paper is accepted into an IGI Global journal, they option to have their paper published under a traditional publishing model or as OA.

Step 4: **IGI Global Will Deduct APC Cost from OA Subsidies Fund:** If the author decides to publish under OA, the OA APC fee will be deducted from the OA subsidies fund.

Step 5: **Author's Work Becomes Freely Available:** The patron's work will be freely available under CC BY copyright license, enabling them to share it freely with the academic community.

Note: This fund will be offered on an annual basis and will renew as the subscription is renewed for each year thereafter. IGI Global will manage the fund and award the APC waivers unless the librarian has a preference as to how the funds should be managed.

Hear From the Experts on This Initiative:

"I'm very happy to have been able to make one of my recent research contributions *freely available* along with having access to the *valuable resources* found within IGI Global's InfoSci-Journals database."

– **Prof. Stuart Palmer**, Deakin University, Australia

"Receiving the support from IGI Global's OA Fee Waiver Initiative *encourages me to continue my research work without any hesitation*."

– **Prof. Wenlong Liu**, College of Economics and Management at Nanjing University of Aeronautics & Astronautics, China

For More Information, Scan the QR Code or Contact:
IGI Global's Digital Resources Team at eresources@igi-global.com.

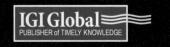

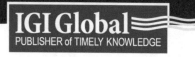
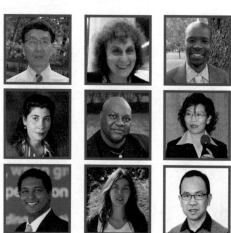
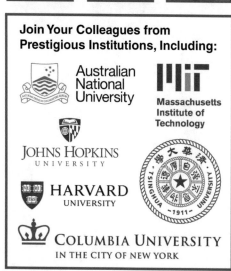

Printed in the United States
by Baker & Taylor Publisher Services